DEPARTMENT OF HEALTH

ON THE STATE OF
THE PUBLIC HEALTH

THE ANNUAL REPORT OF
THE CHIEF MEDICAL OFFICER OF
THE DEPARTMENT OF HEALTH
FOR THE YEAR 1997

)ffice

D0315083

CONTENTS

INTRODUCTION

Rt Hon Frank Dobson MP
Secretary of State for Health

Sir,

I have pleasure in submitting my Report on the State of the Public Health for 1997, together with some comments on the more important developments and events in the first half of 1998. This Report is the 140th of the series which began in 1858.

I am pleased to report that health has continued to improve overall during the year. Infant mortality reached its lowest recorded rate and perinatal mortality also fell in 1997. Progress continued to be made towards more integrated working to maintain the public health, and for more efficient communications between all those involved. The importance of an underlying strategy to enhance public health, not just to treat illness, has been further emphasised by the appointment last year of a Minister for Public Health, and the publication of a Green Paper, *Our Healthier Nation*[1], with the aim to tackle the underlying causes of ill-health and to break the cycle of social and economic deprivation and social exclusion.

As I have discussed in previous years, this Report is not simply a document of record, but must also try to interpret and to explain changes in those factors that are known to influence and to determine health, and should identify areas where improvements could be made. In recent Reports, I have highlighted some issues for special mention, with the intention that they would be followed up: topics identified in earlier years have been acted on and progress is discussed in this Report. As well as a broader discussion of the 150th anniversary of the 1848 Public Health Act[2], and of the public health challenges as we approach the 21st Century, four other key issues are identified for particular attention during the coming year: health and the environment, screening, autism and diabetes mellitus. It is hoped that over the next year these topics will stimulate interest. The multidisciplinary nature of health care has also been addressed by the Chief Nursing Officer and her colleagues on the theme of joint working for health.

As you will be aware, I am retiring as Chief Medical Officer at the end of September 1998, and this is the last Report that I have the honour to present, the first being that for the year 1991. Changes in disease trends often take many years to become apparent, but some striking changes may occur over shorter periods of time. Even over the relatively short period between 1991 and 1997, many of the key indices of health presented in the annual reports of the Chief Medical Officer have shown significant improvements. For example, the infant mortality rate has fallen from 7.3 per 1,000 live births to its lowest ever level of 5.9 per 1,000 live births in 1997 (see Appendix Table A.5). There has also been a substantial fall in post-neonatal mortality (deaths between 28 days and one year-of-age) over this period, from 3.0 to 2.0 per 1,000 live births; much of this fall is attributable to fewer deaths from sudden infant death syndrome (SIDS). More generally, average expectation of life has improved, from 73.4 years in 1991 to 74.6 years in 1996 among males, and from 78.9 years to 79.7 years in females. This improvement reflects substantial reductions in mortality rates which, allowing for changes in age structure, have fallen between 1991 and 1997 by over 11% among males and by 7% in females. Nevertheless, although improvements have been apparent among most age-groups in both sexes, there has been much less progress in the 15-44 years age-group for men and women alike (see page 72): a number of factors have contributed to adverse trends since the mid-1980s, including, in men particularly, the impact of deaths associated with HIV infection and suicides, although the rising trend of suicide deaths evident during the 1980s in young adult men does now appear to have halted.

Falls in deaths occurring under the age of 65 years have been particularly encouraging: these mortality rates fell by over 14% in males and 11% among females between 1991 and 1997. Important reductions have occurred in women of this age-group for both lung and breast cancer (both down by over 15%). Deaths from coronary heart disease (CHD) have continued to fall, the death rate for males and females for all ages combined being 20% lower in 1997 than it was in 1991. In 1991, the number of deaths from CHD exceeded those from cancer by over 5,000 but, by 1997, cancer deaths exceeded CHD deaths by over 12,000. It is also encouraging to note that rates of change in these falls in mortality have increased. For breast cancer, age-standardised mortality rates for women aged 45-64 years changed little between 1980 and 1986 compared with a fall of over 17% between 1990 and 1996; for CHD, the fall in age-standardised mortality rates for men and women aged 45-64 years was around 13% between 1980 and 1986 compared with almost 30% between 1990 and 1996.

Preventive interventions are critical to the future health of the population. Improvements in immunisation rates are therefore encouraging - uptake rates for diphtheria, tetanus and polio up from 92% in 1990/91 to 96% in 1996/97; and for pertussis, up from 84% in 1990/91 to 94% in 1996/97 (see Appendix Table A.9). There have also been substantial improvements during the early 1990s in coverage rates for cervical screening[3].

However adverse trends in some key determinants of future disease are of particular concern: the proportion of the adult population aged 16-64 years who are obese has risen from 13% among males and 15% in females in 1991/92[4], to

16% in males and 17% among females in 1996[5]; and the proportion of children aged 11-15 years who are regular cigarette smokers has risen from 10% in 1990 to 13% in 1996[6].

I wish to acknowledge the help and support given to me by numerous colleagues in the Department of Health and the Office for National Statistics, as well as other Government Departments and Agencies, in the preparation of this Report, and the assistance of The Stationery Office, Norwich, which arranged the printing and publication, and to thank the Report's editor, Dr Mark Powlson, and his staff in the Medical Editorial Unit, for their work in producing this Report and its six predecessors during my tenure as Chief Medical Officer. In the preparation of this Report, I am also particularly grateful for help outside Government from Dr Sally Sheard of the Department of Public Health at the University of Liverpool, and Professor George Alberti, President of the Royal College of Physicians of London, for their contributions in my personal introduction on historical aspects of the 1848 Public Health Act[2] and diabetes mellitus, respectively.

As I leave the Department to return to academic life as Vice-Chancellor and Warden at the University of Durham, I take with me many very fond memories of colleagues within the Department, elsewhere in Government, and throughout the National Health Service (NHS). The occasion of the NHS's 50th anniversary brought home how remarkable that organisation is - mainly due to the people who work in it, and for it. I am happy to have had the opportunity to make a contribution to it in various capacities, and shall continue to try to do so, albeit in a different role.

I am, Sir,
Your obedient servant

Sir Kenneth Calman

September 1998

LONG-TERM STRATEGIC AIMS

Previous Reports[7,8,9,10,11] set out a series of long-term strategic aims which also underpin the content of this Report:

- To promote efforts to ensure health for all;

- To achieve the targets in a strategy for public health;

- To involve patients and the public in choices and decision-making;

- To establish an effective intelligence and information system for public health and clinical practice;

- To ensure a health service based on an assessment of health needs, quality of care and effectiveness of outcome; *and*

- To provide a highly professional team of staff with strong education, research and ethical standards.

These six points continue to provide the strategic direction and intent of the Report.

PUBLIC HEALTH: 1848-1998

The 1848 Public Health Act and its aftermath

The 1848 Act for Promoting the Public Health[2] was the culmination of several years of national and local pressure to improve the condition of the urban environment and the health of the population. From 1844, the Health of Towns Association provided evidence of the link between ill-health and insanitary living conditions. This supplemented the research of Mr (later Sir) Edwin Chadwick, who was central to the demands for sanitary reform, masterminding the Royal Commission on the Sanitary State of Large Towns between 1843 and 1845. In the 1840s, many diseases were thought to be spread by gases given off by decaying matter, and this theory focused public health activity upon 'deposits and decomposition'. Thus, initially, an engineering solution was sought for this medical problem, with the building of sewers, water works, water closets and the arrangement of street cleaning and refuse collection.

Liverpool had achieved an effective public health legislation through its pioneering Sanatory Act[12] in 1846, which was the model for a public health bill introduced by Lord Morpeth into Parliament in 1847. This failed due to the political climate of the times (there was much debate about Ireland and the implementation of a new Poor Law Act[13]); although major sections of the Bill were dropped to try to get it enacted, it was eventually abandoned with a promise to reintroduce it in the 1848 Session. A second Public Health Bill was introduced to Parliament by Lord Morpeth; by the time it received Royal Assent on 31 August 1848, it had succumbed to substantial changes demanded by various opponents within and outside Parliament.

The 1848 Public Health Act[2] established a General Board of Health based in London with three permanent members: Lord Ashley, Earl of Shaftesbury, as President; Lord Morpeth, Earl of Carlisle; and Mr Edwin Chadwick, a lawyer, who was the only salaried Board member. The Board empowered local authorities to form Local Boards of Health to manage sewers, drains, water supplies, gas works, refuse and sewerage systems, to regulate offensive trades, to remove nuisances, to control cellar dwellings and houses unfit for human habitation, and to provide burial grounds, recreation areas, parks, public baths - powers which were backed up with the right to levy local rates and to purchase land. London operated independently of the Public Health Act, through its own Act of 1848 to form the Metropolitan Commissioners of Sewers[14]. At this time London had no constitutional or administrative unity, being comprised of 300 parishes, improvement commissions and boards of trustees working under some 250 Local Acts. Chadwick favoured the abolition of all these agencies and their replacement with an all-embracing Crown-appointed Commission for London, but was frustrated in this plan by the power of the City Corporation and other vested interests, including the eight private London water companies which he wished to buy out.

The 1848 Public Health Act[2] failed to achieve the objectives of Chadwick and his allies for a number of reasons. Some of the key clauses had to be modified to get the Bill passed in the House of Lords and the final Act was more permissive than had been intended. Local Boards of Health were not compulsory and required a preliminary inquiry based on the petition of at least 10% of the ratepaying population, which was in practice difficult to arrange. Alternatively, in districts where the annual mortality rate exceeded 23 per 1,000, the General Board of Health could impose a Local Board of Health. However, Dr (later Sir) John Simon, London's first Medical Officer of Health and subsequently Medical Officer to the Privy Council and Local Government Board (effectively England's first Chief Medical Officer) considered this coercive power to work against the Board, and that this clause could not in practice be made to work. Between 1848 and 1853, the General Board of Health had received only 284 applications for permission to form Local Boards, and only 168 voluntary Boards were created. By 1858 in Lancashire, for example, only 400,000 of a total population of 2,500,000 were served by a public health board. Some of the Local Boards which were formed were nothing more than the adoption of the title by the existing local corporation, which did not establish new services nor appoint Medical Officers of Health and Borough Engineers.

Chadwick, who had been born at the very start of the 19th Century in 1800, nearly lived to its conclusion. He died in 1890, and thus witnessed the progress made by public health in the years after his close involvement, and his reluctant eclipse. His unpopularity in various quarters had forced his resignation in 1854, and the General Board of Health was stood down in 1858. It had been hoped that the Board would provide a national voice for public health issues, but this had been restricted by a reluctance to appear to be seen to interfere in local affairs. However, the public health activity of central Government was reinstated within the Medical Department of the Privy Council in 1858, where Dr John Simon was appointed as Medical Officer. He worked with minimal power: to inspect and report, although he had direct control of the vaccination service. Initially, he was the only employee at the Medical Department, yet through his innovative adoption of the legislation he had a staff of some 30 inspectors by 1872, who prepared the thorough scientific reports needed to press for further public health legislation; this Report is the 140th of the annual series which he began in 1858.

Despite the limitations of the 1848 Act[2], significant progress was made in the arena of public health in the 1850s and 1860s through a series of associated Acts of Parliament related to nuisance removal, and through the Local Government Act of 1858[15], which permitted compulsory property purchase for sanitary purposes. The Sanitary Act of 1866[16] marked Simon's triumph over the restrictions of centralised bureaucracy and introduced a degree of compulsion for local authorities which Chadwick would have been proud of. Yet it failed to unite the multifarious post-1848 legislation, and within two years the Royal Commission on Sanitary Administration had been formed partly as a result of pressure from the prominent statistician William Farr and his associates at the Social Science Association. The outcome of the Commission was the 'great' Public Health Act of 1875[17] which made compulsory the appointment of a Medical Officer of Health in every sanitary district in England and Wales, thus building on the reorganisation of local government which had been accomplished through the Local Government Act 1871[18], and the Public Health Act 1872[19], which had created a national network of rural and urban sanitary authorities.

Simon resigned in 1876, unhappy with the Local Government Board's lack of zeal (duties having been transferred to it from the Privy Council), and the failure of Government to respond to his request for a Ministry of Health with its own

Cabinet Minister. His dissatisfaction was not shared by the doctors who filled over 1,000 new posts formed through the compulsory appointment of Medical Officers of Health to all sanitary authorities in 1872, and who helped to monitor, regulate and advance public health in the late 19th Century. Their role was reinforced through the creation of the Society of Medical Officers of Health in 1889, but their status as civil servants formed the basis for future disputes with the rest of the medical profession in the years to come.

In the last quarter of the 19th Century the discipline of public health was also moulded by scientific and medical developments, particularly bacteriology. The development of the 'germ theory' in the 1880s, and the discovery of the organisms for various infectious diseases in the 1890s, re-emphasised the inspectoral role of the Medical Officers of Health and their staff, who now had the weight of laboratory diagnosis behind their actions. Thus, by the end of that Century, Medical Officers of Health managed a considerable range of services across a wide medical and environmental spectrum - including what would be regarded as 'medical' establishments such as isolation hospitals (soon to metamorphose into general municipal hospitals) and tuberculosis sanatoria, but also public baths and wash-houses, cemeteries and crematoria, infant milk depots and child welfare centres.

The territory of public health had greatly expanded from its original sanitary base, but had not actually required much specific legislation after the Acts of the 1870s. By the first decade of the 20th Century, Medical Officers of Health were voicing opinions on preventive health which stressed the importance of the actions of the individual, particularly through personal and domestic hygiene. It was thus only a relatively small step to the recognition that Britain required a comprehensive health system integrating preventive and curative services alike. The locally based Medical Officers of Health argued that their knowledge and geographical structure would be the obvious delivery system. However, the adoption of the German model of social insurance in Britain through the National Insurance Act 1911[20] made the creation of such a system impossible, and they found that their work was dominated by managerial responsibilities rather than their old investigative and community-based activities.

The creation of the Ministry of Health in 1919[21] was the consolidating action which had, in the opinion of so many 19th Century reformers, been needed for so long. The then Chief Medical Officer, Sir George Newman, continued to make a personal annual report in the tradition established by Simon in 1858, but now it was to a Minister of Health with the authority and finance, and responsibility, to build a new public health for the 20th Century. That responsibility remains as we progress into the 21st Century.

Health trends over the past 150 years

The past 150 years have seen very substantial changes in the population both in terms of demography and levels of health. Considerable caution is necessary in interpreting trends since the 19th Century because of possible under-registration of births and deaths at this time, and problems of comparability of terms such as the cause of death over such a long period; for the purpose of this analysis, figures are based on England and Wales rather than England alone.

Over this period, the population has grown from under 18 million people in 1848[22] to 52 million in 1996[23]. Furthermore, this increase in population has been accompanied by major changes in the age structure of the population. Thus, in the 1851 Census the proportion of the population aged under 20 years was 46%[24], a striking contrast with the equivalent figure in 1996 of 25%[25]. Conversely, the proportion of the population aged over 75 years has grown over this period from around 1% in the mid-19th Century to around 7% now. Such differences are a result of changes in fertility and mortality.

Fertility increased during the mid-1800s to reach a peak around 1880[24]. At that time, average family size was of more than five children[26]. Fertility rates then fell reasonably consistently until the early 1940s apart from a temporary increase after World War I. A more sustained increase after World War II resulted in a peak in the mid-1960s, after which fertility declined to the relatively low levels which now occur.

Declining mortality rates have been associated with major improvements in the average expectation of life at birth. In the mid-1800s, life expectancy for males was less than 40 years[27], compared with 74.4 years in 1995[28]. Most of this improvement in life expectancy has been seen during the 20th Century - life expectancy in 1901 was still only 45 years among males and 49 years in females[26]. The different patterns of mortality can also be illustrated by the changing distribution of deaths at particular ages: in the mid-19th Century, 54% of deaths occurred under the age of 25 years, 26% between the ages of 25 and 64 years and 19% over the age of 65 years[26]; equivalent figures in 1997 were 2%, 15% and 83%, respectively[29].

In the mid-19th Century, many deaths occurred during the first year of life - more than 150 deaths per 1,000 live births[30] (representing over 20% of all deaths). Major causes included infectious diseases, convulsions, prematurity, congenital abnormalities and asphyxia[31]. In 1997, infant deaths numbered less than 4,000 and accounted for less than 1% of all deaths[29]. Infant mortality started to fall at the turn of the Century, since when rates have declined reasonably consistently.

Mortality associated with pregnancy and childbirth caused substantial numbers of deaths in 1848 and this level of mortality - much of it caused by puerperal septic disease - did not decline markedly until the late 1930s. Over the past 50 years, such deaths have fallen from about 4 per 1,000 births to 6 per 100,000 births[32].

The major impact of infectious disease in the last Century is shown by the toll of deaths attributed to it in the mid-1800s. An analysis of deaths in 1848-72[31] indicated that one death in every three was attributed to infection. The highest individual cause of such deaths was respiratory tuberculosis, which was responsible for one-third of all deaths from infectious disease and alone accounted for over 10% of all deaths; non-respiratory tuberculosis accounted for a further 3% of all deaths. The steep decline in tuberculosis mortality did not begin until the late 1940s, and it is not surprising that even in 1919 tuberculosis was described by the then Chief Medical Officer, Sir George Newman, as "one of the most formidable enemies of the race"[33]. Other infectious diseases which resulted in many deaths in the mid- to late-1800s included scarlet fever, diphtheria and typhus; severe cholera epidemics occurred in 1849, 1854 and 1866.

Changes in ascertainment and recording of diseases over lengthy time periods make assessment of changing patterns of disease over time rather hazardous. However, some evidence of the growing burden of deaths attributable to chronic diseases is provided by analysis of major causes of death. In 1848-72, apoplexy (stroke) accounted for about 4%, and all other circulatory diseases under 6%, of all deaths; in 1997, the equivalent figures[29] were 10% and 31%, respectively. Similarly 'cancer' in 1848-72 accounted for less than 1% of all male deaths and about 2% of all female deaths, although death certification practices and diagnostic patterns may well have contributed to the relatively low figures; in 1997, cancer was responsible for 26% of all deaths among males and 22% in females.

Reflections on the 1848 Public Health Act by the Chief Medical Officer

The 1848 Public Health Act[2] was a landmark in the improvement of health in England. Re-reading it closely shows that it covers almost all aspects of public health with the exception, perhaps, of air quality. Organisational aspects of improving health, food safety, housing quality, occupational health, health and safety, and some aspects of lifestyle are all covered. In spite of its rather archaic language, it makes exciting reading; and, as one can see from the historical analysis above describing its introduction, many concerns then still remain with us.

What then has changed in public health over the last 150 years, and do we need a new Act to continue to improve health in England? Health has improved immeasurably in all parameters studied. Lifespan, mortality rates, and quality of life have all improved considerably. Yet problems remain: the mortality rates in young men are still too high; there is still excess winter mortality, which is not so marked in other countries with similar weather; inequalities in health exist, and may even have become more marked over recent years; the role of women still needs strengthening; mental health problems remain a considerable challenge; and environmental problems, although different, are a continuing cause for concern.

So what then might be done to continue to improve health in England? For the last six years I have published as part of the Chief Medical Officer's Annual Report *On The State of the Public Health* a series of principles which set the tone for assessing health issues and my response to new problems. They have been expanded recently in book form[34]. How do they match against current health issues?

Health for all: This aim reflects the need for all citizens in the country to be treated equally, as an issue of social justice. The inequalities in health which exist reflect a need to consider issues such as poverty, unemployment, housing and the environment. There are no simple solutions, and a range of policies are required to make a fairer society and reduce inequalities.

A strategy for public health: The 'Health of the Nation' and now 'Our Healthier Nation' initiatives provide the vehicle for a strategic approach, across Government, to improve health. By selecting key areas, and setting national targets which can be monitored on a regular basis, such an approach allows a wide range of interests to work together to a common agenda. This partnership approach is critical. The Chief Medical Officer's Project to Strengthen the Public Health Function has identified ways in which this strategic view can be put into practice. There is a need for both capacity and capability, and for a multidisciplinary organisation which brings together in a powerful coalition all those concerned with improving the health of the people of England. The 1848 Act[2] had a Board of Health, a high-level committee to oversee the changes proposed. Perhaps something similar would be useful now. In terms of the NHS, the development of National Service Frameworks will provide some of the strategic input into providing a service to the whole community with equality of access and of quality of care: for example, the cancer service framework shows how this might be done, and what the difficulties are.

Public and patient involvement: This is central to improving health and health care. Interestingly it was not a major feature of the 1848 Act[2]. We need to explore better ways to ensure full public participation into the process of changing health. The public are allies to the professions, not the reverse. Over the past few years, public and patient involvement has grown, and this is to be welcomed. But there is a consequent need for those who have responsibility for health and health care to ensure that they communicate effectively with the public on a whole range of issues - in particular, the communication of risk. There is an equivalent need for the public to understand the complexities and uncertainties associated with decision-making in health and health care.

Intelligence and surveillance: It is not possible to continue to improve public health unless the facilities exist to ensure that we know what is happening and what is changing. This can range from the collection of statistics on cancer registration to horizon scanning for new approaches to treatment. Infectious disease surveillance provides an excellent example of a national system which is able to identify outbreaks and new organisms emerging. Assessment of the health impact of policies across Government and considering the longer term consequences of new developments is also part of this process.

The need for a strong evidence base: This is now at the heart of the process of improving health and should be widely welcomed. Much evidence on how to improve health and the quality of care provided already exists. The generation of the evidence, and appropriate implementation in the community or by the professions, remain a challenge.

The importance of education, research and ethical considerations: Many of the improvements listed above could occur if the professions and the public recognised the importance of education and the role of learning in changing attitudes and behaviour. From a medical point of view, medical education, and the changes which have been introduced over the past few years, have had as their purpose the improvement in the quality of care provided. In a similar manner, the public understanding of science has assisted the way in which the public have recognised some of the complexities of clinical practice. Research is fundamental to improving health and there is a need to continue to invest in new methods of care or understanding of disease mechanisms. The National Health Service (NHS) research and development (R&D) programme, coupled with the Research Councils and the medical research charities, provides a remarkable resource to develop the research agenda. Ethical issues will remain central to improving health, and the value base which is adopted will set the overall framework for decision-making. New methods of treatment and investigation raise new moral dilemmas, and each requires careful and public consideration.

So do we need a new Public Health Act? Much of what has been discussed above needs no legislative framework; it requires the implementation of what is already known. In some areas, notably in the field of infectious disease, there is a case for clearer legislation. Across Government, legislation on the environment and food safety are under way and will bring a sharper focus to health issues. Perhaps there is no need for more. Above all, however, it should never be forgotten that public health 'belongs' to the public - and not health professionals (nor indeed politicians). Accordingly, they need the best possible, and readily comprehensible, advice, education and encouragement.

HEALTH IN ENGLAND

Key indicators of the overall health of the population indicate that the substantial health gains of recent years have been maintained during 1997. The infant mortality rate for 1997 reached its lowest ever level of 5.9 per 1,000 live births. The perinatal mortality (stillbirths plus deaths under one week-of-age) also fell in 1997 to 8.4 per 1,000 total births. Provisional mortality rates for 1997 (all ages combined, adjusted for differences in age structure) fell in men and women compared with 1996 rates.

Many factors have contributed to falling mortality rates over recent years and there have been substantial reductions in deaths from several key causes of death. Mortality rates from all cancers combined, for example, have fallen significantly - particularly among men; this could reflect a falling incidence of disease, improved survival, or a combination of these. A recent publication by the Office for National Statistics (ONS) jointly with the Imperial Cancer Research Fund[35] presented trends in cancer survival for people diagnosed with cancer in 1981 compared with those diagnosed in 1989. For all cancers combined (excluding non-melanoma skin cancer), there has been a small but definite increase in survival, with 'five-year relative survival' increasing from 25% in individuals diagnosed in 1981 to 30% in 1989. A number of individual cancers showed particular improvements in 'five-year relative survival' with increases (in percentage points) of seven for breast cancer, 13 for malignant melanoma, and seven for colorectal cancer. For some other cancers such as lung, prostate and stomach there was little or no improvement in five-year survival over this period, and much remains to be done in the areas of prevention and treatment of cancer.

Despite overall improvements in many key indicators of the health of the population, it remains of much concern that substantial inequalities in health persist; indeed, for some health measures the gap between socio-economic groups has widened. Data on health inequalities in this country have been presented in a recent publication from the ONS[36]. Estimates based on the ONS Longitudinal Study indicate marked inequalities in life expectancy by social class: for the period 1987-91 there was a five-year difference in the expectation of life at birth between men in social classes I and II (75 years) compared with social classes IV and V (70 years); for women, the differential was three years (80 years compared with 77 years). Addressing substantial differences such as these represents a major challenge.

Research findings published in October 1997[37,38] provided convincing evidence that the agent which causes new variant Creutzfeldt-Jakob disease (nvCJD) is the same as that which causes bovine spongiform encephalopathy (BSE). However, these findings do not indicate the mechanism by which human beings acquire the disease. It is still widely thought that the most likely route of infection is the ingestion of contaminated bovine offals before the ban on specified bovine offals (SBOs) took effect[39], but there is still no evidence to indicate the routes of exposure by which human beings may be vulnerable to BSE infectivity. The need to maintain a precautionary approach to minimise the risk from BSE is clearly underlined by these findings.

Although there is no current epidemiological evidence of transmission of CJD or nvCJD through blood or blood products, the limited data available indicate that the pathogenesis of nvCJD may possibly involve a more pronounced lymphoreticular phase than classic CJD. The confidence of the public in the safety of blood and blood products is clearly of great importance, and further precautionary measures were announced in February 1998[40]. In May 1998[41], the Committee on Safety of Medicines (CSM) advised that manufactured blood products should not be sourced from United Kingdom (UK) plasma at present; the use of leucodepletion for all blood destined for transfusion is being explored.

Since 31 December 1997 (see page 212), a further four cases of nvCJD have been identified, making a total of 27 up to the end of June 1998.

In early 1998, media reports and public concern were stimulated by a small study of 12 patients which claimed a possible association between measles, mumps and rubella (MMR) vaccine and Crohn's disease and autistic spectrum disorders[42]. Reports of these purported associations have caused parents considerable anxiety, and although coverage levels for routinely recommended immunisations in general remain very high (see page 203), those for MMR are lower. After taking advice from the Joint Committee on Vaccination and Immunisation and the Committee on Safety of Medicines, the Chief Medical Officer asked the Medical Research Council (MRC) to convene a meeting to consider these issues, at which proponents of such associations were given full opportunity to present their data. The MRC expert group concluded that: the available virological and epidemiological evidence does not support a causal role for persistent measles virus infection in Crohn's disease; there is no evidence to indicate any link between MMR vaccination and bowel disease and autism; and there is therefore no reason for a change in the current MMR immunisation policy. These conclusions, and background data, were sent to doctors in March 1998[43]. Early estimates of MMR coverage indicate a possible fall in vaccination uptake over this period, although this has not yet been confirmed; information materials for parents are being prepared to address these concerns.

THE STRATEGY FOR HEALTH

On 5 February 1998, the Government published proposals for a new health strategy for England in a Green Paper, *Our Healthier Nation*[1]. The strategy's twin headline aims are "to improve the health of the population as a whole by increasing the length of people's lives and the number of years people spend free from illness; and to improve the health of the worst off in society and narrow the health gap".

The strategy addresses quality of life as well as length of life, and aims to bring the experience of the worst off closer to that of the best, in a context of continuous overall improvement. The Green Paper recognises that a range of factors influence health: some are fixed, such as genetic inheritance, gender, and date of birth; others, particularly social, environmental and lifestyle factors, and the quality and availability of health care and other services, can be influenced for the better. The Green Paper recognises three levels for such influence - central Government and national organisations, local organisations, and individuals; it also emphasises the need for shared responsibility and partnership across these three levels.

At national level, this means recognising the effect on health of policies across a range of Government Departments and Agencies. While the Department of Health (DH) and the NHS have an important role to play, other Departments' policies such as the integrated transport policy, and the 'Excellence in Schools' and 'Welfare to Work' initiatives will all have an impact on health.

The Green Paper calls for these connections to be made at local level too. It says that health and local authorities should work in partnership with each other and with others, such as local businesses and the voluntary sector. Between this national and local effort, *Our Healthier Nation* aims to create the climate where individuals are empowered and informed to choose healthy lifestyle options for themselves and their families.

The Green Paper identifies four national priority areas and proposes a target for each: "By the year 2010, to reduce the death rate from heart disease and stroke and related illnesses amongst people aged under 65 years by at least a further third; to reduce accidents by at least a fifth; to reduce the death rate from cancer amongst people aged under 65 years by at least a further fifth; to reduce the death rate from suicide and undetermined injury by at least a further sixth"[1]. It proposes that, at local level, health improvement programmes should also include local targets to reflect specific local priorities. The 'Our Healthier Nation' initiative recognises that health needs are not distributed uniformly across the country, and that the health strategy must be sufficiently flexible to address local issues to improve the nation's health. To reinforce the priority areas, *Our Healthier Nation* proposes three settings as a focus for action: schools, workplaces and neighbourhoods. These concentrate attention on the three main population groups of children, those of working age, and older people.

Consultation on the Green Paper ran to 30 April. As part of this process, eight consultation days were held around the country, one in each of the NHS regions; each allowed a wide range of people from health authorities, local authorities and other backgrounds an opportunity to share their views on the proposals in the Green Paper. Ms Tessa Jowell MP, the Minister of State for Public Health, attended each event, accompanied at a number by Ministers from other Government Departments. A meeting was also held for leaders and chief executives of local authorities, to complement a meeting held for health authority chairmen and chairwomen and chief executives, held in November 1997.

The consultation prompted over 5,500 responses, the overwhelming majority broadly supportive of the Green Paper's proposals[1]. The detailed comments submitted will form an important part of the development of the *Our Healthier Nation* White Paper. Other important pieces of work will contribute to the White Paper, notably the Independent Inquiry into Inequalities in Health chaired by Sir Donald Acheson, formerly Chief Medical Officer of the Department of Health; the Chief Medical Officer's Project to Strengthen the Public Health Function; and the Independent Review of the 'Health of the Nation' initiative.

As the 'Our Healthier Nation' initiative develops, efforts will be made to ensure consistency and complementarity with the implementation of the White Paper *The new NHS: modern, dependable*[44]. Health improvement programmes, set out in *The new NHS*[44], will be the major vehicle to deliver *Our Healthier Nation*[1] targets and will provide the framework needed at a local level to encourage a co-ordinated approach to improve health and health care. The 11 health action zones established this year, and the planned development of a network of healthy living centres will also help with implementation of the 'Our Healthier Nation' initiative, and the achievement of its aims to improve public health and to reduce health inequalities.

Publication of the *Our Healthier Nation* White Paper is planned for later this year.

JOINT WORKING FOR HEALTH

Public health has long been acknowledged as a multidisciplinary activity that involves many professional groups working in various sectors[45]. All now have a key role in taking forward the Government's public health policy[1].

The 1848 Public Health Act[2] has special significance for environmental health officers, as it launched their profession - first known as inspectors of nuisances, later sanitary inspectors, then public health inspectors and, since 1980, environmental health officers. The principal founder of the public health movement, Sir Edwin Chadwick, placed great importance on the role of these officials, who initially worked mainly in local government. However, their expertise in environmental health has achieved growing recognition, and a substantial proportion of the profession now works in industry, voluntary services, Government Departments and, increasingly, in various forms of consultancy within the UK and overseas. The Chartered Institute of Environmental Health, the professional body for environmental health officers, envisages a continuing evolution of the profession to complement the skills of specialists from other backgrounds in meeting challenges in hygiene and environmental health.

Health visiting started in the mid-1800s, with concern focused on the protection of mother and child. In 1862, the first recorded health visitor was employed in Salford, and in 1892 special training for health visitors was introduced. In 1977, the Council for Education and Training of Health Visitors produced four guiding principles of health visiting which reflected the way the profession had developed a broader focus: to uncover unmet health needs, not just measure ill-health; to raise awareness of health as a first step in engaging people to discuss their own health needs; to influence local and national planning and policy by collective and collaborative action; and to facilitate health-enhancing activities through the combination of environmental change, preventive activities and therapeutic intervention. Nowadays, health visitors' extensive local knowledge of the local environment, culture, communities, individuals and families places them in an unique position to deliver public health objectives where people live - at the level of communities and local groups.

Historically, school nurses have dedicated their time to screening children to identify health problems, particularly those which may influence development or may affect the child's ability to take full advantage of educational opportunities. However, there is now greater diversity in the work of school nurses, with a greater proportion of their time being given to health promotion activities with individual children, and as part of a general approach to health within schools.

The first infection control nurse was appointed in April 1959 during an outbreak of staphylococcal infection at Torbay Hospital. The valuable contribution to the quality of patient care made by the development of this nursing role was soon recognised, and within the next 20 years the specialist role of infection control nurses became well established. Once exclusively working in hospitals, an increasing number of infection control nurses now work in community settings.

Challenging times and a rapidly changing environment saw the therapy professions become a reality around the turn of the last Century. However, the main lever to future development was the effect of two World Wars and the subsequent need for a fit, healthy workforce, in which physiotherapy and occupational therapy in particular had a major role. These professionals now help to develop healthy children, advise on healthy workplaces and help to recover or maintain independence for elderly people, and they have been joined by other professionals trained in speech and language therapy, dietetics and podiatry to provide a comprehensive rehabilitation service to promote healthy living and a healthy environment.

Effective multidisciplinary teamwork by health care professionals is important not just for treatment, but also for health promotion and prevention of illness in various settings, not just within the health care sector.

PROGRESS ON ACTION POINTS IN PREVIOUS REPORTS

Each year, topics which have been highlighted in recent Reports are reviewed and any action noted. In this Report, all topics raised since this initiative was started by the Chief Medical Officer in 1991 are revisited.

Progress on topics identified in 1991

Health of black and ethnic minority groups: This issue, the subject of the special chapter in the 1991 Report[46], continues to be a high priority to the Department and an important consideration in the development of health policy. The importance of health needs assessment of people from minority ethnic groups in the light of the White Paper *The new NHS: modern, dependable*[44] and the Green Paper *Our Healthier Nation*[1] was emphasised to the NHS in July[47], and in the book *Assessing health needs of people from minority ethnic groups*[48].

Communicable diseases: As noted above, communicable diseases were a major factor behind the setting up of the 1848 Public Health Act[2] and much subsequent activity in the field of public health; current work is described elsewhere in this personal introduction, and in Chapter 6, Chapter 7 (food poisoning) and Chapter 4 (in relation to climate change).

Clinical audit and outcomes of health care: Following a tendering exercise, the Central Health Outcomes Unit (CHOU), which was set up by DH in 1993, moved in Summer 1998 to be jointly based at the London School of Hygiene and

Tropical Medicine and the University of Oxford. Its programme to develop health outcomes assessment will continue to evolve and will include: publication of an electronic compendium of existing clinical and health outcome indicators; development and evaluation of new outcome indicators; development of critical reviews and a repository of outcome measurement techniques; development of relevant methods, data systems, skills and expertise; and promotion and facilitation of the use of health outcomes assessment. Much of this programme will build on previous work by the CHOU.

Medical education and manpower: The structure of the Advisory Group on Medical and Dental Education, Training and Staffing (AGMETS) was changed in June 1997 and has a more strategic focus on the needs of the NHS to help to shape the future strategic direction of medical and dental education, training and workforce policies. The Medical Workforce Standing Advisory Committee has recommended an increase in the annual intake to UK medical schools. The White Paper *The new NHS: modern, dependable*[44] gave increased emphasis on the responsibility of the NHS and all who work within it to improve the quality of NHS patient services, in which a new system of clinical governance will be introduced to ensure that clinical standards are met within a single, coherent local programme for quality improvement. A consultation document was issued in July 1998[49].

Progress on topics identified in 1992

Health of men: Men's life expectancy is improving but they are still more likely to die prematurely than women, and men in lower social classes are at particularly high risk. In May 1998, two health promotion leaflets were published - one aimed at older men in lower social classes[50], and the other at younger men[51].

Cigarette smoking in children: Regular smoking prevalence among 11-15-year-olds rose from 12% in 1994 to 13% in 1996; by the age of 15 years, about three of every ten children smoke at least one cigarette a week[6]. This disappointing trend is being vigorously addressed. On 22 June 1998, the European Union (EU) Council of Ministers formally adopted the Directive to ban tobacco advertising and sponsorship which was voted through the EU Parliament in May. Details of the implementation of the tobacco advertising Directive in UK law will be incorporated into the White Paper on tobacco control due to be published in late 1998. The first report of the Scientific Committee on Tobacco and Health was published in March 1998[52].

Mentally disordered offenders: The development of a research strategy for forensic mental health continues, in conjunction with other Departments and Agencies. A key policy area is that of antisocial personality disorder.

Verocytotoxin-producing Escherichia coli: Between 1996 and 1997, there \
an increase of almost 65% in isolations of verocytotoxin-producing *Escherichia coli* (VTEC) O157 from clinical samples, with over 1,000 isolates being reported from England and Wales. A number of outbreaks occurred. As in previous years, food was an important vehicle, but one outbreak was thought to be due to contact with contaminated mud, and there were several outbreaks among children who visited open farms. An expert group was convened to give advice on the management of one of these open farm outbreaks. As a result of these events, the Health and Safety Executive (HSE) has recently updated its guidance to farmers and teachers on how to minimise the risk of exposure to pathogens at open farms[53].

Progress on topics identified in 1992

Health of adolescents: Activities to promote the health of young people continue to develop, with a particular focus on healthy schools, as proposed in the Green Paper *Our Healthier Nation*[1]. In May 1998, Ministers from DH and the Department for Education and Employment (DfEE) jointly launched a 'healthy schools' initiative, with the development of a National Healthy Schools Award, which will recognise commitment to an ethos of positive health, social and personal development. A National Advisory Group on personal social and health education was established to make recommendations to the Qualifications and Curriculum Authority.

Asthma: Asthma and other chronic respiratory disease was first in the list of possible local target areas in the Green Paper *Our Healthier Nation*[1], which reflects the high priority that DH continues to give to services for people with these conditions. Further health promotion activity will be considered in the light of market research carried out in Spring 1998. The possible effects of air pollution are discussed elsewhere in this Report (see page 123). Work continues with health professional organisations, patient bodies and the pharmaceutical industry to inform professionals and the public alike about the changeover to chlorofluorocarbon (CFC)-free metered-dose inhalers[54].

Genetic factors and disease: Developments in genetic science have highlighted the growing importance of genetic technology in diagnosis and treatment, and the importance of NHS clinical genetics services and their scientific and laboratory support. The establishment of the Gene Therapy Advisory Committee (GTAC) and the Advisory Committee on Genetic Testing (ACGT) have ensured that the social, ethical and scientific implications of genetics in these areas are considered. Genetics will play an increasing role in health care into the next millennium, and will also continue to attract widespread interest; clinicians and the public alike will need to develop their understanding of this science and its implications.

terns of infectious diseases: The 1993 Report[55] emphasised the
| for vigilance, and a public health infrastructure, to keep abreast
he occurrence of infectious diseases. It is now more fashionable
new, emerging and re-emerging infectious disease', but the
ame - there is no room for complacency. Since 1993, there have
...... notable successes, due to the availability of new technologies or the
prompt recognition and response to changing patterns of incidence. Meningitis
in children due to *Haemophilus influenzae* type b (Hib), for instance, has been
virtually eliminated in the UK since the inclusion of Hib vaccine in the childhood
immunisation programme in 1992; a projected measles outbreak was averted by
the prompt institution of a national measles immunisation campaign in 1994; and
the introduction of combination drug therapies for HIV/AIDS patients has
significantly delayed disease progression and mortality. On the other hand, foodborne infections continue to increase; the global burden caused by infectious
diseases such as tuberculosis, malaria and HIV/AIDS is rising, and increased
resistance of micro-organisms to antimicrobial agents threatens to jeopardise the
ability to treat them. National and international efforts to address these issues are
described in various sections of this report.

Health in the workplace: The special chapter in the report for 1994[56] outlined
some of the important effects of work on health, the effects of health on work
and the value of health promotion in the workplace. The new health strategy
Green Paper, *Our Healthier Nation*[1], identifies the workplace as a key setting to
achieve its aims. The HSE worked closely with DH to develop this aspect of the
strategy and the Health and Safety Commission will advise Ministers on a
flexible framework of occupational health support for small and medium-sized
enterprises; development work includes a joint DH/HSE conference. In Summer
1998, the HSE will publish a discussion document on developing an occupational
health strategy for Britain. The health of the NHS workforce has been identified
as a key priority within the NHS, and a guidance document[57] on the management
of health, safety and welfare issues for NHS staff was published by the NHS
Executive in April 1998.

Equity and equality: The 1994 Report[58] discussed the important issues of equity
and equality. These issues remain at the heart of improving health and health
care. Inequalities in health, and their modification, are now recognised to be of
major importance in achieving health gain. During 1997, the Office for National
Statistics (ONS) produced a report[36] on inequalities in health which set out the
differences in health between social classes for various illnesses; many of these
differences had not improved over the years. Inequalities also exist in the
outcomes of health care for many procedures and treatments[59], and this issue will
be taken forward as part of the health service reforms outlined in the White Paper
The new NHS: modern, dependable[44]. Sir Donald Acheson, formerly Chief

Medical Officer of the Department of Health, has been commissioned to prepare a report on inequalities in health which will be available in late-1998 and which will contribute to the development of the White Paper on the 'Our Healthier Nation' initiative[1].

Food poisoning: Following two years in which notifications of food poisoning remained relatively stable, there was an increase in notifications of just under 13% in 1997. *Campylobacter* was the commonest bacterial isolate reported by laboratories, increasing by nearly 16%, whilst laboratory reports of *Salmonella* isolates increased by some 5%. The reported number of *Salmonella enteritidis* isolates continued to increase, and phage type 4 remained the most common phage type (see page 218). This increase in *Salmonella* isolates, and the findings of a survey of shell eggs from the UK carried out by the Public Health Laboratory Service (PHLS), which indicated that the level of contamination with *Salmonella enteritidis* has not changed significantly since 1991, gives cause for concern and the Advisory Committee on the Microbiological Safety of Food (ACMSF) has set up a working group to investigate these issues. By contrast, reported isolates of *Salmonella typhimurium* fell by nearly 20%. As a result of concerns expressed in an earlier report by the Royal Commission on Environmental Pollution[60], Government Departments had commissioned a review of the scientific basis for current controls on the agricultural use of sewage sludge, which was published in June 1998[61]. This review provides a basis for Government action in response to views of the Select Committee for the Environment, Transport and the Regions on sewage treatment and disposal. Parliamentary interest in food safety is underlined by the recent publication of a report on food safety from the Select Committee on Agriculture[62]. In part, this is a response to proposals for a Food Standards Agency which were the subject of a White Paper[63] published on 16 January 1998. Following public consultation on the White Paper, a draft Bill to establish the Agency has been prepared.

Drug and solvent misuse: The Government published its new drugs strategy, *Tackling drugs to build a better Britain*[64] in April 1998. Results of the DH-funded National Treatment Outcome Research Study, launched on 10 June 1998 by Ms Tessa Jowell MP, Minister of State for Public Health, indicated the benefits of drug treatment services in respect of individuals' drug use, risk-taking behaviour, and general health. These findings will inform the commissioning of services for drug misusers by health authorities.

Progress on action points identified in 1995

Risk communication and the language of risk: As discussed in the last two Reports[66,67], public reactions to risk can seem surprising, but are not totally unpredictable. Effective communication is necessarily a two-way process, requiring openness in the policy process; and good risk communication requires a coherent strategy, rather than ad-hoc reaction to events. While the challenges to effective communication of risk remain great, progress has been made to put these principles into practice. For example, the Advisory Committee system is being made more transparent, with publication of material on some dedicated websites. This progress has been informed by wider exchanges of views involving Government, the NHS, academia, industry and non-Governmental organisations[68]. Meanwhile, investigation into risk and its communication is to be stimulated by a substantial new DH research programme. The internal DH programme of staff development exercises, case studies and support for current episodes has continued, and a guidance booklet[69] was published in late 1997. The specific area of food safety has seen the establishment of the Joint Food Safety and Standards Group (JFSSG) as the precursor to a Food Standards Agency (see page 218), and a small Risk Communication Unit has already been set up. Cross-Departmental liaison continues via the Inter-Departmental Group on Public Health and the Inter-Departmental Liaison Group on Risk Assessment, which has established a risk communication sub-group chaired by DH.

Mental health: Progress during 1997, following the special chapter on mental health in the 1995 Report[70], is described on pages 93 and 168. Mental health has been chosen for development of one of the first two National Service Frameworks set out in the White Paper *The new NHS: modern, dependable*[44]. The Independent Reference Group, set up in Autumn 1997, has met regularly and has achieved its initial task to review closure plans for the remaining long-stay psychiatric institutions; its role as a reference group will continue and expand. A seminar on dual diagnosis and the management of complex needs was held in March 1998, and has led to further collaborative work within the Department. In acknowledgement of the major role played by primary care in the provision of mental health care, an audit has been commissioned into the mental health component of vocational training schemes for general practitioners, to assess the extent to which the training is relevant to primary rather than secondary care. Support is also being provided in the development of the mental health aspects of Health Action Zones. The Mental Health Partnership Fund supports innovative projects which are developed in partnership with other providers of care.

Antibiotic-resistant micro-organisms: Since this topic was raised in the 1995 Report[71], as an area of growing importance that required further work, it has increasingly been emphasised in national and international health agendas alike (see page 211). Some of the initiatives have progressed during the first half of 1998. The House of Lords Select Committee on Science and Technology published the report of its Inquiry into resistance to antibiotics and other antimicrobial agents in April 1998[72], based on written and oral evidence from over 100 individuals and organisations, and visits to meet national and international experts in the field. The Committee's recommendations are wide-ranging and are being carefully considered by the Government. In May 1998, the World Health Assembly noted concern about the rapid emergence and spread of human pathogens resistant to available antibiotics and the extensive use of antibiotics in food production which may further accelerate the development of such resistance, and passed a Resolution urging Member States to take various actions to improve surveillance; to encourage the prudent use of antimicrobial agents in human beings and animals alike; to achieve better infection control; and to educate health professionals and the public[73]. It urged the Director-General of the World Health Organization (WHO) to support countries in their efforts to control antimicrobial resistance and to encourage promotion of research and the development of novel antimicrobial agents. The WHO Emerging and other communicable diseases (EMC) Division has published a report on the current status of antimicrobial resistance surveillance in Europe[74] and an outline control strategy[75], which covers areas already identified as crucial for a UK strategy to contain, as far as possible, the development of antimicrobial resistance.

Information technology: During the year, a substantial exercise was undertaken by DH to hear what the NHS feels are its information requirements. The findings show that real benefits come when information technology (IT) is used to support the clinical process - not only within organisations, but also in supporting communications between them. The Clinical Systems Group (see page 247) found that whilst major IT issues need to be addressed, the primary requirement is to improve cultural and technical aspects of clinical information standards. Important progress has made to resolve the tensions that exist between the needs for agreed and appropriate standards of professional practice for information handling (particularly when person-identifiable), and the widest possible use of IT to benefit clinical practice and research. The Caldicott and Bellingham Committees (see pages 149 and 247) have shown the need for effective partnerships between health care and IT professionals. Another factor which is becoming increasingly apparent is that increased use and availability of IT will have a profound effect on patient and public awareness of health care issues, with the potential for great benefits in terms of health education and promotion, but also for considerable anxieties and inappropriate use of health care services if inaccurate or misleading information is promulgated. *Improving clinical communications*[76], produced by the Clinical Systems Group, contains three studies that illustrate these general observations.

HIV infection and AIDS: Antiretroviral combination drug therapy has continued to delay the progression to a diagnosis of AIDS in HIV-infected people and to reduce mortality due to AIDS (see page 189). The long-term benefits of combination therapy are unknown, and there are still uncertainties about the best time to start 'highly active antiretroviral therapy' (HAART), in view of concerns about patient compliance with the complex drug regimens, reports of drug resistance and side-effects such as lipodystrophy and diabetes mellitus. However, HAART significantly decreases the amount of circulating virus, increases CD4 cell counts and improves quality of life, such that many patients can return to work. Combination therapies also significantly reduce the incidence of opportunistic infections in patients with HIV/AIDS, which raises questions about whether or not to continue with antimicrobial prophylaxis in patients for whom combination therapy is proving effective[77].

Progress on topics identified during 1996

The potential for health: In last year's Report[78] the potential for health for the people of England which might result from the use and implementation of existing knowledge was discussed. A model of health was proposed which took into account a wide range of factors which might influence health and health care, and emphasised the need for a long-term strategic approach to health problems. The *Our Healthier Nation* Green Paper[1] provides such a long-term approach, and considers a wide range of factors which influence health. In the subsequent White Paper, which will be published in Autumn 1998, targets will be set. The model emphasised the importance of people in making decisions and in involving them in improving health, and noted the importance of surveillance of health and of monitoring outcomes; education and research were seen to be central, and ethical issues and values set the context for achieving changes in health. It is important to develop such models of health and to learn from testing these concepts in real life. The conceptual framework synthesises all factors that determine health and influence health care; the potential for health can only be realised if we put into practice what is already known and allow patients and the public to be involved in the process. Promotion of public health may be perceived to be a severe, often admonitory task, concerned more with stricture than encouragement. But being healthy is a very positive thing to be, and it should be enjoyable and rewarding both to have a healthy lifestyle and to try to promote good health.

Health of disabled people: Much work continues to be done to improve services for disabled people and to raise awareness about their individual needs, as highlighted in last year's Annual Report[79]. To underline its commitment to disabled people, the Government has announced the implementation of Section 21 of the Disability Discrimination Act 1995[80], concerned with access to goods and services for disabled people in the private and public sectors alike. It will be implemented in two stages: first, from October 1999, providers of services will have to take reasonable steps to ensure that disabled people are able to use those services - which may involve changes in working practices, the provision of auxiliary aids, and overcoming physical barriers to disabled people. Secondly, from the year 2004, providers of services will have to take reasonable steps to remove, or substantially reduce, those physical barriers. The challenge of meeting the needs of disabled people will continue to be a priority for national and local agencies. Progress will not be sustainable if agencies act in isolation of other agencies or of disabled people themselves. The emphasis on working through partnerships to achieve goals continues to be highlighted both nationally across Government Departments and locally between different agencies, and increasingly involves disabled people and their carers and families.

Consent: Highlighted in last year's Report[81], consent issues have remained a focus of public and professional interest and concern. In December 1997, the Lord Chancellor's Department issued a consultation paper *Who decides?*[82], which built on earlier work of the Law Commission[83] and sought views on reform of the law governing decision-making on the health, welfare and financial affairs of mentally incapacitated adults. In relation to health, the consultation paper sought detailed views on the law governing advance statements in respect of treatment; procedures which may give rise to particular concern, including sterilisation and non-therapeutic research; and the creation of a power of attorney to enable a person to choose who should take decisions concerning their health and welfare when they could no longer do so themselves. Consultation closed on 31 March 1998. After a case which established that written consent is necessary for the storage or posthumous use of gametes in assisted reproduction[84], a review of consent procedures for the removal, storage and use of gametes is being conducted by Professor Sheila McLean, Professor of Law and Ethics in Medicine at the University of Glasgow, on behalf of UK Health Ministers. A consultation paper, *Consent and the law*[85], issued in September 1997, reviewed and sought opinions on the current state of the law in this area, including the implications of relevant European legal provisions, and on whether reform was indicated.

Domestic violence: As highlighted in last year's Report[86], action to combat domestic violence continues to be accorded high priority. DH has worked closely with the Home Office and the Women's Unit, which also have responsibilities in this area, to ensure an inter-Departmental approach for an effective long-term strategy; a joint publicity campaign will be launched in 1999. Many women who have experienced domestic violence seek treatment in the NHS. All staff in primary care, accident and emergency, obstetrics and gynaecology and mental health services especially need to be aware that women whom they see may have experienced domestic violence. On 6 November 1997, the Department wrote to the NHS to encourage health professionals to be alert to the possibility of abuse when they see women who have symptoms which are consistent with domestic violence[87], and provided information about the new civil remedies introduced by Part IV of the Family Law Act 1996[88], which came into operation on 1 October 1997, as well as some examples of good practice. In June 1997, the Department sent a training pack to all directors of social services; *Making an impact: children and domestic violence*[89] aims to help social services staff in the context of Part IV of the Family Law Act 1996[88] and the framework for child protection. A number of medical and nursing Royal Colleges and other professional organisations have issued, or are in the process of issuing, new or updated guidance to their members in respect of domestic violence.

Air quality and health: Publication of the report *Quantification of the effects of air pollutants on health in the United Kingdom*[90] by the Committee on the Medical Effects of Air Pollutants (COMEAP) in January 1998 represents an important step forward in assessment of the extent of the effects of air pollution on health. The report applied, cautiously, such relations as were available to link concentrations of pollutants and effects on the health of the UK population. Numbers of deaths and hospital admissions from respiratory disease brought forward by exposure to particles, sulphur dioxide and ozone were estimated. Considerable uncertainty surrounded the estimates for ozone because of difficulties in ascertaining a threshold of effect; however, for particles some 8,000 deaths and 10,000 admissions annually appear to be associated with exposure (all estimates relate to urban areas only in Great Britain). An expert group was set up in September 1997 to look at the feasibility of estimating the impact of these effects in financial terms - an important initiative which, if successful, will contribute to the cost-benefit analysis of the National Air Quality Strategy[91] (see page 123).

NEW TOPICS IDENTIFIED DURING 1997

Each year a small number of issues are identified as topics of particular importance, to be followed up in subsequent Reports. It should be recognised that the actions needed to ensure progress on these topics may be the responsibility of a wide range of organisations and individuals.

Health and the environment

The special chapter in this year's Report (see page 108) focuses on the environment and its impact on health, especially how possible climate change may influence some of these effects. The link between the environment and health has been recognised for many years[2]. More recently, there has been increasing awareness of the interconnection between our environment and quality of life, and that changes in the environment may lead to ill-health[92,93,94,95]. This was recognised nationally by the publication of the UK National Environmental Health Action Plan (NEHAP)[96], part of the internationally agreed Environment and Health Action Plan for Europe (EHAPE), a principal feature of which was that Environment and Health Departments in individual countries would work together to prepare national action plans. The UK was one of six countries to produce pilot plans in order to assist other countries to prepare their own.

Sustainable development recognises the need for technological development, but without environmental damage that might adversely affect the quality of life now, and for generations to come, and with the inclusion of all sectors of society[97,98,99].

The key to the implementation of many improvements to the environment and health is through action at a local level, and much is already being done through 'Local Agenda 21'- a comprehensive action plan at the local level for sustainable development into the 21st Century. The activities often deliver health benefits as well as environmental ones, and involvement in the partnerships and planning stimulates the development of a healthier community.

But there are also global challenges to the environment and so, potentially, to human health. One of these is climate change due to human activity, which has great potential to affect health[100]. This needs to be tackled internationally through agreements such as the Kyoto agreement, where most developed nations committed themselves to reduce their emissions of 'greenhouse gases'. Environmental factors and their impact on health need to be tackled at every appropriate level - invidually, locally, nationally and internationally.

Autism

Since the term autism was first used by Kanner in 1943[101] to describe children who had serious difficulties in relating to people, problems in the development of normal language and ritualistic and obsessional behaviours, the recognition and understanding of this condition has increased considerably and the diagnostic criteria have broadened, particularly since Asperger syndrome was recognised as a related disorder. The autistic spectrum has widened and within it subgroups are emerging, although current attempts to identify these are considered unsatisfactory[102]. The true incidence of autistic spectrum disorders is uncertain because diagnostic criteria have changed and health and educational services have become more able to recognise individuals who are mildly or atypically affected[103]. Moreover, limitations of current survey methods make it difficult to detect trends[104].

Detailed information about the modes of presentation, prognostic indicators and the usual course of this condition is limited. The usual age of first concern is between the first and second birthday[105]. Sometimes it is possible to identify earlier signs[106], but in some children there is apparently normal development followed by speech loss[107]. Follow-up studies indicate that around 60% of autistic subjects remain severely handicapped in adult life and require high levels of support and care; most of these individuals have a learning disability in addition to their autistic disability. Higher scores on intelligence quotient (IQ) tests, communicative speech and appropriate play are considered to be prognostic of a better outcome[108,109].

The aetiology of autistic spectrum disorders is far from clear but there is no evidence that psychodynamic family factors contribute, as was initially supposed[110]. However, there is evidence that brain dysfunction is present and that genetic factors play a part in many cases[111,112]. The mechanism and nature of this brain dysfunction has been the subject of many hypotheses and much research: core deficit hypotheses include lack of 'theory of mind'[113] and cerebellar, limbic and other neural pathways[114,115,116] have been implicated in some, but not all, necropsy and neuroimaging studies; there are also several neurobiological theories[116]. There is a growing suspicion that autism is not a unitary condition, but a number of related disorders with considerable overlap.

In view of the uncertainty about the relative contributions of various possible aetiologies, variations in the course of the condition, and diagnostic drift over past 50 years, it is not surprising that many interventions that have been put forward as beneficial for autism have proved difficult to evaluate properly in terms of long-term outcome. Research into various approaches to behaviour modification, based on modern learning theory and structured teaching, have shown some promising results, but are hard to compare because of different approaches and different measures of outcome[117,118,119,120].

There is much more to be learnt about this serious disorder. Early recognition of autism, which is becoming more possible, will be a key factor; identification of the most effective form of management of the disorder requires further research. The DfEE is funding a review on research interventions for children with autism which should be published in late 1998 and will inform the commissioning of future research.

Screening

Screening for disease is the systematic application of a test or inquiry to identify individuals at sufficient risk of a specific disorder to warrant further investigation or direct preventive action, among persons who have not sought medical attention on account of symptoms of that disorder.

In a speech at the launch of the *Journal of Medical Screening* in 1995, the Chief Medical Officer outlined a new strategy for screening, policy-making and quality management.

A National Screening Committee was set up with the remit to advise on:

- the case for implementation of new population screening programmes not presently purchased by the NHS;

- the implementation of screening technologies of proven effectiveness, but which require controlled and well-managed introduction; *and*

28

- the case for continuing, modifying or withdrawing existing population screening programmes, in particular programmes inadequately evaluated or of doubtful effectiveness, quality or value.

The Committee produced its first annual report in 1998[121] which is also available on the Departmental Web site at http://www.open.gov.uk/doh/nsc/nsch.htm.

The National Screening Committee makes its decisions principally on evidence produced by the Population Screening Panel of the Department's Health Technology Assessment Programme. As discussed later (see page 150), in its first year the National Screening Committee has: drawn up an inventory of 200 potential and almost 100 existing screening programmes; revised the criteria that were used for 30 years to appraise new screening tests; set up sub-groups to co-ordinate policy-making and quality management for antenatal screening and child health screening; examined the evidence for screening for prostatic cancer, leading to Departmental guidance that screening should not, at present, be introduced; recommended screening antenatally for hepatitis B susceptibility; organised workshops to appraise the evidence on colorectal cancer screening; reviewed the quality assurance system for neonatal metabolic disease screening for hypothyroidism and phenylketonuria; and published ethical principles for considering screening.

The Committee's forward agenda is even more ambitious. Building on the solid foundations of its first year and the hard work of many contributors, the Committee will be taking innovative approaches to a wide range of problematic screening issues. A 'Quality management for screening' project will make recommendations about a strategic national framework for quality assurance of all screening programmes to ensure a coherent, co-ordinated and effective approach. Evaluative pilot studies for colorectal cancer screening and *Chlamydia trachomatis* will inform consideration of feasibility, cost-effectiveness and public acceptability for national programmes. The antenatal screening and child health screening expert sub-groups will examine the range of tests undertaken on expectant mothers and the newborn, testing them against the evidence and establishing new quality standards. New challenges also face the Committee, such as screening for diabetes mellitus or ovarian cancer, where the NHS is looking for advice. There are, of course, many other issues that require debate and leadership, such as the role of primary care in screening; informed choice for consumers; and the emergence of the new genetic testing. The National Screening Committee will work with others to advance thinking in all these areas.

The National Screening Committee is a UK Committee involving all four Health Departments. Screening is an important public health service - but the potential benefit that the early detection of disease offers can only be realised if policy-making takes into account not only the benefits but also the potential adverse effects and opportunity costs of screening and if the screening programme, when operational, is part of a system of quality assurance, with explicit standards and an information system to allow the programme to compare its performance with those standards and act with authority if the screening programme does not meet them.

Diabetes mellitus

Diabetes mellitus (DM) is a common chronic disorder with high morbidity and increased mortality. It exists in two main forms: type 1 DM, which occurs primarily among younger people; and type 2 DM which is much commoner and can be symptomless for many years, found usually in older people[122]. Type 1 DM is caused by autoimmune destruction of the insulin-producing cells of the pancreas, and patients require insulin treatment. The precise causes of type 2 DM are less well established, although patients are characterised by resistance to the actions of insulin with insufficient insulin secretion to overcome this resistance. Type 2 DM is associated with obesity, physical inactivity, ethnicity and increasing age, as well as being associated with other cardiovascular risk-factors, such as hypertension and high blood triglyceride concentrations.

The most recent estimates indicate that, in 1997, there were 199,000 people with type 1 and 1,078,000 with type 2 DM[123,124] in the UK, amounting in total to about 2% of the population. A recent survey in Newcastle upon Tyne found that 4.8% of caucasian adults aged 25-74 years had type 2 DM[125]. A high proportion (perhaps up to 50%) of those with type 2 DM are not diagnosed until complications of the disease, such as retinopathy, are already present. A much higher proportion of people of Asian Indian and of Afro-Caribbean origin have type 2 DM; in the Newcastle study[125], 17.9% of Asian Indians aged 25-74 years were found to have the disorder, with a further 18.7% having impaired glucose tolerance, which implies a 30-50% higher risk of the development of DM in 5-10 years[126]. Both types of diabetes mellitus are rising rapidly world wide, and it is estimated that there will be nearly three million people with type 2 DM in the UK by the year 2010[123].

Diabetes mellitus causes particular damage to eyes, kidneys and nerves via effects on the microvascular circulation. It is the commonest cause of blindness under the age of 65 years, and is a leading cause of renal failure and the need for dialysis and transplantation[127]. There is a two to five-fold increased risk of myocardial infarction and stroke, and it also causes peripheral vascular disease, particularly in the arteries of the legs, which, together with neuropathy, can lead to foot gangrene; the risk of amputation is increased 15-fold among people with DM. Most of these complications can be prevented by good control of blood glucose. In type 1 DM, improved control decreases retinopathy by 60%[128].

Earlier detection is also required, particularly for symptomless type 2 diabetes, which may be present for four to seven years on average before diagnosis[129], to minimise complications. The economic burden of DM is high, with 5-10% of hospital costs in the UK being attributed to DM and its complications - some £1,400 million at 1996 prices[130,131].

The twin cornerstones of treatment of type 2 DM are patient education and lifestyle (diet and exercise) modification[132]. Diets are designed to attain normal body weight and to be high in unrefined carbohydrates and low in fat. To convert this advice into action has been of limited success, and better ways to get this message across are needed. Drug treatment is therefore often necessary - usually via agents which increase insulin secretion (eg, sulphonylureas) and those which diminish insulin resistance (eg, metformin). Insulin therapy is required in virtually all type 1 diabetic patients, and in type 2 diabetic subjects who have not achieved adequate blood glucose concentrations on other forms of therapy. Patient self-management is extremely important, aided by monitoring of their own blood glucose.

Traditionally, care for DM has been delivered in hospital diabetic clinics, but over recent years there has been increased emphasis on management of type 2 diabetes in primary care. Improvements in the standard of care have been stimulated by the WHO Europe St Vincent programme[133] and the British Diabetic Association, which has led to the establishment of local diabetes services advisory groups (LDSAGs) in many districts, involving primary and secondary care physicians, diabetes specialist nurses, chiropodists, dietitians, patients and public health doctors[134]. The LDSAGs can review the whole of a district's services and fit in ideally with the concept of Health Improvement Programmes; one of the Health Action Zones will also focus on diabetes care. Multidisciplinary working has also improved diabetes care, as has the development of dedicated centres in many districts which act as focal points of care. Secondary and tertiary prevention are vital elements of treatment - to prevent the development of complications and to stop the complications, if present, from causing major complications.

The recent widespread introduction of protocols and guidelines[132,135] and the establishment of standards[136] have also begun to have an impact, and will be given added impetus by the National Institute for Clinical Excellence. Similarly, improved training of physicians and nurses alike is having a beneficial effect.

Several aspects of diabetes care need more attention in the future. Better planning and integration of multidisciplinary diabetes services across districts and regions is vital. Prevention of type 2 DM through lifestyle modification is feasible and requires much more effort to decrease the overall personal and economic burden; it is worth stressing that the same modifications will help to prevent heart disease. Selective screening to detect those at high risk (ethnic minorities, those with a positive family history, the very obese and older people) may help to pre-empt the development of complications. Finally, the introduction of schemes for the accreditation of diabetes care services should ensure uniformly high standards of care.

EXECUTIVE SUMMARY

VITAL STATISTICS

Population size

The estimated resident population of England at 30 June 1997 was 49.3 million, an increase of 0.2 million (0.4%) compared with 1996 and of 3.8% compared with 1987.

Age and sex structure of the resident population

There has been a striking increase in the number of adults aged 25-34, 35-44, and 45-54 years over the past 10 years. Elderly people (those aged 65 years and over) and, in particular, very elderly people (those aged 85 years and over) still continue to increase in number.

Fertility statistics

In 1996, 773,600 conceptions occurred to women resident in England, a 3% increase from the figure in 1995 (750,000), with an overall rate of 76.1 per 1,000 women aged 15-44 years. During 1996, there were 9.3 conceptions per 1,000 girls aged 13-15 years in England, compared with 8.5 per 1,000 in 1995 and 8.3 per 1,000 in 1994. In 1997, there were 607,200 live births in England - 1.1% fewer than in 1996; the total period fertility rate in 1997 was 1.71 compared with 1.73 in 1996. During 1996, 160,629 abortions were performed on women resident in England, an increase of 9% compared with 1995.

Trends in reporting congenital abnormalities

In 1997, the notification rate for live births with congenital abnormalities fell to 79.2 per 10,000 live births, 5% lower than in 1996 and 8% lower than in 1992 (see Appendix Table A.6).

Mortality

Provisional statistics for 1997 indicate that 3,591 babies died in England before the age of one year, compared with 3,725 in 1996, and that the infant mortality rate was 5.9 per 1,000 live births (the lowest ever recorded). Based on provisional statistics, there were 3,250 stillbirths in England in 1997 compared with 3,345 in 1996; the stillbirth rate per 1,000 total births fell from 5.4 in 1996 to 5.3 in 1997. Provisional data for England in 1997 indicate 1,734 deaths among children aged 1-15 years, compared with 1,712 in 1996. Deaths registered in England decreased from 526,650 in 1996 to 521,958 in 1997, a fall of 1%.

33

Prevalence of disease in the community

Between 1994 and 1996, the proportion of the population prescribed drugs for asthma rose by 4% among males and 7% in females. The same period saw a 15% increase in the proportion of women and a 19% increase in the proportion of men aged 15 years and over who were prescribed antidepressants.

Trends in cancer incidence and mortality

The age-standardised incidence rate for all malignant neoplasms combined (excluding non-melanoma skin cancer) rose by nearly 10% among males and by over 20% in females between 1979 and 1992. Among males, the largest percentage increases were in cancer of the pleura and in malignant melanoma; among females, the largest percentage increases were in non-Hodgkin's lymphoma and in malignant melanoma.

THE NATION'S HEALTH

Basic sources of information

The Health Survey for England[5] is an annual national survey of those living in private households. In 1997, it focused on the health of children and young people as well as covering core topics in the adult population.

Substance misuse

The Government appointed a UK Anti-Drugs Co-ordinator to advise on a new strategy. The Department continues to monitor the availability of appropriate, effective and cost-effective services for drug misusers. Evidence provided through this work will contribute towards the work of the UK Anti-Drugs Co-ordinator and his deputy in reviewing the Government's drugs strategy. The Department continued its contract with the Health Education Authority (HEA) for a drugs and solvents prevention campaign and with Network Scotland to provide a free 24-hour National Drugs Helpline. A Ministerial Group on Alcopops was established to draw together activity to combat under-age alcohol misuse.

Smoking

Smoking prevalence continued to rise in young people[6] and previous falls have levelled off among adults. The European Directive to ban cigarette advertising was agreed by Health Ministers. New research on passive smoking indicated increased risks among adults and in children[137,138,139].

Nutrition

The Committee on Medical Aspects of Food and Nutrition Policy (COMA) prepared a statement on selenium levels in the UK diet[140], and finalised its report on nutritional aspects of the development of cancer[141]. DH commissioned a review of the effectiveness of interventions for obesity[142,143] and nine research projects. The National Network of Breast-feeding Co-ordinators continued to promote breast-feeding within and outside the NHS. Reports of the 1995 Infant Feeding Survey[144] and of the Survey of Infant Feeding in Asian Families[145] were published.

Health of children

In Spring 1997, the House of Commons Select Committee on Health published four reports on the general health status of children[146,147,148,149]. The Government response was published in November[150].

Health of adolescents

Activities to promote the health of young people continued during 1997, with a particular focus on health in schools. DH and the DfEE worked together to develop policy on healthy schools.

Health of women

During the year, DH announced the development of additional health promotion materials for women in older and younger age-groups.

Health of men

Work during the year focused on areas identified as key factors in the improvement of public health.

Health of black and ethnic minorities

An international conference on 'Health gain for black and ethnic communities' took place in September. In October, the National Institute for Ethnic Studies in Health and Social Policy published a report[151].

Health in the workplace

The Health and Safety Executive continued to build on the success of its 'Good health is good business' campaign. More than 80% of NHS Trusts and health authorities are now involved in the 'Health at work in the NHS' project.

Health of people in later life

DH worked to improve services to promote independence for older people by the development of joint investment plans for continuing and community care, and of recuperation and rehabilitation services for older people.

Mental health

Mental health continues to be a priority within the NHS, with increased emphasis on mental health promotion and preventive work at national and local levels.

Health of disabled people

Highlighted in last year's Report[79], much work continues to be done to improve services for disabled people and to raise awareness about their individual needs.

THE STRATEGY FOR HEALTH

Introduction

Ms Tessa Jowell MP, Minister of State for Public Health, outlined the key features of the new strategy for health on 7 July[152], and a Green Paper *Our Healthier Nation*[1] will be published for consultation in early 1998 with the view to publication of a White Paper later in that year.

Health of the Nation

The Health of the Nation White Paper[153], launched in 1992, set 27 targets to improve health. Progress on these is reviewed.

Wider determinants of health

Although the effects on health of an individual's age, sex, genetic make-up and lifestyle choices are beyond dispute, the circumstances under which they live, which may not be subject to choice, also have a major impact on their health.

Inequalities in health

Social class inequalities in death rates do not appear to have fallen over the past 40 years[36]. Action to address these inequalities in health will be a major priority.

Health alliances and healthy settings

The concept of alliances for health will be central to health improvement programmes to be established by each health authority in partnership with local interests. Healthy settings provide a helpful focus for health promotion activities - for example in schools and workplaces.

Inter-Departmental co-operation

A new Cabinet sub-committee has been set up to oversee the development, implementation and monitoring of the Government's health strategy, and to co-ordinate the Government's policies on UK-wide issues that affect health.

ENVIRONMENT AND HEALTH

Introduction

Some of the interactions between the environment and health have been recognised for centuries, and there has been a clear legislative link between health and the environment since the 1848 Public Health Act[2]. The special chapter in this year's Report explores various aspects of the wider environment and its impact on health, including how climate change may affect some of these.

National and international issues

Climate change and human health: Human activities are increasing the atmospheric concentrations of 'greenhouse gases', which tend to warm the atmosphere and are thought likely to lead to regional and global changes in climate[154]. Potentially serious impacts of climate change could include an increase in temperature fluctuations, floods, droughts and pest outbreaks, and longer-term effects on ecosystems - which would have direct and indirect effects on health. In view of these concerns, and the need for future data, the Government has established the UK Climate Impacts Programme.

Sustainable development: Sustainable development recognises the need for technological development, but without environmental damage that might adversely affect the quality of life now, and for generations to come, and with the inclusion of all sectors of society.

'Local Agenda 21': This comprehensive action plan for sustainable development into the 21st Century aims to bring together local government, business, voluntary and community sectors to identify what their local communities want and need, and then to co-ordinate delivery by means of local resources, taking account of local interests.

National environmental health action plan: The UK NEHAP[155] builds on existing strategies for sustainable development, concentrating on health implications and environmental policies in their widest sense and following the objectives of the environment and health action plan for Europe.

Lifestyle, environment and health

The concept of environmental health encompasses the workplace or classroom, home and leisure environments, each of which has many components.

Housing: In general, basic housing conditions have improved considerably over the past 50 years, but a minority of houses still pose health and safety risks. The most vulnerable members of society are more likely to live in poor housing[156], and many initiatives are under way to tackle poor housing conditions.

Transport and health: Transport and health are linked in several respects, and initiatives are in place to promote safe cycling and walking as alternatives to using motor vehicles.

Leisure: Leisure pursuits play an important part in health promotion - increased physical exercise and reduction of stress are among the benefits - but environmental hazards associated with such activities should be minimised.

Environmental influences on health

Air pollution: Concentrations of several air pollutants have fallen dramatically in the UK this Century, but the extent of the anticipated improvement has been limited by the growth of traffic-generated air pollution, which is currently a major challenge. Recent initiatives include assessments of the effects of individual pollutants, a national air quality strategy[91] and a handbook on air pollution and health[157]. Indoor air pollution, including environmental tobacco smoke, is also a factor.

Noise: The effects of noise on hearing in occupational settings is established, and research will be commissioned during 1998 into the effects of environmental noise on other aspects of health.

Radiation in the environment: Radon, a natural radioactive gas, is the main source of human exposure to ionising radiation and concentrations in the home are higher in certain parts of the country. Electromagnetic fields have been the subject of public and media fears about potential health effects, although there is no clear causal link to provide a scientific basis for those fears. Excess exposure to ultraviolet radiation from the sun is associated with adverse health effects, particularly the development of skin cancer. Nuclear radiation has known effects on human health, although no causal link has been established between cancer incidence and radioactive material released from nuclear installations in the UK. Research continues into all aspects of radiation in the environment.

Environmental chemicals: As well as general work to establish priorities for public health responses to environmental chemical pollutants, particular attention is being paid to the effects of lead and endocrine disruptors.

Microbiological factors: Reduced rainfall as a result of climate change may have an effect on water quality and waterborne diseases. Pests, such as rats, are also likely to increase with a warmer climate. Foodborne diseases are more common in summer months, and increased temperatures are likely to lead to increased cases of food poisoning. Vector-borne diseases will also be affected by climatic change because of its effects on the life-cycle of the vectors.

Biotechnology developments: Safe uses of biotechnology could foster the aim of sustainable development, but should be regulated and audited to ensure that they are safe, and seen to be safe, as well as ethical.

Monitoring and surveillance of environmental indicators

An understanding of the health implications of climate change and other environmental factors requires the ability to identify changes in health and whether they are linked to local or global environmental changes.

Clusters of disease and the Small Area Health Statistics Unit: Apparent clusters of disease can cause substantial public anxiety and are often speculatively linked with a supposed local environmental hazard. The Small Area Health Statistics Unit investigates claims of unusual clusters of disease or ill-health, particularly in the vicinity of point sources of pollution from chemicals and/or radiation.

Response to specific incidents: In 1997, DH, together with the other UK Health Departments, established a national focus for work on the response to chemical incidents and the surveillance of the health effects of environmental chemicals at the University of Wales Institute, Cardiff.

The way ahead

Continued and enhanced research into the links between environment and health will lead to a better understanding of which factors affect health, how they interact and the size of those effects. The resources and the will needed to maintain and to improve environmental health should not be underestimated, and can only be achieved by collaboration - individually, locally, nationally and internationally.

HEALTH CARE

Role and function of the National Health Service in England

Purpose: The purpose of the NHS is to secure through the resources available the greatest possible improvement in the physical and mental health of the population by: promoting health, preventing ill-health, diagnosing and treating disease and injury, and caring for those with long-term illness and disability.

Policies and strategies: The main Government policies for the NHS have been set out in *The new NHS: modern, dependable*[44] White Paper, which will be followed in early 1998 by the Green Paper *Our Healthier Nation*[1]. DH, along with all Government Departments, is involved in a Comprehensive Spending Review which will inform plans from 1999/2000.

Priority setting: The Government has set out plans to improve national consistency of services and to ensure that there is fair access to services, with a commitment to services being available on the basis of need and not the ability to pay.

Research and development: The R&D strategy has two complementary programmes: the policy research programme, which provides a knowledge base for strategic matters across the Department and is developing a co-ordinated approach to public health research; and the NHS R&D Programme, which is priority-led, with a key role in evidence-based health care. A new funding system for NHS R&D is now in place.

Role of the NHS in maintaining public health

Public health and the NHS: In the White Paper *The new NHS: modern, dependable*[44,] the NHS has a key role in moves to improve the nation's health.

Chief Medical Officer's project to strengthen the public health function: The Chief Medical Officer's project to strengthen the public health function linked directly to, and supported, activity on the Green Paper *Our Healthier Nation*[1] and the White Paper *The new NHS: modern, dependable*[44], and will inform preparation on the 'Our Healthier Nation' initiative.

Health care needs assessment: A second health care needs assessment series was published in January[158]. Work started on a third series of these epidemiologically based reviews, and on updating the first series.

National Casemix Office and NHS Centre for Coding and Classification: The National Casemix Office and the Centre for Coding and Classification continued to develop terms that support clinicians, and groupings of activity data for analysis and management purposes.

National Screening Committee: The National Screening Committee advises UK Ministers and Departments of Health on the need for the introduction, review, modification or cessation of national population screening programmes.

Quality of service and effectiveness of care: Improvement of the quality and clinical effectiveness of services continues to be a fundamental aim for the NHS, as recognised in the NHS White Paper *The new NHS: modern, dependable*[44], which sets out a range of initiatives which together put quality of care firmly at the heart of the new NHS.

Clinical and health outcomes: Nine of the ten multidisciplinary working groups set up to develop new outcome indicators submitted their reports. The NHS Executive published a consultation document on a first set of 15 clinical indicators[159]. Following evaluation, an outcomes assessment system, 'Functional Assessment of Care Environments', was made available for use by the NHS to assess outcomes among people with mental illness, learning disabilities and older people.

Regional epidemiological services for communicable disease: Surveillance, prevention and control of communicable disease remains a fundamental public health task. A national Service Level Agreement, which came into effect on 1 April 1996 between the NHS Executive and the Public Health Laboratory Service (PHLS), has continued.

Primary health care

Organisation of primary care: Opportunities for locally sensitive organisation of primary care services increased in 1997, based on the 1996 White Papers *Choice and opportunity*[160] and *Primary care: delivering the future*[161], and the 1997 White Paper *The new NHS: modern, dependable*[44].

Development of emergency services in the community: The Chief Medical Officer's review of emergency services in the community was published in September[162]. Pilot studies of emergency telephone helplines were prepared. The spread of the co-operative movement for general practitioner (GP) out-of-hours services continued.

Health promotion in general practice: New arrangements came into force for health promotion activity, which will be subject to review.

Review of continuing professional development: A review of continuing professional development in general practice, led by the Chief Medical Officer, will be published in Spring 1998.

Prescribing: There have been further initiatives to ensure that prescribing becomes more clinically effective and more cost-effective.

Specialised clinical services

Specialised services: The National Specialist Commissioning Advisory Group commissioned three new established services, and identified two for evaluation.

Cancer: Further implementation of a policy framework for the commissioning of cancer services[163] continued; an additional £10 million were made available for breast care services, and further evidence-based guidance for commissioners of health care[164] was published.

National Confidential Enquiry into Perioperative Deaths: The National Confidential Enquiry into Perioperative Deaths continued its work to raise professional and organisational standards of surgery, and published two reports[165,166].

Safety and Efficacy Register of New Interventional Procedures: The Safety and Efficacy Register of New Interventional Procedures considered 67 procedures during the year.

Osteoporosis: DH began work on a new strategy for osteoporosis in consultation with clinicians and health care managers.

Transplantation: During the year, 2,293 cadaveric organ transplants were performed in England. The number of patients who might benefit from transplants continued to rise. By December 1997, over 4.65 million people had registered with the NHS Organ Donor Register.

National renal review: Work continues to improve access to services for patients with end-stage renal failure[167].

Statins and coronary heart disease: In August, the Standing Medical Advisory Committee issued a statement on the use of statins in the treatment of patients with coronary heart disease[168].

Adult intensive care: Recent policy initiatives on adult intensive care include the introduction of a national intensive care bed register and the mandatory collection of a standardised national data set on activity in intensive and high-dependency care units.

Emergency care services: An additional £269 million made available for the NHS in England in October, together with better planning and closer co-operation with social services departments, helped to ease pressures on the health and social care systems during the winter.

Ambulance performance standards review: Four ambulance services started to prioritise calls in April, followed by a further five in October.

Palliative care: The Department is committed to the benefits of specialist palliative care for patients with cancer and other life-threatening illnesses, and for their carers and families.

Diabetes mellitus: DH issued service guidance, *Key features of a good diabetes service*[169], to the NHS in November. Clinical guidelines on non-insulin-dependent DM, and Effective Health Care Bulletins, have been commissioned.

Asthma: DH is working with other interested parties to inform health professionals and the public about the change to CFC-free inhalers.

Mental health

Mental health promotion: In partnership with 6,000 local agencies and 50 national organisations, the HEA's World Mental Health Day campaign works to increase public understanding of mental health, to reduce stigma and to support those working to promote mental health locally, and to increase understanding of these issues in the media.

Mental health in primary care: Mental health problems in primary care are common[170]. During the year a toolkit for primary care mental health was published[171], innovative practices shared, training of GPs was audited and the development of primary mental health care further explored.

Occupational mental health: Work continued to increase employers' awareness of occupational mental health issues and to encourage further action.

Psychological treatment services: Following publication of the NHS Executive's strategic review of psychotherapy services in September 1996[172], regional conferences were held, an independent review of funding for psychotherapy training was commissioned[173], and education and training planning guidance was issued in October[174].

Child and adolescent mental health: Awareness of the needs of children and young people with mental health problems continues to increase. Work to improve child and adolescent mental health services continued throughout the year, and will be further enhanced when the outcome of three major studies are published over the next two years.

National Confidential Inquiry into Suicide and Homicide by People with Mental Illness: The Inquiry is conducting a national audit of suicides and homicides by people who have a history of contact with mental health services; a progress report was published on 12 December[175].

Specialised mental illness services: DH remains committed to comprehensive, locally based services in which the needs of individuals are provided by multidisciplinary teams that work in partnership, with initiatives to improve the quality and efficiency of, and public confidence and partnerships in, the provision of care for individuals with severe mental illness, along with an increased focus on prevention. The problem of co-morbidity of substance misuse and severe mental illness is a particular challenge.

Services for mentally disordered offenders: Research and training in forensic mental health services are key areas for the High Security Psychiatric Services Commissioning Board. Antisocial personality disorder is a key policy area for DH and the Home Office, reflected in the Board's R&D strategy.

Mental health legislation: The Mental Health Act 1983[176] provides the statutory power for the formal detention of mentally disordered patients who meet the criteria laid down in the Act.

Maternity and child health services

Implementation of 'Changing Childbirth': Continued promotion of continuity and choice in maternity services was supported by education and training initiatives.

Confidential Enquiry into Stillbirths and Deaths in Infancy (CESDI): The CESDI report for 1995, published in July 1997[177], made a number of observations about inadequate clinical and post-mortem practices, identified from the examination of cases for that year.

Folic acid and the prevention of neural tube defects: The HEA's campaign to promote the benefits of increasing folic acid intake around the time of conception continued.

Sudden infant death syndrome: Since the 1991 launch of DH's campaign to reduce the number of cot deaths, the number of such deaths has more than halved.

Prophylaxis of vitamin K deficiency bleeding in infants: An expert group was convened to consider all evidence related to the use of prophylaxis for vitamin K deficiency bleeding in infants, and is expected to report in 1998.

Retinopathy of prematurity: The multidisciplinary research project set up to assess and to improve the care of infants with retinopathy of prematurity continues.

Paediatric intensive care: The report *Paediatric intensive care: a framework for the future*[178], published in July, together with an accompanying report on nursing standards, education and workforce planning, *A bridge to the future*[179], outline policies to improve paediatric intensive care that are now being implemented.

Disability

General aspects of disability: Last year's Report[79] included a special chapter on the health of disabled people. The *Health Survey for England 1995* provided further data on self-reported disability: some 18% of males and females aged over 16 years who were living in private households had some degree of moderate or serious disability; 4% of men and 5% of women had a serious disability.

Types of disability: All aspects of disability - physical, sensory, learning and mental - need to be taken into account when assessing care needs and service provision.

Re-ablement: The joint initiative on the co-ordination of rehabilitation services for disabled people held four regional seminars during the year; a report is in preparation. Measures to help people with a disability or long-term illness to find or to remain in work were taken forward. The health care needs of disabled people, and their carers, were further examined.

Complementary medicine

Progress continues towards implementation of the statutory regulation of osteopaths and chiropractors.

Prison health care

Noteworthy developments in prison health care were made during the year, particularly in respect of training, mental health and health promotion.

COMMUNICABLE DISEASES

HIV infection and AIDS

The pattern of HIV infection was similar to that in previous years, but a significant change was seen for AIDS cases. During 1997, the number of AIDS cases reported fell by 26% compared with 1996, probably due to the uptake of new combination drug therapies which delay progression to a diagnosis of AIDS. Monotherapy with anti-HIV drugs has been found to lose therapeutic benefit due to the development of viral resistance, and clinical guidelines published in April[180] recommended treatment with a combination of antiretroviral drugs. However, none of the treatments yet identified represent a cure for HIV infection, and it is possible that HIV will eventually develop resistance to the combinations of drugs currently in use. Public health measures to prevent the spread of infection still remain crucial to the control of the HIV virus.

Other sexually transmitted infections

Over 420,000 new cases were seen at genito-urinary medicine (GUM) clinics during 1996. Total diagnoses of acute sexually transmitted infections rose by 7% between 1995 and 1996[ref]. Diagnoses of gonorrhoea, uncomplicated *Chlamydia* and genital warts rose by 17%, 11% and 5%, respectively, during the same period.

Chlamydia

The Expert Advisory Group on *Chlamydia trachomatis* agreed that action was required to reduce the morbidity associated with this infection[181]. A key conclusion was that health gains would result from the screening of symptomless, sexually active young women.

Immunisation

Immunisation coverage has remained at extremely high levels, although there has been a small but concerning decline in measles, mumps and rubella (MMR) vaccine coverage.

Viral hepatitis

During 1997, the PHLS Communicable Disease Surveillance Centre received reports from laboratories of 1,260 confirmed cases of hepatitis A and 616 confirmed cases of acute hepatitis B in England.

Influenza

The UK Health Departments issued their contingency plans for pandemic influenza in March[182]. In December, an outbreak of influenza in Hong Kong, due to an avian (H_5N_1) influenza virus not previously known to infect man, raised concerns about a possible pandemic. In the event, no person-to-person transmission was confirmed and the outbreak was brought to an end following the widespread cull of chickens in Hong Kong.

Meningitis

Since 1995, there has been an increase in the incidence of meningococcal disease, which has continued into 1997, although data for late 1997 indicate that the incidence has now started to fall.

Tuberculosis

New notifications for tuberculosis remained fairly steady. Forty-nine per cent of patients studied in the 1993 survey of tuberculosis notifications had been born abroad, with important differences in trends between ethnic groups; a further survey is planned in 1998.

Hospital-acquired infection

Interest in hospital-acquired infection continued to increase. A national surveillance scheme has been established and a DH-funded audit of surveillance and policies for infection control[183] was published in May.

Antimicrobial-resistant infection

Several committees undertook work which will help to define future strategy to limit the further development, and spread, of antimicrobial resistance.

New variant Creutzfeldt-Jakob disease and transmissible spongiform encephalopathies

The Spongiform Encephalopathy Advisory Committee (SEAC) has concluded that the most likely explanation for the cases of nvCJD to date is exposure to BSE before the introduction of the specified bovine offals ban in 1989. Research findings published in October[37,38] were considered by the SEAC, which concluded that they provided convincing evidence that the agent which causes nvCJD in human beings is the same as that which causes BSE in cattle. The findings do not, however, identify the means by which patients become infected.

Emerging and re-emerging infectious diseases

Several notable outbreaks of what are now referred to as new, emerging and re-emerging infectious diseases occurred in various parts of the world, with improved co-ordination of international responses.

Travel-related and tropical diseases

The number of cases of malaria imported into the UK continues to cause concern. New guidelines for the prevention of malaria in travellers from the UK were published[184], and an information leaflet produced for travellers[185]. An updated Memorandum on leprosy was also issued[186].

FOOD SAFETY

Introduction of the Food Standards Agency

During the year, the Government undertook work in preparation for the establishment of a Food Standards Agency.

Foodborne and waterborne diseases

Following two years of relative stability, food poisoning notifications made to the PHLS rose by nearly 13% compared with 1996. The number of *Salmonella* isolates rose, and *Campylobacter* isolates rose by nearly 16%. There was a striking increase of isolates of VTEC O157 of over 60%. The ACMSF's working group on foodborne viral infections should report in 1998; another working group has considered microbial antibiotic resistance in relation to the food chain.

Biotechnology and novel foods

A statutory EU pre-market clearance system was introduced on 15 May for novel foods and food ingredients.

Toxicological safety

The Committee on Toxicity of Chemicals in Food, Consumer Products and the Environment (COT) continued to provide expert advice to Government Departments on the safety of chemicals in food and the environment.

Pesticides

In March, the Advisory Committee on Pesticides published the results of a survey of organophosphorus and carbamate residues in a range of individual fruits and vegetables[187]. The results of a survey of organochlorine residues in human fat samples were also published[188].

Veterinary products

The Veterinary Products Committee and its Medical and Scientific Panel have considered the safety of organophosphorus (OP) sheep dips during the year and epidemiological research on the subject continued. A Working Group established by the Royal Colleges of Physicians and Psychiatrists met several times during the year. DH continued to advise upon human safety aspects of veterinary medicine and animal feed ingredients in the UK and the EU.

EDUCATION, TRAINING AND STAFFING

Junior doctors' hours

The reduction of working hours for junior doctors remains a priority for NHS Trusts, as does the provision of adequate on-call accommodation and catering services. Reports in September showed full compliance with hours targets in over 80% of junior doctors' posts.

Advisory Group on Medical and Dental Education, Training and Staffing, the Specialty Workforce Advisory Group and the Medical Workforce Standing Advisory Committee

The format of the AGMETS was changed in June to give the Group a more strategic focus and to increase its relevance to the needs of the health service. The Medical Workforce Standing Advisory Committee's third report[189] recommended a 20% increase in medical student intake. For 1997/98, the Specialty Workforce Advisory Group recommended an additional 850 training placements for higher specialist trainees.

Postgraduate medical training

The introduction of the new specialist registrar (SpR) grade was completed on 31 March when the final group of 14 specialties completed transition into the new grade. Work continued to put in place arrangements for summative assessment of vocational training in general practice, which will be a legal requirement from 30 January 1998.

Equal opportunities

Guidelines for NHS employers incorporate good practice in equal opportunities in all areas, including race, sex and disability 'Family friendly' employment policies are being encouraged to help doctors balance the demands of their career with other responsibilities.

Retention of doctors

The proportion of medical graduates who do not practise medicine five years after qualification appears to be between 5-9% in cohort studies, and this rate does not appear to have greatly changed over recent years.

Undergraduate medical and dental education

Good progress continues to be made to strengthen the partnership between the NHS and providers of higher education.

Maintaining medical excellence

Progress continued towards the implementation of the recommendations of *Maintaining medical excellence*[190]. The British Association of Medical Managers issued a resource pack *When things go wrong*[191] to all medical directors which provided practical disciplinary advice.

Training developments for wider professional staff

A more integrated approach to the planning and development of health professionals is being encouraged by the NHS Executive. This will emphasise the need for lifelong learning to support clinical governance in the NHS within a sound regulatory framework. The structure and function of the scientific and technical workforce is also under review.

OTHER TOPICS OF INTEREST IN 1997

Medicines Control Agency

Role and performance: The Medicines Control Agency (MCA) safeguards public health by ensuring that all medicines for use in human beings meet appropriate standards for safety, quality and efficacy. Despite an increased workload, the Agency met almost all of its key targets during the year.

Legal reclassification of medicinal products: Three substances were reclassified as prescription-only medicines, one reclassified to pharmacy sale and existing exemptions were widened for four substances; several substances (some in combinations) were added to the General Sale List.

Drug safety issues: A meta-analysis of studies of hormone replacement therapy (HRT) and breast cancer did not markedly alter current perspectives on the risk:benefit ratio of HRT. Terfenadine was restricted to prescription-only use. Concerns about hepatotoxicity led to the withdrawal of troglitazone, a drug introduced for the treatment of diabetes mellitus. The anorectic agents fenfluramine and dexfenfluramine were withdrawn because of evidence of an association with valvular heart disorders.

Pharmaceutical developments in the European Union: The MCA participated in the discussions concerning removal of specified-risk materials from medicinal products and legislative developments in respect of clinical trials, starting materials and fees payable to the European Medicines Evaluation Agency.

Medical Devices Agency

The Medical Devices Agency is an Executive Agency of DH. Its role is to ensure that all medical devices used in the UK meet appropriate standards of safety, quality and performance. The Agency achieves this role through implementation of the EU Medical Devices Directives, a reporting system for device-related adverse incidents, an evaluation programme of a wide range of medical devices and the publication of safety and guidance information.

National Blood Authority

A review of the services provided by the Merseyside Blood Centre, which may have wider implications for the National Blood Service, was initiated and an interim report was produced in September. Concerns about the theoretical risk of transmission of nvCJD through blood and blood products were a major focus of activity.

National Biological Standards Board

The National Biological Standards Board has had a statutory duty to assure the quality of biological substances used in medicine. The National Institute for Biological Standards and Control is a WHO International Laboratory for Biological Standards and prepares and distributes the bulk of the world's international standards and reference materials.

National Radiological Protection Board

The National Radiological Protection Board has the responsibility to acquire and advance knowledge about the protection of mankind from radiation hazards (for both ionising and non-ionising radiation), and to provide information and advice to support protection from radiation hazards. During the year it issued advice on emergency reference levels of dose in emergency planning and response[192], the relative biological effectiveness of neutrons for the induction of cancer[193], chromosome 2 hypersensitivity and clonal development in murine radiation acute myeloid leukaemia[194], carcinogenic response at low doses and dose rates[195], and assessment of skin doses from exposure to ionising radiation[196].

United Kingdom Transplant Support Service Authority

The UK Transplant Support Service Authority was established in 1991 to facilitate the matching and allocation of organs for transplantation; it maintains the NHS organ donor register.

Public Health Laboratory Service Board

The core purpose of the Public Health Laboratory Service (PHLS) is to protect the population from infection. During 1997, a new structure was established to enhance delivery of services in London.

Microbiological Research Authority

The Microbiological Research Authority is a Special Health Authority which directs the work of the Centre for Applied Microbiology and Research.

Gulf War syndrome

The clinical assessment of individual Gulf War veterans continued throughout the year, and a programme of epidemiological research projects, overseen by the Medical Research Council (MRC), was launched.

Bioethics

Research ethics committees: Multi-centre research ethics committees were established and arrangements made to review the research ethics committee system.

Bioethics in Europe: The Council of Europe and the United Nations Educational, Scientific and Cultural Organization (UNESCO) both adopted provisions to prohibit the cloning of human individuals.

Human genetics and the Human Genetics Advisory Commission: The Human Genetics Advisory Commission (HGAC) first met in February. During the year, the HGAC issued a report on the insurance implications of genetic testing[197] and worked towards a consultation paper on the issues arising from mammalian cloning.

Advisory Committee on Genetic Testing: The ACGT issued a code of practice and guidance on human genetic testing services supplied direct to the public[198], and a consultation document on genetic testing for late-onset disorders[199].

Gene Therapy Advisory Committee: During the year the GTAC met five times and approved six gene therapy research protocols.

Assisted conception: Aspects of infertility and related services continued to arouse substantial public interest.

Protection and use of patient information: The Caldicott report made recommendations in relation to the use of patient-identifiable information.

Consent issues: The legal position of people incapable of giving consent before examination or treatment saw important developments in case law and the publication of a Green Paper[82,85].

Complaints

The new NHS complaints procedure introduced in April 1996 is now established.

Research and development

The Department's R&D strategy promotes strong links with the science base, other major research funders in this country, and with EU research and technology programmes.

Use of information technology in clinical care

Work to implement the existing information management technology strategy continued, and some major parts of the technical infrastructure are now in place; the strategy was reviewed during the year.

Dental health

Dental health of the nation: There has been a fall in the number of 12-year-old children with dental decay. Those with dental caries have more teeth affected but fewer filled, and wide regional variations persist.

General dental services: The Government has taken steps to improve access to dentistry. Proposals for the provision of personal dental services were received.

Community dental services: The role of the community dental services was redefined to include provision of services for patients who have difficulty in obtaining treatment from the general dental services, as well as for those who would not otherwise seek it.

Hospital dental services: The number of hospital dentists rose by 2%. There were 636,039 new referrals and 1,929,951 repeat attendances to outpatient clinics in 1996/97.

Continuing education and training for dentists: There was an increase in the number of trainees in regionally based vocational training schemes between September 1996 and September 1997. The National Centre for the Continuing Professional Education of Dentists was established.

Dental research: The fourth national survey of adult dental health was commissioned. The NHS research and development programme in primary dental care invited applications for research.

INTERNATIONAL HEALTH

England, Europe and health

The UK shares many health challenges with the rest of Europe, and the opportunity to work together on common problems brings substantial benefits. European programmes and initiatives allow countries to pool their experience and knowledge, and to take advantage of the greater resources that international co-operation brings into play.

The European Union: During 1997, the European Community (EC) continued its programme of public health initiatives. The Health Council met in June and December; it adopted conclusions on the EU-United States Task Force on communicable diseases, and agreed resolutions on the European Commission's report on the state of women's health, migrant doctors, health-related aspects of drug use, and cross-border co-operation on the supply of organs and tissues of human origin. The High Level Committee on Health met twice during the year.

Council of Europe: The Council's European Health Committee took forward work on several fronts including transplantation and equity in health care.

Relations with Central and Eastern Europe: Work continued in relation to applications to join an enlarged EU.

The Commonwealth

Dr Jeremy Metters, the Deputy Chief Medical Officer, led the British delegation to the Commonwealth Health Ministers' meeting on 4 May.

World Health Organization

European Regional Committee: The Chief Medical Officer led the UK delegation to the 47th session of the European Regional Committee.

Executive Board: The Chief Medical Officer is a member of the Executive Board and attended its meetings in January and May. At the January meeting, the Chief Medical Officer gave a presentation to the Board on a future 'Health for All' strategy.

World Health Assembly: The UK delegation to the 50th World Health Assembly was led by the Deputy Chief Medical Officer.

References

1. Department of Health. *Our Healthier Nation: a contract for health*. London: Stationery Office, 1998 (Cm. 3852).
2. *An Act for Promoting the Public Health 1848*. London: HMSO, 1848 (11+12 Vict. c.lxiii).
3. Department of Health. *Cervical screening programme, England: 1996-97*. London: Department of Health, 1997 (Statistical Bulletin 1997/27).
4. Breeze E, Maidment A, Bennett N, Flatley J, Carey S. *Health Survey for England 1992*. London: HMSO, 1994.
5. Prescott-Clarke P, Primatesta P. *Health Survey for England 1996*. London: Stationery Office, 1998.
6. Office for National Statistics. *Smoking among secondary school children in 1996: England*. London: Stationery Office, 1997.

7.   Department of Health. *On the State of the Public Health: the annual report of the Chief Medical Officer of the Department of Health for the year 1992.* London: HMSO, 1993; 2.

8.   Department of Health. *On the State of the Public Health: the annual report of the Chief Medical Officer of the Department of Health for the year 1993.* London: HMSO, 1994; 2.

9.   Department of Health. *On the State of the Public Health: the annual report of the Chief Medical Officer of the Department of Health for the year 1994.* London: HMSO, 1995; 2.

10.   Department of Health. *On the State of the Public Health: the annual report of the Chief Medical Officer of the Department of Health for the year 1995.* London: HMSO, 1996; 2.

11.   Department of Health. *On the State of the Public Health: the annual report of the Chief Medical Officer of the Department of Health for the year 1996.* London: Stationery Office, 1997; 2.

12.   *An Act for the Improvement of the Sewerage and Drainage of the Borough of Liverpool and for making further provision for the Sanatory Regulation of said Borough 1846.* London: HMSO, 1846 (9+10 Vict c.cxxvii).

13.   *The 1834 Poor Law Amendment Act 1847.* London: HMSO, 1847 (4+5 W.4.c.76).

14.   *An Act to Consolidate and Continue in Force for Two Years and to the then Next Session of Parliament the Metropolitan Commission of Sewers Act 1848.* London: HMSO, 1848 (11+12 Vict c.112).

15.   *The Local Government Act 1858.* London: HMSO, 1858 (21+22 Vict c.98).

16.   *An Act to Amend the Law relating to the Public Health 1866.* London: HMSO, 1866 (29+30 Vict c.79).

17.   *An Act for Consolidating and Amending the Acts relating to Public Health in England 1875.* London: HMSO, 1875 (38+39 Vict c.55).

18.   *An Act for Constituting a Local Government Board and Vesting therein certain functions of the Secretary of State and Privy Council concerning the Public Health and Local Government, together with the powers and duties of the Poor Law Board 1871.* London: HMSO, 1871 (34+35 Vict c.70).

19.   *The Public Health Act 1872.* London: HMSO, 1872 (35+36 Vict c.79).

20.   *An Act to provide against Loss of Health and for the Prevention and Cure of Sickness and for Insurance against Unemployment, and for purposes incidental thereto 1911.* London: HMSO, 1911 (1+2 Geo.5 c.55).

21.   *An Act to establish a Ministry of Health to exercise in England and Wales powers with respect to Health and Local Government, and confer upon the Chief Secretary certain powers with respect to Health in Ireland, and purposes connected therewith 1919.* London: HMSO, 1919 (9+10 Geo.5 c.21).

22.   Registrar General of Births, Deaths and Marriages in England. *Twenty-second annual report of the Registrar General.* London: HMSO, 1861.

23.   Office for National Statistics. *Key population and vital statistics: 1996.* London: Stationery Office, 1998 (Series VS; no.23, PP1; no. 19).

24.   Botting B, ed. *The health of our children: the Registrar General's decennial supplement for England and Wales: Office for National Statistics.* London: HMSO, 1995 (Series DS; no. 11).

25.   Office for National Statistics. *Mortality statistics: cause: review of the Registrar General: England and Wales: 1996.* London: Stationery Office, 1998 (Series DH2; no. 23).

26.   Charlton J, Murphy M, eds. *The health of adult Britain 1841-1994: vol 1: Office for National Statistics.* London: Stationery Office, 1997 (Series DS; no. 12).

27.   Office for National Statistics. *Mortality statistics: general, 1993, 1994, 1995.* London: Stationery Office, 1997 (Series DH1; no. 28).

28.   Office for National Statistics. Expectation of life (in years) at birth and selected ages. *Population Trends* 1998; **92**: 65.

29.   Office for National Statistics. *Deaths registered in 1997 by cause, and by area of residence.* London: Office for National Statistics, 1998 (Population and Health Monitor; DH2 98/1).

30.   Office of Population Censuses and Surveys. *Mortality statistics: serial tables: 1841-1990.* London: HMSO, 1992 (Series DH1; no. 25).

31.   Logan WPD. Mortality in England and Wales from 1848 to 1947. *Population Studies* 1950; **4**: 132-78.

32. Markowe HLJ. Health trends in the past 75 years. *Health Trends* 1994; **26**: 98-105.

33. Ministry of Health. *On the State of the Public Health: the Annual Report of the Chief Medical Officer of the Ministry of Health for the year 1919.* London: HMSO, 1920 (Cm. 978).

34. Calman KC. *The potential for health.* Oxford: Oxford University Press, 1998.

35. Office for National Statistics, Imperial Cancer Research Fund. *Cancer survival in England and Wales: 1981 and 1989 registrations.* London: Office for National Statistics, 1998 (Population and Health Monitor MB1 98/1).

36. Drever F, Whitehead M, eds. *Health inequalities: decennial supplement: Office for National Statistics.* London: Stationery Office, 1997 (Series DS; no. 15).

37. Bruce ME, Will RG, Ironside JW, et al. Transmissions to mice indicate that 'new variant' CJD is caused by the BSE agent. *Nature* 1997; **389**: 498-501.

38. Hill AF, Desbrulais M, Joiner S, et al. The same prion strain causes nvCJD and BSE. *Nature* 1997; **389**: 448-50.

39. Department of Health. *On the State of the Public Health: the annual report of the Chief Medical Officer of the Department of Health for the year 1996.* London: Stationery Office, 1997; 3-4, 239-42.

40. Department of Health. *Further precautionary measures on blood products announced.* London: Department of Health, 1998 (Press Release: H98/076).

41. Department of Health. *Committee on Safety of Medicines completes review of blood products.* London: Department of Health, 1998 (Press Release: H98/182).

42. Wakefield AJ, Murch S, Anthony A, et al. Ileal lymphoid nodular hyperplasia, non-specific colitis and pervasive developmental disorder in children. *Lancet* 1998; **351**: 637-41.

43. Department of Health. *Measles, measles mumps rubella (MMR) vaccine, Crohn's disease and autism.* London: Department of Health, 1998 (Professional Letter: PL/CMO(98)2).

44. Department of Health. *The new NHS: modern, dependable.* London: Stationery Office, 1997 (Cm. 3807).

45. Department of Health. *On the State of the Public Health: the annual report of the Chief Medical Officer of the Department of Health for the year 1996.* London: Stationery Office, 1997; 5-7.

46. Department of Health. *On the State of the Public Health: the annual report of the Chief Medical Officer of the Department of Health for the year 1991.* London: HMSO, 1992; 8-9, 54-77.

47. Department of Health NHS Executive. *Assessing health needs of people from minority ethnic groups.* London: Department of Health, 1998 (Health Service Circular: HSC(98)999).

48. Rawaf S, Bahl V. *Assessing health needs of people from minority ethnic groups.* London: Royal College of Physicians of London, 1998.

49. Department of Health. *A first class service.* London: Department of Health, 1998.

50. Department of Health. *Life begins at forty: health tips for older men.* London: Department of Health, 1998.

51. Health Education Authority. *Healthy living for men.* London: Health Education Authority, 1998.

52. Scientific Committee on Tobacco and Health. *First report.* London: Stationery Office, 1998.

53. Health and Safety Executive. *Avoiding ill health at open farms: advice to farmers (with teachers' supplement).* London: Health and Safety Executive, 1998 (HSE Agriculture Information Sheet; no. 23).

54. Department of Health. Propellant changes in metered-dose inhalers. *CMO's Update* 1998; **17**: 1.

55. Department of Health. *On the State of the Public Health: the annual report of the Chief Medical Officer of the Department of Health for the year 1993.* London: HMSO, 1994; 6.

56. Department of Health. *On the State of the Public Health: the annual report of the Chief Medical Officer of the Department of Health for the year 1994.* London: HMSO, 1995; 7, 88-127.

57. Department of Health NHS Executive. *The management of health, safety and welfare issues for NHS staff.* Leeds: Department of Health, 1998.

58. Department of Health. *On the State of the Public Health: the annual report of the Chief Medical Officer of the Department of Health for the year 1994.* London: HMSO, 1995; 7-8.

59. Department of Health. *Variations in health: what can the Department of Health and the NHS do?* London: Department of Health, 1995.

60. Royal Commission on Environmental Pollution. *Sustainable use of soil.* London: HMSO, 1996 (Cm. 3165).

61. Carrington EG, Davis RD, Pike EB. *Review of the scientific evidence relating to the controls on the agricultural use of sewage sludge.* London: Department of the Environment, Transport and the Regions, 1998 (DETR 4415/3, DETR 4454/4).

62. House of Commons Select Committee on Agriculture. *Food safety: fourth report: Session 1997-98.* London: HMSO, 1998 (HC 331-I).

63. Ministry of Agriculture, Fisheries and Food, Joint Food Safety and Standards Group, Department of Health. *The Food Standards Agency: a force for change.* London: Stationery Office, 1998 (Cm. 3830).

64. President of the Council's Office. *Tackling drugs to build a better Britain.* London: Stationery Office, 1998 (Cm. 3945).

65. Department of Health. *First full report of largest UK drug study published: National Treatment Outcome Research Study for drug treatment services.* London: Department of Health, 1998 (Press Release: H98/226).

66. Department of Health. *On the State of the Public Health: the annual report of the Chief Medical Officer of the Department of Health for the year 1995.* London: HMSO, 1996; 8-13.

67. Department of Health. *On the State of the Public Health: the annual report of the Chief Medical Officer of the Department of Health for the year 1996.* London: Stationery Office, 1997; 10-12.

68. Bennett PG, Calman KC, eds. *Risk communication and public health.* Oxford: Oxford University Press (in press).

69. Department of Health. *Communicating about risks to public health: pointers to good practice.* London: Department of Health, 1997.

70. Department of Health. *On the State of the Public Health: the annual report of the Chief Medical Officer of the Department of Health for the year 1995.* London: HMSO, 1996; 13-4, 95-126.

71. Department of Health. *On the State of the Public Health: the annual report of the Chief Medical Officer of the Department of Health for the year 1995.* London: HMSO, 1996; 14-6.

72. House of Lords Science and Technology Committee. *Resistance to antibiotics and other antimicrobial agents: seventh report from the Science and Technology Committee: Session 1997-98.* London: Stationery Office, 1998 (HL 81; vol I). Chair: Lord Soulsby of Swaffham Prior.

73. World Health Assembly. *Emerging and other communicable diseases: antimicrobial resistance.* Geneva: World Health Organization, 1998.

74. World Health Organization. *The current status of antimicrobial resistance surveillance in Europe: report of a WHO workshop held in collaboration with the Italian Associazione Culturale Microbiologia Medica, Verona, Italy, 12 December 1997.* Geneva: World Health Organization, 1998 (WHO/EMC/BAC/98.1).

75. Williams RJ, Heymann DL. Containment of antibiotic resistance. *Science* 1998; **279:** 1153-4.

76. Clinical Systems Group. *Improving clinical communications.* Leeds: Department of Health, 1998.

77. Chaisson R, Bishai W, Marco M. The decrease in incidence and changing spectrum of opportunistic infections in the era of highly active antiretroviral therapy. *Eur AIDS Treatment News* 1998: 11-3.

78. Department of Health. *On the State of the Public Health: the annual report of the Chief Medical Officer of the Department of Health for the year 1996.* London: Stationery Office, 1997; 14-20.

79. Department of Health. *On the State of the Public Health: the annual report of the Chief Medical Officer of the Department of Health for the year 1996.* London: Stationery Office, 1997; 20, 104-45.

80. *The Disability Discrimination Act 1995.* London: HMSO, 1995.

81. Department of Health. *On the State of the Public Health: the annual report of the Chief Medical Officer of the Department of Health for the year 1996.* London: Stationery Office, 1997; 21-3.

82. Lord Chancellor's Department. *Who decides?: making decisions on behalf of mentally incapacitated adults.* London: Stationery Office, 1997.

83. Law Commission. *Mental incapacity.* London: HMSO, 1995 (Law Com; no. 231).

84. R v Human Fertilisation and Embryology Authority, Ex parte Diane Blood [1997] 2 All ER 687.

85. McLean S. *Consent and the law: review of the current provisions in the Human Fertilisation and Embryology Act 1990 for UK Health Ministers.* London: Department of Health, 1997.

86. Department of Health. *On the State of the Public Health: the annual report of the Chief Medical Officer of the Department of Health for the year 1996.* London: Stationery Office, 1997; 23-4

87. Department of Health NHS Executive. *Domestic violence.* London: Department of Health, 1997.

88. *The Family Law Act 1996.* London: HMSO, 1996.

89. Department of Health. *Making an impact: children and domestic violence.* London: Department of Health, 1997.

90. Committee on the Medical Effects of Air Pollutants, Department of Health. *Quantification of the effects of air pollutants on health in the United Kingdom.* London: Stationery Office, 1998. Chair: Professor Stephen Holgate.

91. Department of the Environment. *The United Kingdom National Air Quality Strategy.* London: Stationery Office, 1997.

92. Department of the Environment, Transport and the Regions. *The potential effects of ozone depletion in the United Kingdom.* London: Stationery Office, 1996.

93. McMichael AJ, Haines A. Global climate change: the potential effects on health. *BMJ* 1997; **315:** 805-9.

94. United Kingdom Climate Change Impact Review Group. *Review of the potential effects of climate change in the UK.* London: HMSO, 1996.

95. Palutikof JP, Subak S, Agnew MD, eds. *Economic impacts of the hot summer and unusually warm year of 1995.* London: Department of the Environment, Transport and the Regions, 1997.

96. Department of the Environment, Department of Health. *United Kingdom national environmental health action plan.* London: HMSO, 1996.

97. Department of Health. *On the State of the Public Health: the annual report of the Chief Medical Officer of the Department of Health for the year 1992.* London: HMSO, 1993; 171-2.

98. Department of the Environment, Transport and the Regions. *Opportunities for change: consultation paper on a revised UK strategy for sustainable development.* London: Department of the Environment, Transport and the Regions, 1998.

99. Local Government Association. *Sustainable local communities for the 21st Century.* London: Local Government Association, 1998.

100. World Health Organization. *Potential health effects of climatic change.* Geneva: World Health Organization, 1990.

101. Kanner L. Autistic disturbance of affective contact. *Nervous Child* 1943; **2:** 217-50.

102. Wing L. The autistic spectrum. *Lancet* 1997; **350:** 1761-6.

103. Wing L. Autistic spectrum disorders: no evidence for or against an increase in prevalence. *BMJ* 1996; **312:** 327-8.

104. Fombonne E. Is the prevalence of autism increasing? *J Autism Dev Disord* 1996; **26:** 673-6.

105. De Giacomo A, Fombonne E. Parental recognition of developmental abnormalities in autism. *Eur Child Adolescent Psychiatry* (in press).

106. Osterling J, Dawson G. Early recognition of children with autism: a study of first birthday home videotapes. *J Autism Dev Disord* 1994; **24:** 247-57.

107. Rogers SJ, DiLalla DL. Age of symptom onset in young children with pervasive developmental disorders. *J Am Acad Child Adolesc Psychiatry* 1990; **29:** 863-72.

108. Rutter M. Autistic children: infancy to adulthood. *Semin Psychiatry* 1970; **2**: 435-50.

109. DeMyer MK, Barton S, DeMyer WE, et al. Prognosis in autism: a follow-up study. *J Autism Childh Schizophr* 1973; **3**: 199-246.

110. Cantwell DP, Baker L. *Research concerning families of children with autism.* In: Schopler E, Mesibov GB, eds. *The effects of autism on the family.* New York: Plenum Press, 1984; 41-63.

111. Rutter M, Schopler E. Autism and pervasive developmental disorders: concepts and diagnostic issues. *J Autism Dev Disord* 1987; **17**: 159-86.

112. Bailey A, Le Couteur A, Gottesman I, et al. Autism as a strongly genetic disorder: evidence from a British twin study. *Psycholog Med* 1995; **25**: 63-77.

113. Bowler B. 'Theory of mind' in Asperger's syndrome. *J Child Psychol Psychiatry* 1992; **33**: 877-93.

114. Denckla M. Brain mechanisms. *J Autism Dev Disord* 1996; **26**: 134-8.

115. Aitken K. Examining the evidence for a common structural basis to autism. *Dev Med Child Neurol* 1991; **33**: 930-4.

116. Bauman ML, Kemper TL, eds. *The neurobiology of autism.* Baltimore: Johns Hopkins University Press, 1994.

117. DeMyer MK, Hingtgen JN, Jackson RK. Infantile autism reviewed: a decade of research. *Schizophr Bull* 1981; **7**: 388-451.

118. Rutter M. The treatment of autistic children. *J Child Psychol Psychiatry* 1985; **26**: 193-214.

119. Smith T. *Autism.* In: Giles TR, ed. *Handbook of effective psychotherapy.* New York: Plenum Press, 1993.

120. Howlin P. Prognosis in autism: do specialist treatments affect long-term outcome? *Eur Child Adolesc Psychiatry* 1997; **6**: 55-72.

121. National Screening Committee. *First report of the National Screening Committee.* Milton Keynes: National Screening Committee, 1998.

122. Alberti KGMM, Zimmet P, for the WHO Consultation. Definition, diagnosis and classification of diabetes mellitus and its complications: part 1: diagnosis and classification of diabetes mellitus: provisional report of a WHO consultation. *Diabetic Med* 1998; **15**: 539-58.

123. Amos AF, McCarty DJ, Zimmet P. The rising global burden of diabetes and its complications: estimates and projections to the year 2010. *Diabetic Med* 1997; **14 (suppl 5)**: S57-85.

124. Yudkin J, Forrest R, Jackson C, Burnett S, Gould M. The prevalence of diabetes and impaired glucose tolerance in a British population. *Diabetes Care* 1993; **16**: 1530.

125. Unwin N, Alberti KGMM, Bhopal R, Harland J, Watson W, White M. Comparison of the current WHO and new ADA criteria for the diagnosis of diabetes mellitus in three ethnic groups in the UK. *Diabetic Med* 1998; **15**: 554-7.

126. Alberti KGMM. The clinical implications of impaired glucose tolerance. *Diabetic Med* 1996; **13**: 927-37.

127. British Diabetic Association. *Diabetes in the United Kingdom.* London: British Diabetic Association, 1996.

128. The Diabetes Control and Complications Trial Research Group. The effect of intensive treatment of diabetes on the development and progression of long-term complications in insulin-dependent diabetes mellitus. *N Engl J Med* 1993; **329**: 977-86.

129. Harris MI, Klein R, Welborn TA, Knuiman MW. Onset of NIDDM occurs at least 4-7 years before clinical diagnosis. *Diabetes Care* 1992; **15**: 815-9.

130. Marks L. *Counting the cost: the real impact of non-insulin-dependent diabetes.* London: British Diabetic Association, 1996.

131. Currie CJ, Kraus D, Morgan CL, Gill L, Stott NCH, Peters JR. NHS acute expenditure for diabetes: the present, future and excess inpatient cost of care. *Diabetic Med* 1997; **14**: 686-92.

132. Report of a Joint Working Party of the British Diabetic Association, the Research Unit of the Royal College of Physicians of London and the Royal College of General Practitioners. Guidelines for good practice in the diagnosis and treatment of non-insulin-dependent diabetes mellitus. *J R Coll Physicians Lond* 1993; **27**: 259-66.

133. Department of Health, British Diabetic Association. *St Vincent Joint Task Force for Diabetes: the report.* London: Department of Health, 1995.

134. British Diabetic Association. *Guidance on local diabetes services advisory groups.* London: British Diabetic Association, 1995.

135. British Diabetic Association. *Recommendations for the management of diabetes in primary care.* London: British Diabetic Association, 1997.

136. Clinical Standards Advisory Group. *Standards of clinical care for people with diabetes.* London, HMSO, 1994.

137. Strachan DP, Cook DG. Parental smoking and lower respiratory illness in infancy and early childhood. In: Britton JR, Weiss ST, eds. Health effects of passive smoking: 1. *Thorax* 1997; **52**: 905-14.

138. Anderson HR, Cook DG. Passive smoking and sudden infant death syndrome: review of the epidemiological evidence. In: Britton JR, Weiss ST, eds. Health effects of passive smoking: 2. *Thorax* 1997; **52**: 1003-9.

139. Cook DG, Strachan DP. Parental smoking and prevalence of respiratory symptoms and asthma in school age children. In: Britton JR, Weiss ST, eds. Health effects of passive smoking: 1. *Thorax* 1997; **52**: 1081-94.

140. Ministry of Agriculture, Fisheries and Food, Department of Health. Selenium: *COMA statement: reports the conclusions of COMA on the nutritional implications of selenium intakes.* London: Ministry of Agriculture, Fisheries and Food, Department of Health, 1998 (Food Safety Information Bulletin; no. 93).

141. Department of Health, Jackson MA. *Nutritional aspects of the development of cancer: report of the working group on diet and cancer.* London: Stationery Office, 1998 (Report on Health and Social Subjects; no. 48).

142. Glennie A-M, O'Meara S. *A systematic review of interventions in the treatment and prevention of obesity.* York: NHS Centre for Reviews and Dissemination, University of York, 1997 (CRD report; no. 10).

143. NHS Centre for Reviews and Dissemination, University of York. The prevention and treatment of obesity. *Effective Health Care* 1997; **3**: 1-12.

144. Foster K, Lader D, Cheesbrough S. *Infant feeding 1995: results from a survey carried out in England by the Social Survey Division of the Office for National Statistics on behalf of the UK Health Departments.* London: Stationery Office, 1997.

145. Thomas M, Avery V. *Infant feeding in Asian families: early feeding practices and growth: a survey carried out in England by the Social Survey Division of the Office for National Statistics on behalf of the Department of Health.* London: Stationery Office, 1997.

146. House of Commons Health Committee. *The specific health needs of children and young people: report from the Health Committee: Session 1996-97.* London: Stationery Office, 1997 (HC 307-I). Chair: Mrs Marion Roe.

147. House of Commons Health Committee. *Health services for children and young people in the community, home and school: report from the Health Committee: Session 1996-97.* London: Stationery Office, 1997 (HC 314-I). Chair: Mrs Marion Roe.

148. House of Commons Health Committee. *Hospital services for children and young people: report from the Health Committee: Session 1996-97.* London: Stationery Office, 1997 (HC 128-I). Chair: Mrs Marion Roe.

149. House of Commons Health Committee. *Child and adolescent mental health services: report from the Health Committee: Session 1996-97.* London: Stationery Office, 1997 (HC 26-I). Chair: Mrs Marion Roe.

150. Department of Health. *Government response to the reports of the Health Committee on health services for children and young people: Session 1996-97.* London: Stationery Office, 1997 (Cm. 3793).

151. National Institute for Ethnic Studies in Health and Social Policy. *Ethnic diversity in England and Wales: an analysis by health authorities based on the 1991 Census.* London: National Institute for Ethnic Studies in Health and Social Policy, 1997.

152. Department of Health. *Public health strategy launched to tackle root causes of ill-health.* London: Department of Health, 1997 (Press Release: H97/197).

153. Department of Health. *The Health of the Nation: a strategy for health in England.* London: HMSO, 1992 (Cm. 1986).

154. Houghton JT, Meirafilho LG, Callander BA, Harris N, Kattenberg A, Maskell K, eds. *Climate change 1995: the science of climate change.* Cambridge: Cambridge University Press, 1995.

155. Department of the Environment, Department of Health. *United Kingdom national environmental health action plan.* London: HMSO, 1996.

156. Department of the Environment, Transport and the Regions. *English House Condition Survey 1996.* London: Department of the Environment, Transport and the Regions, 1998.

157. Department of Health, Committee on the Medical Effects of Air Pollutants. *Handbook on air pollution and health.* London: Stationery Office, 1997. Chair: Professor Stephen Holgate.

158. Stevens A, Raftery J, eds. *Health care needs assessment: the epidemiologically based needs assessment reviews: second series.* Oxford: Radcliffe Medical, 1997.

159. NHS Executive. *Clinical indicators for the NHS: 1994-95: a consultation document.* Leeds: NHS Executive, 1997.

160. Department of Health, Scottish Office, Welsh Office. *Choice and opportunity: primary care: the future.* London: Stationery Office, 1996 (Cm. 3390).

161. Department of Health. *Primary care: delivering the future.* London: Stationery Office, 1996 (Cm. 3512).

162. Department of Health NHS Executive. *Developing emergency services in the community (vols 1 and 2).* London: Department of Health, 1996. Chair: Sir Kenneth Calman.

163. Department of Health, Welsh Office. *A policy framework for commissioning cancer services: a report by the Expert Advisory Group on Cancer to the Chief Medical Officers of England and Wales: guidance for purchasers and providers of care.* London: Department of Health, 1995.

164. Department of Health. *Improving outcomes in colorectal cancer: guidance on commissioning cancer services.* Leeds: Department of Health, 1997.

165. Gallimore SC, Hoile RW, Ingram GS, Sherry KM. *The report of the National Confidential Enquiry into Perioperative Deaths 1994/1995 (1 April 1994 to 31 March 1995).* London: National Confidential Enquiry into Perioperative Deaths, 1997.

166. Campling EA, Devlin HB, Hoile RW, Ingram GS, Lunn JN. *Who operates when? A report by the National Confidential Enquiry into Perioperative Deaths (1 April 1995 to 31 March 1996).* London: National Confidential Enquiry into Perioperative Deaths, 1997.

167. Department of Health. *Report of the Health Care Strategy Unit: review of renal services: evidence for the review.* London: Department of Health, 1994.

168. Department of Health NHS Executive. *SMAC statement on use of statins.* Leeds: Department of Health, 1997 (Executive Letter: EL(97)41).

169. Department of Health. *Key features of a good diabetes service.* London: Department of Health, 1997 (Health Service Guidelines: HSG(97)45).

170. McCormick A, Fleming D, Charlton J. *Morbidity statistics from general practice: fourth national study: 1991-1992.* London: HMSO, 1995 (Series MB5; no. 3).

171. Armstrong E, ed. *The primary mental health toolkit.* Wetherby (West Yorkshire): Department of Health, 1997.

172. Parry G, Richardson A. *NHS psychotherapy services in England: review of strategic policy.* London: NHS Executive, 1996.

173. Damon S. *Commissioning and funding of training in psychotherapies for the NHS in England.* London: Department of Health, 1997.

174. Department of Health. *Education and training: planning guidance.* Leeds: Department of Health, 1997 (Executive Letter: EL(97)58).

175. Appleby L. *National Confidential Inquiry into Suicide and Homicide by People with Mental Illness: progress report 1997.* London: Department of Health, 1997.

176. *The Mental Health Act 1983.* London: HMSO, 1983.

177. Confidential Enquiry into Stillbirths and Deaths in Infancy. *4th annual report: 1 January - 31 December 1995: concentrating on intrapartum related deaths 1994-95.* London: Maternal and Child Health Research Consortium, 1997.

178. Department of Health NHS Executive, Health Services Directorate. *Paediatric intensive care: a framework for the future.* Leeds: Department of Health, 1997.

179. Department of Health NHS Executive. *A bridge to the future: report of the Chief Nursing Officer's Taskforce: nursing standards, education and workforce planning in paediatric intensive care.* Leeds: Department of Health, 1997.

180. British HIV Association Guidelines Co-ordinating Committee. British HIV Association guidelines for antiretroviral treatment of HIV seropositive individuals. *Lancet* 1997; **349:** 1086-92.

181. Department of Health Expert Advisory Group on *Chlamydia trachomatis. Chlamydia trachomatis: summary and conclusions of the Chief Medical Officer's Expert Advisory Group.* London: Department of Health, 1998.

182. UK Health Departments. *Multiphase contingency plan for pandemic influenza.* London: Department of Health, 1997.

183. Charlett A, Cole N, Cookson B, et al. *Hospital-acquired infection: surveillance, policies and practice.* London: Public Health Laboratory Service, 1997.

184. Bradley DJ, Warhurst DC. Guidelines for the prevention of malaria in travellers from the United Kingdom. *Commun Dis Rep CDR Rev* 1997; **7:** R137-52.

185. Department of Health. *Visiting Africa, Asia, South America? Think malaria.* London: Department of Health, 1997.

186. Department of Health, Welsh Office. *Memorandum on leprosy.* London: Department of Health, 1997.

187. Advisory Committee on Pesticides. *Unit to unit variation of pesticide residues in fruit and vegetables.* London: Advisory Committee on Pesticides, 1997.

188. Ministry of Agriculture, Fisheries and Food, Health and Safety Executive. *Annual report of the Working Party on Pesticide Residues: 1996: supplement to the Pesticides Register 1997.* London: Ministry of Agriculture, Fisheries and Food, 1997.

189. Department of Health Medical Workforce Standing Advisory Committee. *Planning the medical workforce: third report.* London: Department of Health, 1997.

190. Department of Health. *Maintaining medical excellence: review of guidance on doctors' performance: final report.* Leeds: Department of Health, 1995.

191. British Association of Medical Managers. *When things go wrong: practical steps for dealing with the problem doctor.* Cheadle (Cheshire): British Association of Medical Managers, 1997.

192. National Radiological Protection Board. *Intervention for recovery after accidents: application of emergency reference levels of dose in emergency planning and response: identification and investigation of abnormally high gamma dose rates.* Chilton (Oxon): National Radiological Protection Board, 1997 (Doc. NRPB 8; no. 1).

193. National Radiological Protection Board. *Relative biological effectiveness of neutrons for stochastic effects.* Chilton (Oxon): National Radiological Protection Board, 1997 (Doc. NRPB 8; no. 2).

194. Bouffler SD, Meijne EIM, Morris DJ, Papworth D. Chromosome 2 hypersensitivity and clonal development in murine radiation acute myeloid leukaemia. *Int J Radiat Biol* 1997; **72:** 181-9.

195. Cox R. *Carcinogenic response at low doses and dose rates: fundamental issues and judgment.* In: Goodhead DT, ed. *Proceedings of the 12th symposium on microdosimetry.* Cambridge: Royal Society of Chemistry, 1997; 225-7.

196. Little MP, Charles MW, Hopewell JW, et al. *Assessment of skin doses.* London: Stationery Office, 1997 (Doc. NRPB 8; no. 3).

197. Human Genetics Advisory Commission. *The implications of genetic testing for insurance.* London: Human Genetics Advisory Commission, 1997.

198. Advisory Committee on Genetic Testing. *Code of practice and guidance on human genetic testing services supplied direct to the public.* London: Department of Health, 1997.

199. Advisory Committee on Genetic Testing. *Consultation report on genetic testing for late-onset disorders.* London: Department of Health, 1997.

Communications from the Chief Medical Officer to the medical profession and others during 1997

Copies of CMO Letters and *CMO's Update* may be obtained from: Department of Health Mailings, PO Box 410, Wetherby, West Yorkshire LS23 7LN.

CMO Letters

Meningococcal infection: meningitis and septicaemia (Professional Letter: PL/CMO(97)1) (3 January).
Urgent communications (Professional Letter: PL/CMO(97)2) (3 February).
Avian (H_5N_1) influenza in Hong Kong (Professional Letter: PL/CMO(97)3) (17 December).

CMO's Update

CMO's Update 13 (February). Includes: Specialist registrar training; Chronic fatigue syndrome or myalgic encephalomyelitis; Acute low back pain; News in brief: How to get the best from maternity services, Pupils with medical needs; Review of psychotherapy services; Unlinked anonymous HIV surveys; Mental health education in primary care; Influenza immunisation policy; Advice to pregnant women during the lambing season; New variant of Creutzfeldt-Jakob disease; Food hygiene; Carbon monoxide; Transplant activity and outcome; Congenital limb reduction defects; Nutritional assessment of infant formulas.

CMO's Update 14 (May). Includes: National focus for work on response to chemical incidents and surveillance of health effects of environmental chemicals; Biotechnology and sustainable development; Overseas doctors; Planning for an influenza pandemic; Hib and DTP vaccines; Involving patients in general practice issues; Certification of elimination of poliomyelitis; New variant of Creutzfeldt-Jakob disease; Viral haemorrhagic fevers; Purchasing effective treatment and care for drug misusers; Review of prescribing; Palliative care services for children; Health Survey for England; Mental health of older people.

CMO's Update 15 (August). Includes: Influenza immunisation; Prevention of malaria; Leprosy Memorandum; Post-exposure prophylaxis for occupational exposure to HIV in health care workers; Statins and coronary heart disease; 'Saventrine' tablets withdrawal; New variant of Creutzfeldt-Jakob disease; Primary mental health care toolkit; Multi-centre research ethics committees;

Recommendations on general clinical training; Advisory Group on Confidentiality; Oilseed rape allergenicity and irritancy; Legal rulings on surgical interventions in pregnancy; Reporting cases of drug misuse to Regional Drug Misuse Databases.

CMO's Update 16 (November). Includes: On the State of the Public Health; Gulf Veterans' Medical Assessment Programme; Carbon monoxide; Mobile telephones and medical devices; Health strategy Green Paper; Meningococcal infection; Personal medical services pilot schemes; Future patterns of care; Air pollution and health; Clinical effectiveness; Developing emergency services in the community; Transplant activity and outcome; Helping practices to help themselves; New variant of Creutzfeldt-Jakob disease; Review of the law on communicable disease; New guidelines for prevention of malaria; Surveillance of measles 1995-97; National Survey of Tuberculosis; Clinical guidelines and independent appraisal; Advisory Committee on Genetic Testing; Removal and storage of testicular tissue from young boys.

Public Health Link

Copies of Public Health Link communications can be obtained from: The Chief Medical Officer, Richmond House, 79 Whitehall, London SW1A 2NS.

Electronic cascade messages

'Milumil' infant milk powder: product withdrawal (CEM/CMO(97)1) (8 January).
Bogus doctor (CEM/CMO(97)2) (24 February).
Pharmaceutical product batch recall: 'Phenergan' elixir batch no. 78357 (CEM/CMO(97)3) (5 April).
Review of dioxins and PCBs (CEM/CMO(97)4) (14 May).
Safety of vitamin B6 dietary supplements and licensed medicines (CEM/CMO(97)5) (3 July).
Reassurance about MMR vaccine (CEM/CMO(97)6) (1 August).
Withdrawal of fenfluramine ('Ponderax') and dexfenfluramine ('Adifax'): effects on heart valves (CEM/CMO(97)7) (16 September).
HRT and breast cancer (CEM/CMO(97)8) (9 October).

CMO's Internet homepage

Recent communications from the Chief Medical Officer can be found on the Internet at: http://www.open.gov.uk/doh/cmo/cmoh.htm.

CHAPTER 1

VITAL STATISTICS

(a)   Population size

The estimated resident population of England at 30 June 1997 was 49.3 million, an increase of 0.2 million (0.4%) compared with 1996 and of 3.8% compared with 1987.

(b)   Age and sex structure of the resident population

Figure 1.1 shows the changes in the age and sex structure of the population of England between 1987 and 1997. There has been a striking increase in the 25-34 years, 35-44 years, and 45-54 years age-groups, reflecting the post-war and the mid-1960s 'baby-booms'. There has also been a steep fall in the number of 15-24-year-olds over the last decade, as the 'baby-boomers' born in the mid-1960s move into the older age-groups, combined with a fall in fertility rates in the late 1970s. Similar factors explain the drop in the number of 55-64-year-olds between 1987 and 1997, as those people born after World War I move into the 65-74 years age-group, combined with very low fertility rates in the 1930s. The numbers of people aged over 65 years, and in particular those aged over 85 years, still continue to increase.

Figure 1.1: *The changing age structure in England, 1987 and 1997*

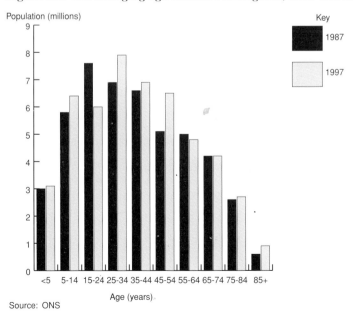

Source: ONS

Figure 1.2: *The age structure of the population, England and Wales, 1948 and*
1997

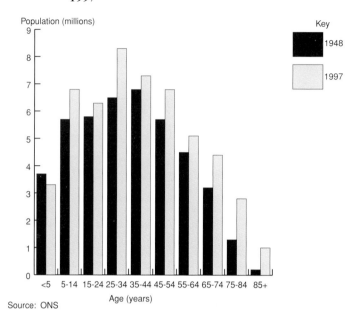

Source: ONS

Figure 1.2 shows the changes in the age structure of the population of England
and Wales between 1948 and 1997. The most striking changes are seen in the
25-34 years and 65 years and over age-groups, accounted for by the 'baby boom'
of the 1960s, and the post-World-War-I 'baby boom' combined with increased
life expectancy, respectively.

(c)   Fertility statistics

Conceptions

Data on conceptions relate to pregnancies that led to a birth or to a legal
termination under the Abortion Act 1967[1,2]; they exclude spontaneous and illegal
abortions. In 1996, 773,600 conceptions occurred to women resident in England,
a 3% increase from the figure in 1995 (750,000), with an overall rate of 76.1 per
1,000 women aged 15-44 years (a 3% increase compared with the rate in 1995).

Conceptions to girls aged under 16 years

In 1996, there were 9.3 conceptions per 1,000 girls aged 13-15 years in England,
compared with 8.5 per 1,000 in 1995 and 8.3 per 1,000 in 1994. Figure 1.3
shows the trends in underage conceptions by outcome in England since 1974.

66

Figure 1.3: *Underage conceptions per 1,000 women aged 13-15 years by outcome,England, 1974-96*

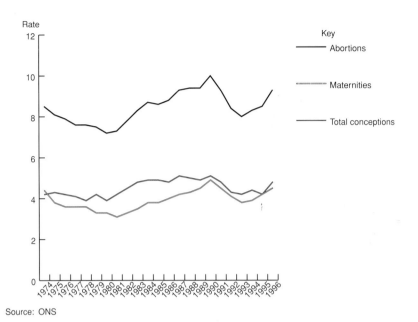

Source: ONS

Figure 1.4: *Total period fertility rate (TPFR), England, 1971-97*

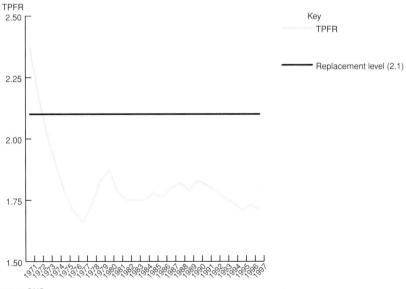

Source: ONS

Figure 1.5: *Live births outside marriage as a percentage of all live births, England, 1987-97*

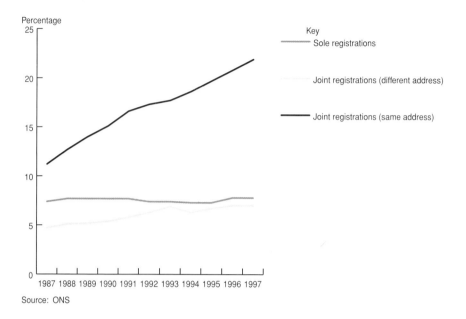

Source: ONS

Total live births

In 1997, there were 607,200 live births in England - 1.1% fewer than in 1996 (see Table 1.1). In England, the total period fertility rate (TPFR, a measure of the average number of children that would be born per woman if current age-specific fertility rates continued throughout her childbearing years) was 1.71 in 1997 compared to 1.73 in 1996. The TPFR for England has now remained below 2.1, the level that would give long-term 'natural' replacement of the population, since 1973 (see Figure 1.4).

The proportion of live births outside marriage has increased rapidly from 9.8% of all live births in England in 1977 to 36.7% in 1997. Most of this rise can be attributed to a growing number of births outside marriage registered by both parents. Figure 1.5 shows the trends in births outside marriage in England and Wales by type of registration over the past decade. Births outside marriage that were solely registered remained relatively stable, at 7-8% of all births; however, the proportion of births outside marriage that were registered by both parents rose from 16% of all births in 1987 to 29% in 1997. Three-quarters of these births were registered by parents living at the same address, and presumably cohabiting.

68

Table 1.1: *Live births and proportion of live births outside marriage, crude birth rate, general and total period fertility rates, and sex ratio, England, 1987, 1996 and 1997*

Year of birth	Live births	Crude birth rate*	General fertility rate†	Total period fertility rate (TPFR)	Percentage of live births outside marriage	Sex ratio
1987	643330	13.6	62.0	1.81	23.2	105.3
1996	614184	12.5	60.4	1.73	35.5	105.5
1997	607216	12.4‡	59.7‡	1.71‡	36.7	105.1

* Births per 1,000 population of all ages.
† Births per 1,000 females aged 15-44 years.
‡ Provisional (based on 1996 population figures).
Note: Sex ratio represents number of male births per 100 female births.

Source: ONS

Abortions

In 1996, 160,629 abortions were performed under the Abortion Act 1967[1,2] for women who were resident in England, an increase of 9% compared with 1995. This is the first increase in the annual number of abortions since 1990, and may be a consequence of the announcement in October 1995 of an association between oral contraceptives that contain gestodene or desogestrel and venous thromboembolism[3,4].

In each year between 1990 to 1996, the highest quarterly abortion rate has been recorded in the March quarter and, since 1989, the lowest quarterly abortion rate has been recorded in the December quarter. Use of quarterly moving averages to smooth out variations shows an increase which started between the March and June 1996 quarters and which, since then, has remained at a significantly higher level (see Figure 1.6).

References

1. *The Abortion Act 1967.* London: HMSO, 1967.
2. *The Abortion Act 1967 (as amended by Statutory Instrument: SI 480c10).* London: HMSO, 1991.
3. Committee on Safety of Medicines. *Combined oral contraceptives and thromboembolism.* London: Committee on Safety of Medicines, 1995.
4. Department of Health. *On the State of the Public Health: the annual report of the Chief Medical Officer of the Department of Health for the year 1995.* London: HMSO, 1996; 9-10, 204.

Figure 1.6: *Quarterly moving average abortion rates per 1,000 women aged 14-49 years, England, 1985-97*

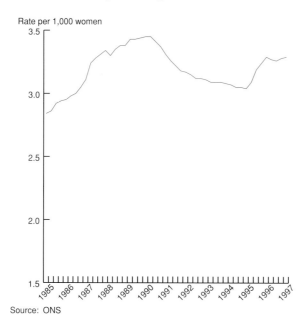

Source: ONS

(d)   Trends in reporting congenital abnormalities

Appendix Table A.6 shows the number of babies notified who had selected congenital abnormalities. In 1997, the notification rate for live births with congenital abnormalities fell to 79.2 per 10,000 live births, 5% lower than in 1996 and 8% lower than in 1992.

An exclusion list was introduced in January 1990 to identify minor anomalies which should no longer be notified. As a result, the total number of notifications received fell by 4,058 (34%) between 1989 and 1990. This fall was accounted for entirely by a decrease in notifications of live births with anomalies. Four groups shown in Table A.6 were affected by the exclusion list: ear and eye anomalies, cardiovascular anomalies, hypospadias and talipes. For these groups, the comments in the following paragraphs are restricted to the changes that took place between 1991 and 1997; for the remainder, the comments refer to the changes between 1987 and 1997.

Since 1987, there has been a reduction in the rate of central nervous system anomalies for live births (from 6.2 to 2.4 per 10,000 births) and stillbirths (from 1.2 to 0.6 per 10,000 total births). Conditions such as hydrocephalus and anencephaly, which are within the group most likely to be detected prenatally by diagnostic ultrasound or alphafetoprotein screening, have shown the largest fall. Similar decreases have been reported in other countries.

70

Between 1987 and 1997, the rate (per 10,000 live births) for cleft lip/palate anomalies has fallen from 12.1 to 8.6. Since 1992, the rate (per 10,000 live births) for ear and eye anomalies has changed very little from 3.2 to 3.3, for hypospadias/episadias has fallen from 8.0 to 7.2 and for talipes has fallen from 11.3 to 9.3.

(e)   Mortality

(i)   *Infant and perinatal mortality*

Provisional statistics for 1997 indicate that 3,591 babies died in England before the age of one year, compared with 3,725 in 1996. The infant mortality rate fell to 5.9 per 1,000 live-births, the lowest ever recorded.

Based on provisional statistics, there were 3,250 stillbirths in England in 1997 compared with 3,345 in 1996. The stillbirth rate fell from 5.4 to 5.3 per 1,000 total births between 1996 and 1997 (see Figure 1.7).

(ii)   *Childhood mortality*

Provisional statistics for 1997 in England indicate that 1,734 children died between the ages of 1 and 15 years (inclusive), compared with 1,712 in 1996.

Figure 1.7: *Stillbirths and infant mortality rates, England, 1987-97*

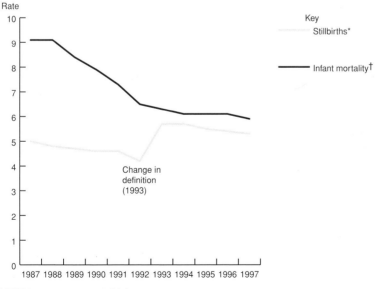

*Stillbirth rates per 1,000 total births
†Infant mortality rates per 1,000 live births

Source: ONS

71

(iii)   Adult mortality

Deaths registered in England decreased from 526,650 in 1996 to 521,598 in 1997, a fall of 1.0%. For most age-groups, mortality rates fell during the 1980s among males and females alike, but a 7.5% increase was seen for men aged 15-44 years between 1985 and 1990; the mortality rate among men in this age-group fell between 1990 and 1993, and has since remained fairly stable[1].

Socio-economic differences

During the 1980s, the life expectancy of men in the non-manual social classes (I, II and IIIN) improved more than that of manual workers (IIIM, IV and V); in the years 1987-91, there was a five-year difference in life expectancy at birth between men in social classes I and II (75 years) compared with social classes IV and V (70 years). Changes in male death rates by social class and employment status between 1976 and 1992 are shown in Appendix Table A.12; in each social class, the death rate among employed men was lower than that in unemployed men. Relative differences between manual and non-manual social classes widened in the late 1980s among employed and unemployed men alike, but more so for those who were unemployed. Regional differences in death rates among men are shown in Figure 1.8; again, clear social class gradients in mortality exist in the North, North West, South West and South East regions of England.

Examination of social class differences in mortality among women is more difficult than for men because fewer data are available; housing tenure statistics indicate that mortality rates are highest among women who live in local authority housing and lowest in women who live in owner-occupied accommodation.

Social class differences have also now emerged among people born in the Caribbean and Indian sub-Continent (see Appendix Table A.13), although trends are hard to ascertain.

Suicides and undetermined deaths

A recent study of trends in suicide in England and Wales between 1982 and 1996[2] indicated that the total number of suicides and undetermined deaths among those aged 15 years and over fell from 5,655 in 1982 to 4,872 in 1996. In 1982, men accounted for just under two-thirds of all suicides, but by 1996 this proportion had reached three-quarters. The age-standardised suicide rate for men increased from 191 per million in 1982 to 207 per million in 1988, before falling to 174 per million in 1996 (a fall of 9% between 1982 and 1996). Among women, the age-standardised death rate from suicide fell from 98 per million in 1982 to 56 per million in 1996, a fall of 43%.

Figure 1.8: *Standardised death rates* per 100,000 population, all causes, men aged 40-64 years at death, by social class, 1988-94*

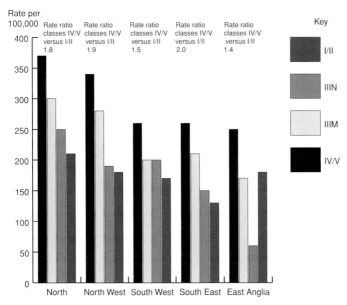

*Standardised to European standard population

Source: *Population Trends*

Figure 1.9: *Age-specific death rates (as three-year rolling averages) from suicide among men, England and Wales, 1983-95*

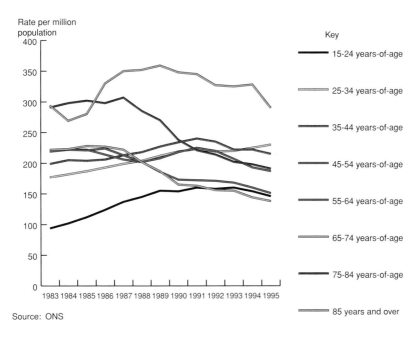

Source: ONS

Figure 1.10: *Age-specific death rates (as three-year rolling averages) from suicide among women, England and Wales, 1983-95*

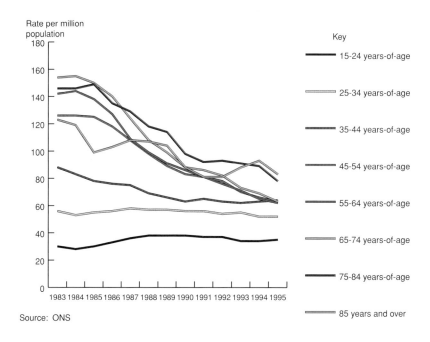

Source: ONS

Figures 1.9 and 1.10 show mortality trends in age-specific suicide rates for men and women, respectively. In 1983, the highest rates for men were found among those aged 45 years and over; however, between 1983 and 1995 male suicide rates fell by 30-40% in the age-groups 55-64, 65-74 and 75-84 years, whereas rates in the 25-34 years age-group rose by 30%. This age-group now has the highest suicide rate for men except for those aged 85 years and over. Rates in the male age-groups of 15-24 and 35-44 years peaked in 1991. For women, suicide rates fell in all age-groups between 1983 and 1995, except for females aged 15-24 years who showed a 16% increase. Although the total number of suicides has decreased in recent years, the contribution of suicides to total years of working life lost has increased, due to an increase in suicide among some younger age-groups. Analyses by method of suicide and occupation indicate a link between suicide rates and access to and knowledge of an effective method of suicide. A fall in male suicide rates from poisoning by 'other gases and vapours' (principally motor vehicle exhaust gas) is the major contributor to the overall fall in male suicide rates during the 1990s. Occupations with the highest ratio of suicide to all-cause mortality, for men and women alike, appear to be associated with access to the means of committing suicide; these include access to guns among farmers, and to drugs among those involved in health or veterinary professions[2].

74

References

1. Department of Health. *On the State of the Public Health: the annual report of the Chief Medical Officer of the Department of Health for the year 1996.* London: Stationery Office, 1997; 65-7.
2. Kelly S, Bunting J. Trends in suicide in England and Wales, 1982-1996. *Population Trends* (in press).

(f)   Prevalence of disease in the community

The General Practice Research Database (GPRD) provides data on over three million patients on consultations, prescriptions and referrals. Between 1994 and 1996, there has been a rise in the proportion of the population prescribed asthma drugs and who had a diagnosis of asthma of 4% among males and 7% in females (see Table 1.2). Over the same period, there has been a 15% increase in the proportion of women and a 19% increase in the proportion of men aged 15 years and over who were prescribed antidepressants. There has also been a 9% increase in the proportion of women and a 10% increase among men aged 35 years and over who had a diagnosis of hypertension and who had been treated with antihypertensive drugs.

(g)   Trends in cancer incidence and mortality

The latest totals of cancer registrations for England and Wales relate to 1992 (see Appendix Tables A.7 and A.8). The age-standardised incidence rates for all malignant neoplasms combined (excluding non-melanoma skin cancer) rose by nearly 10% among males and by over 20% in females between 1979 and 1992. Among males, the largest percentage increase was seen in cancer of the pleura,

Table 1.2: *Prevalence of treated asthma, anxiety/depression, and hypertension per 1,000 patients, males and females, England and Wales, 1994-96*

| | 1994 | | 1995 | | 1996 | |
	Males	Females	Males	Females	Males	Females
Asthma	64.5	63.9	66.2	67.5	66.8	68.6
Anxiety/depression	30.5	71.2	33.1	76.9	36.2	81.9
Hypertension	43.9	48.0	46.0	50.5	48.1	52.5

Prevalence rates age-standardised to European standard population (all ages).

Source: GPRD

with a rise of 240% in the age-standardised incidence rate between 1979 and 1992; the asbestos-related disease mesothelioma accounts for most cases of cancer of the pleura. Non-Hodgkin's lymphoma showed the largest percentage rise among females, with an increase of 88% in the age-standardised incidence rate between 1979 and 1992; in males, the age-standardised incidence rate of non-Hodgkin's lymphoma increased by 74% in this period. Malignant melanoma showed the second largest percentage increase for both sexes over the same period (125% and 71% for males and females, respectively). Figures 1.11 and 1.12 show the percentage change in the directly age-standardised incidence rates for the major sites of cancer between 1979 and 1992, among males and females, respectively, in England and Wales.

Among males, lung cancer, while remaining the most common cancer (23% of all malignancies in 1992), has declined steadily over the past 13 years, and the incidence rate is now 20% below the peak in the late 1970s. As the survival for lung cancer is very short, the trend in incidence is very similar to that for mortality. The incidence of lung cancer in men was substantially higher among manual workers in social classes IIIM, IV and V than in non-manual workers (see Table 1.3). Among men aged under 65 years, the incidence of lung cancer has fallen by a similar amount in all social classes, but in those aged over 65 years, the largest fall in incidence has occurred in the higher social classes. While there has been only a small increase in colorectal cancer, prostate cancer has increased by around 55% since 1979, and is now the second most common cancer in men (16% of all malignancies). Bladder cancer increased during the 1980s, but the rate has stabilised at around 15% above that observed in 1979. There has been a downward trend in the incidence of stomach cancer since at least the early 1970s; mortality from stomach cancer has been falling since the early part of this century.

Among females, breast cancer is by far the most common cancer (28% of registrations in 1992); up to 1988, the rate rose on average by about 2% annually. The subsequent sharper increase appears to be accounted for by the introduction of the national breast screening programme: rates in women aged 50-64 years (the screened age-group) in 1992 were some 28% higher than would have been expected had the pre-screening trend continued. In younger women, the association between social class and breast cancer has been reversed in women over the last 20 years: the incidence of breast cancer in women aged 15-64 years is now lowest among women from social class I, whereas in older women it remains highest among social classes I, II and IIIN. There has been little change in the rate of colorectal cancer in females, among whom it remains the second most common cancer. By the late 1980s, lung cancer (the third most common cancer in women) had risen by almost 30%, but the rate of increase has since

Figure 1.11: *Percentage change in directly age-standardised cancer incidence rates for major cancers, males, England and Wales, 1979-92 (1979=100)*

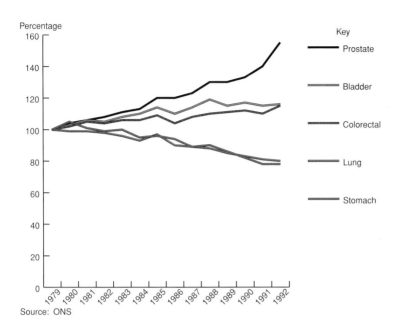

Source: ONS

Figure 1.12: *Percentage change in directly age-standardised cancer incidence rates for major cancers, females, England and Wales, 1979-92 (1979=100)*

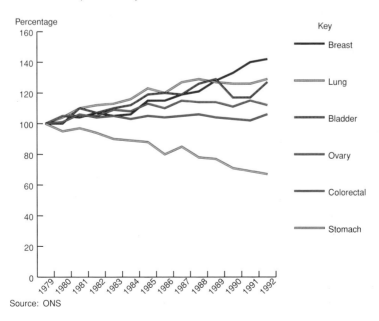

Source: ONS

Table 1.3: *Standardised cancer incidence rates per 100,000 population for lung cancer among men and breast cancer among women, by social class, England and Wales, 1976-80 to 1986-89*

Lung cancer among men

Social class	15-64 years				65 years and over			
	1976-80	1981-85	1986-89	Change (%)	1976-80	1981-85	1986-89	Change (%)
I/II	44	33	27	-39	348	273	230	-34
IIIN	55	49	32	-42	352	292	310	-12
IIIM	70	59	45	-36	468	388	434	-7
IV/V	83	67	52	-37	547	460	426	-22

Breast cancer among women

Social class	15-64 years				65 years and over			
	1976-80	1981-85	1986-89	Change (%)	1976-80	1981-85	1986-89	Change (%)
I/II	81	78	65	-20	225	210	194	-14
IIIN	73	73	85	16	255	221	196	-23
IIIM	79	69	86	9	219	159	176	-20
IV/V	67	66	71	6	186	167	158	-15

Source: ONS

levelled off. The rate of ovarian cancer rose during the mid-1980s, but has since been fairly stable. The striking fall in the rate of stomach cancer among women is similar to that in men, as is the long-term downward trend in mortality from this disease.

CHAPTER 2

THE NATION'S HEALTH

(a)   Basic sources of information

Statistics on morbidity complement standard mortality data. Some useful information is available from routine sources (eg, data on hospital admissions or general practitioner [GP] consultations), but health surveys also provide essential information about the health of the population because they can cover individuals who are not in contact with health or social care services, address a wide range of aspects of health and facilitate the collection of data in a standardised fashion[1].

Health Survey for England

The Health Survey for England, an annual national survey of a representative sample of the population living in private households, focused on cardiovascular disease and its main risk-factors from 1991-94. Since 1993, these Surveys have had a sample size in excess of 15,000, which makes it possible to provide prevalence estimates at regional level. The report of the 1995 Survey[2], published in February, included data on respiratory disease, accidents and disability.

During 1996, the modules on respiratory disease and accidents were repeated and a new module on special measures of general health was included in addition to core data on sociodemographic variables, smoking, alcohol consumption, obesity, and blood pressure. Preliminary analyses indicate, for example, that 77% of men and 75% of women described their health either as "very good" or "good". This proportion varied between social classes, declining progressively from social class I to social class V; this pattern was confirmed by analyses according to 'Acorn' categories (which vary according to level of prosperity), even after adjustment for age, sex and social class. Such findings are of concern given the evidence that self-reported health predicts the likelihood of subsequent death, even after health as assessed in other ways has been allowed for[3].

The combined 1995 and 1996 data also indicate that the annual rate of accidents that led to a medical consultation was 21 per 100 adult men and 15 per 100 adult women. The full report of the 1996 Survey will be published early in 1998[4]. The 1997 Survey focused on the health of children and young people, and the 1998 Survey will return to a focus on cardiovascular disease.

The Health Survey for England is part of a wider Departmental health survey programme which includes, for example, the National Survey of Psychiatric Morbidity and the National Diet and Nutritional Surveys.

References

1. Gupta S. Health surveys as a tool for government: the Health Survey for England as a paradigm case. *Arch Publ Health* 1994; **52**: 99-113.

2. Prescott-Clarke P, Primatesta P, eds. *Health Survey for England 1995: a survey carried out on behalf of the Department of Health (vols 1 and 2).* London: Stationery Office, 1997 (Series HS; no. 5).

3. Idler E, Benyamini Y. Self-rated health and mortality: a review of twenty-seven community studies. *J Health Soc Behav* 1997; **38**: 21-37.

4. Prescott-Clarke P, Primatesta P, eds. *Health Survey for England 1996: a survey carried out on behalf of the Department of Health (vols 1 and 2).* London: Stationery Office (in press) (Series HS; no. 6).

(b) Substance misuse

Drug misuse

The Government continued with the implementation of the third and final year of the anti-drugs strategy 'Tackling Drugs Together'[1]. Mr Keith Hellawell, previously Chief Constable of West Yorkshire, was appointed as the United Kingdom (UK) Anti-Drugs Co-ordinator and asked to advise Government on a new strategy.

The Department of Health (DH) continues to fund the National Treatment Outcome Research Study (NTORS), which is tracking 1,000 drug misusers through various forms of treatment over a five-year period; a one-year follow-up study will be published in April. DH is also funding the new Substance Misuse Advisory Service to provide guidance to health and local authorities on commissioning services for drug and alcohol misusers. A working group chaired by Professor John Strang, Professor of the Psychiatry of Addiction at the University of London, was set up and is currently revising the clinical guidelines for doctors, which were last revised in 1991; new guidelines will be published in late 1998. The Department has also been involved in a number of initiatives in respect of drug misuse services for parents, children and young people, in conjunction with the Local Government Drugs Forum and the Standing Conference on Drug Abuse[2,3].

The Department continued its contract with the Health Education Authority (HEA) for a drugs and solvents prevention campaign, focused on informing young people and parents about the health risks of drug and solvent misuse, particularly ecstasy (methylenedioxymethamphetamine or MDMA), lysergic acid diethylamide (LSD), amphetamines, psilocybin-containing mushrooms and certain volatile substances. This included the publication of a review of the effectiveness of health promotion in preventing substance misuse[4] and the results of a 1995 survey of drug misuse among 11-35-year-olds[5]. DH continued its contract with Network Scotland to provide a free 24-hour National Drugs Helpline (0800 776600) offering confidential information and advice[6,7]. The

Department also funded the Association of Nurses in Substance Abuse to produce three booklets of clinical guidance for nurses who work in substance misuse services[8], with children and young people[9] and in primary care[10].

Alcohol

The Ministerial Group on Alcopops was established in May to draw together Government activity to combat under-age alcohol misuse. The Group announced a package of measures in the Summer to reinforce self-regulatory action being taken by the industry, and will review progress in 1998.

The latest comprehensive survey of young teenagers' drinking habits in England, *Young teenagers and alcohol in 1996*[11] was published in October. Although there has been no increase during the 1990s in the proportion of children aged 11-15 years who drink alcohol at all, those who do drink are drinking more: the average number of units of alcohol drunk in a week by all of the children of this age surveyed had more than doubled between 1990 and 1996 from 0.8 to 1.8 units a week. Although the survey found that the majority of children had drunk little or nothing in the previous seven days (78% had drunk no alcohol) and most of the remainder had drunk only modest amounts, 5% of boys and 3% of girls had consumed 15 or more units in the week preceding the survey.

The preliminary report of the findings of the 1996 General Household Survey (GHS)[12] showed that, in England, among those aged 18 years and over the proportion of men drinking more than 21 units of alcohol a week has remained the same throughout the 1990s (27%), while the proportion of women drinking more than 14 units a week had increased from 11% in 1990 to 14% in 1996. The full report will be published in 1998.

The HEA continued its alcohol health promotion campaign on behalf of the Department. This focused on working with local health promotion organisers to convey to the public the advice on sensible levels of alcohol consumption which were set out in the 1995 inter-Departmental report *Sensible drinking*[13].

References

1. Lord President's Office. *Tackling drugs together: a strategy for England: 1995-1998.* London: HMSO, 1995 (Cm. 2846).
2. Standing Conference on Drug Abuse. *Drug-related early intervention.* London: Standing Conference on Drug Abuse, 1997.
3. Local Government Drugs Forum. *Drug using parents: policy guidelines for inter-agency working.* London: Local Government Association, 1997.
4. Health Education Authority, White D, Pitts M. *Health promotion with young people for the prevention of substance misuse.* London: Health Education Authority, 1997 (Effectiveness Review Series; no. 5).
5. Health Education Authority/BMRB International, Raw M, McNeill A. *Drug use in England: results of the 1995 National Drugs Campaign Survey.* London: Health Education Authority, 1997.

6.   Department of Health Social Services Inspectorate. *Substance misuse and young people: the social services response.* London: Department of Health, 1997 (Executive Letter: EL(97)79).

7.   Local Government Drugs Forum. *Children and young people: guidance for commissioners and providers of substance misuse services from the HAS report.* London: Local Government Association, 1997.

8.   Association of Nurses in Substance Abuse. *Substance use: guidance on good clinical practice for nurses, midwives and health visitors working with alcohol and drug users.* London: Association of Nurses in Substance Abuse, 1997.

9.   Association of Nurses in Substance Abuse. *Substance use: guidance on good clinical practice for nurses, midwives and health visitors working with children and young people.* London: Association of Nurses in Substance Abuse, 1997.

10.   Association of Nurses in Substance Abuse. *Substance use: guidance on good clinical practice for nurses, midwives and health visitors working within primary health care teams.* London: Association of Nurses in Substance Abuse, 1997.

11.   Office for National Statistics. *Young teenagers and alcohol in 1996: England.* London: Stationery Office, 1997.

12.   Office for National Statistics. *Living in Britain: preliminary results from the 1996 General Household Survey.* London: Stationery Office, 1997.

13.   Department of Health. *Sensible drinking: the report of an Inter-Departmental Working Group.* London: Department of Health, 1995.

(c)   Smoking

Figures published during 1997 showed a rise in adult smoking prevalence, which had been declining steadily since 1972. The percentage of males aged 16 years and over who smoked stayed about the same between 1994 and 1996 (at 28%), but the proportion of females aged 16 years and over who smoked increased from 25% to 27% over the same period (see Table 2.1)[1]. It is not known whether the new figures indicate a trend or a short-term fluctuation. Of even greater concern was the trend in smoking among young people: figures published by the ONS[2] showed that regular smoking prevalence among 11-15-year-olds rose from 12% in 1994 to 13% in 1996. By the age of 15 years, about three of every ten children smoke at least one cigarette a week; for girls aged 15 years the prevalence is 33%, and for boys it is 28%.

The Government came to power in May with a manifesto commitment to ban all tobacco advertising. A Tobacco Summit, held in July, was addressed by the Secretary of State for Health and the Minister of State for Public Health, Ms Tessa Jowell MP, and explored important facets of tobacco control in addition to banning advertising.

The draft European Directive to ban tobacco advertising was the subject of intensive negotiations between Member States, culminating in a vote in favour at the December Health Ministers meeting. The draft Directive was then submitted to the European Parliament.

The health effects of passive smoking were highlighted in systematic reviews of existing studies, published in the Autumn. The adjusted estimate for the increased risk of lung cancer in exposed non-smokers was 26%[3], and for

Table 2.1: *Prevalence of cigarette smoking among males and females aged 16 years and over, England, 1974-96*

Year	Males %	Females %	Total %
1974	51	40	45
1976	45	37	41
1978	44	36	40
1980	42	36	39
1982	37	32	35
1984	35	32	33
1986	34	31	32
1988	32	30	31
1990	31	28	29
1992	29	27	28
1994	28	25	26
1996	28	27	28

Note: Percentages rounded to nearest whole figure.

Source: ONS (GHS)

ischaemic heart disease (IHD) was 23%[4], equivalent to several hundred lung cancer deaths per year in the UK, and several thousand deaths annually from IHD. Another series of scientific overviews addressed environmental tobacco smoke (ETS) and the increased risk of childhood respiratory diseases[5,6,7]. It was concluded that infants exposed to parental smoking had more than double the risk of sudden infant death syndrome (SIDS).

The report of the Scientific Committee on Tobacco and Health, which will review the latest scientific evidence on both passive and active smoking, will be published in early 1998[8], and will contribute to the White Paper on tobacco control which is expected later that year.

References

1.   Office for National Statistics. *Living in Britain: preliminary results from the 1996 General Household Survey.* London: Stationery Office, 1997.

2.   Office for National Statistics. *Smoking among secondary school children in 1996: England.* London: Stationery Office, 1997.

3.   Hackshaw AK, Law M, Wald NJ. The accumulated evidence on lung cancer and environmental tobacco smoke. *BMJ* 1997; **315:** 980-8.

4.   Law MR, Morris JK, Wald NJ. Environmental tobacco smoke exposure and ischaemic heart disease: an evaluation of the evidence. *BMJ* 1997; **315:** 973-80.

5.   Strachan DP, Cook DG. Parental smoking and lower respiratory illness in infancy and early childhood. In: Britton JR, Weiss ST, eds. Health effects of passive smoking: 1. *Thorax* 1997; **52:** 905-14.

6.   Anderson HR, Cook DG. Passive smoking and sudden infant death syndrome: review of the epidemiological evidence. In: Britton JR, Weiss ST, eds. Health effects of passive smoking: 2. *Thorax* 1997; **52**: 1003-9.

7.   Cook DG, Strachan DP. Parental smoking and prevalence of respiratory symptoms and asthma in school age children. In: Britton JR, Weiss ST, eds. Health effects of passive smoking: 1. *Thorax* 1997; **52**: 1081-94.

8.   Department of Health, Department of Health and Social Services Northern Ireland, Scottish Office Department of Health, Welsh Office. *Report of the Scientific Committee on Tobacco and Health.* London: Stationery Office (in press).

(d)   Nutrition

During 1997, the Committee on Medical Aspects of Food and Nutrition Policy (COMA) prepared a statement on the implications of lower intake of selenium by the population, to be published in the *Food Safety Information Bulletin*[1], and finalised its report on nutritional aspects of the development of cancer[2].   DH commissioned a review of the effectiveness of interventions for the prevention and treatment of obesity from the National Health Service (NHS) Centre for Reviews and Dissemination[3], which was also published as an Effective Health Care Bulletin[4], and nine research projects as part of its policy research programme.

Promotion of the benefits of breast-feeding continued. The National Network of Breast-feeding Co-ordinators met twice during the year to share experiences and to disseminate good practice on the promotion and protection of breast-feeding throughout the NHS. Another successful National Breast-feeding Awareness Week in May attracted media attention, and was supported by Ms Tessa Jowell MP, Minister of State for Public Health.

The report of the 1995 United Kingdom (UK) survey of infant feeding[5] was published in May; since 1990, rates of breast-feeding at birth have increased in England, Scotland, Wales and particularly Northern Ireland, although rates there remained below the UK average. The report of the survey of infant feeding in Asian families in England showed that mothers from Asian communities in England have higher initial rates of breast-feeding than white mothers living in the same neighbourhood[6]. Analysis of data from the National Diet and Nutrition Survey (NDNS) of people aged 65 years and over continued in preparation for publication of a report in 1998; the field work for the NDNS of people aged 4-18 years continued throughout 1997, and a report is expected in 1999.

References

1.   Ministry of Agriculture, Fisheries and Food, Department of Health. *Selenium: COMA statement: reports the conclusions of COMA on the nutritional implications of selenium intakes.* London: Ministry of Agriculture, Fisheries and Food, Department of Health (in press) (Food Safety Information Bulletin; no. 93).

2.   Department of Health. *Nutritional aspects of the development of cancer: report of the working group on diet and cancer.* London: Stationery Office (in press) (Report on Health and Social Subjects; no. 48).

3. Glennie A-M, O'Meara S. *A systematic review of interventions in the treatment and prevention of obesity.* York: NHS Centre for Reviews and Dissemination, University of York, 1997 (CRD report; no. 10).

4. NHS Centre for Reviews and Dissemination, University of York. The prevention and treatment of obesity. *Effective Health Care* 1997; **3**: 1-12.

5.. Foster K, Lader D, Cheesbrough S. *Infant feeding 1995: results from a survey carried out by the Social Survey Division of the Office for National Statistics on behalf of the UK Health Departments.* London: Stationery Office, 1997.

6. Thomas M, Avery V. *Infant feeding in Asian families: early feeding practices and growth: a survey carried out in England by the Social Survey Division of the Office for National Statistics on behalf of the Department of Health.* London: Stationery Office, 1997.

(e)   Health of children

In the Spring, the House of Commons Select Committee on Health published four reports[1,2,3,4] on the general health status of children, the culmination of a two-year inquiry. The reports - which considered the health needs of healthy children as well as those who are ill; children with disabilities; children with a life-threatening or terminal condition; and children with mental health, emotional and behavioural problems - make a substantial contribution to the debate about children's health. The Committee noted that, although the overall status of children's health is encouraging, with a fall in childhood mortality rates and significant reductions in the incidence and severity of childhood diseases, there is still room for improvement. Healthy children are much more likely to become healthy adults, and there is no room for complacency about children's health.

The Government response, published in November[5], agreed with the Committee that the health needs of children are significantly different from those of adults; that they are a particularly vulnerable group; and that the provision of effective health services for children depends upon a thorough understanding of their particular needs

References

1. House of Commons Health Committee. *The specific health needs of children and young people: report from the Health Committee: Session 1996-97.* London: Stationery Office, 1997 (HC307-I). Chair: Mrs Marion Roe.

2. House of Commons Health Committee. *Health services for children and young people in the community, home and school: report from the Health Committee: Session 1996-97.* London: Stationery Office, 1997 (HC 314-I). Chair: Mrs Marion Roe.

3.. House of Commons Health Committee. *Hospital services for children and young people: report from the Health Committee: Session 1996-97.* London: Stationery Office, 1997 (HC 128-I). Chair: Mrs Marion Roe.

4. House of Commons Health Committee. *Child and adolescent mental health services: report from the Health Committee: Session 1996-97.* London: Stationery Office, 1997 (HC 26-I). Chair: Mrs Marion Roe.

5. Department of Health. *Government response to the reports of the Health Committee on health services for children and young people: Session 1996-97.* London: Stationery Office, 1997 (Cm. 3793).

(f)   Health of adolescents

During the year, activities to promote the health of young people were further developed, with a particular focus on health in schools.

In February, DH and the Department for Education and Employment (DfEE) worked together to produce a newsletter on education and health, issued to all schools[1]. DH and the DfEE continued to work together throughout the year to develop policy on healthy schools, and both Departments contributed to the section on healthy schools in the DfEE White Paper *Excellence in schools*[2], which noted the importance of good education for children on the wrong side of the 'health divide' and expressed a commitment to help all schools to become healthy schools. DH also contributed to the DfEE Green Paper *Excellence for all children: meeting special education needs*[3]. A joint seminar on a proposed national healthy schools award was organised for February 1998.

During the year, DH supported the peer education programme run by Youth Clubs UK, the Cities in Schools (UK) health education programme and the National Pyramid Trust's development project. Findings from the European Network of Health Promoting Schools' project in England were published and the HEA are developing a resource pack for use by schools based on this research. The Young Peoples' Health Network commissioned projects on the development of models to evaluate health promotion work for young people and to involve young people themselves in health promotion.

The 1997 Health Survey for England included a boosted sample of children and young people to provide up-to-date information on young people's health and baseline data against which future trends may be interpreted.

Initiatives to reduce unwanted teenage conceptions continued throughout the year and the Contraceptive Education Service, delivered by the Family Planning Association and the HEA, entered the second year of its three-year contract.

The 'Sexwise' telephone helpline, which offers a free, confidential service to enable young people to speak to a trained adviser about sex and personal relationships, continued to grow in popularity.

England has one of the highest rates of teenage conceptions in the developed world; conceptions among 13-15-year-olds have risen for 12 of the past 16 years for which figures are available (1980-96), and have risen for the past three years in succession. In November, Ms Tessa Jowell MP, Minister of State for Public

Health, announced that the Government would set up four task groups to tackle the challenge of unintended pregnancies, particularly among girls aged under 16 years[4]; the HEA is conducting a consultation exercise on a national programme and young people and parents will be involved throughout the process. A national initiative should be launched in late 1998.

References

1.   Department of Health. Educating for better health: the health of the young nation. *Target* 1997; **22**: 1-4.
2.   Department for Education and Employment. *Excellence in schools.* London: Stationery Office, 1997 (Cm. 3681).
3.   Department for Education and Employment. *Excellence for all children: meeting special educational needs.* London: Stationery Office, 1997 (Cm. 3785).
4.   Department of Health. *Tessa Jowell announces action plan on teenage pregnancy.* London: Department of Health, 1997 (Press Release: H97/360).

(g)   Health of women

DH continues to develop health promotion initiatives for women, and is preparing information aimed specifically at older and younger age-groups to build on the success of its free booklet, *Well women today and tomorrow: health tips for the over 35s*[1], launched in June 1996. Work continued on health promotion initiatives relevant to women in respect of smoking, alcohol consumption, sexual health and exercise, in conjunction with the HEA and the media.

The Government is committed to a major inter-Departmental initiative to tackle domestic violence, in which DH will play a key role. The Department recognises the need for health professionals to be appropriately trained to offer help to women victims of domestic violence[2]. In September, a comprehensive circular was sent to local authorities[3], copied to health authorities, setting out the changes introduced by the Family Law Act 1996[4]. In November, the Department wrote to health authorities and NHS Trusts to raise health professionals' awareness of domestic violence[5]. DH is also working with professional groups such as the Royal College of Obstetricians and Gynaecologists, the Royal College of Nursing and the Royal College of Midwives, all of whom are working to produce guidelines to help their members to deal effectively with women who have experienced such violence.

The Government also continues to work towards the eradication of female genital mutilation, a practice that has been illegal in the UK since the Prohibition of Female Circumcision Act 1985[6], and increased its financial support to the Foundation for Women's Health, Research and Development.

References

1.   Department of Health. *Well women: today and tomorrow: health tips for the over 35s.* London: Department of Health, 1996.
2.   Department of Health. *On the State of the Public Health: the annual report of the Chief Medical Officer of the Department of Health for the year 1996.* London: Stationery Office, 1997; 23-4.
3.   Department of Health. *Family homes and domestic violence.* London: Department of Health, 1997 (Local Authority Circular: LAC(97)15).
4.   *The Family Law Act 1996.* London: HMSO, 1996.
5.   Department of Health. *Domestic violence.* London: Department of Health, 1997.
6.   *The Prohibition of Female Circumcision Act 1985.* London: HMSO, 1985.

(h)   Health of men

Since men's health was highlighted in the 1992 Report[1], increased interest and attention have been paid to this topic. Average male life expectancy in England was 74.6 years in 1996, compared with 72.1 years in 1986.

Key areas identified for improvement of the public health - such as those in relation to the workplace, suicides and inequalities - should have a major impact on men's health[2,3]. During the year, the Department continued to talk to organisations and media about issues relevant to the promotion of health among men to assess the most effective ways to target health promotion messages to this audience.

The workplace provides an important setting for the dissemination of health promotion messages to men, and the work of the Workplace Health Advisory Team, launched in June, will help to take forward this work (see page 91).

The research project 'Alive and kicking' by the Community Education Development Centre, funded by the Department, completed its work in March. This project involved working with football leagues in Coventry and Leamington Spa to raise awareness of healthy lifestyles among the players in local teams, and proved to be a rewarding and innovative experience for players and advisers alike[4].

Men's health was also emphasised in other initiatives, such as the Royal College of Nursing's 'Men's health forum', which published an audit of health care organisations specifically designed or targeted at men[5], and a conference on ways to improve men's health and wellbeing was organised by the Kirklees men's health network.

The Department has developed a leaflet to promote men's health, targeted at men in lower social classes aged over 40 years, to be published in early 1998, and the HEA has prepared a general leaflet on health advice for younger men for distribution in Spring 1998.

89

References

1. Department of Health. *On the State of the Public Health: the annual report of the Chief Medical Officer of the Department of Health for the year 1992.* London: HMSO, 1993; 5, 79-106.
2. Department of Health. *The Health of the nation: a strategy for health in England.* London: HMSO, 1992 (Cm. 1986).
3. Department of Health. *Our Healthier Nation: a contract for health.* London: Stationery Office (in press) (Cm. 3852).
4. Community Education Development Centre. *Alive and kicking.* Coventry: Community Education Development Centre, 1997.
5. Royal College of Nursing. *Men's health audit.* London: Royal College of Nursing, 1997.

(i)   Health of black and ethnic minorities

An international conference between the UK and the United States of America (USA), 'Health gain for black and minority ethnic communities' took place on 16-18 September. The conference's aims were:

- to share UK and USA experience in meeting the health needs of black and minority ethnic groups;

- to establish a collaborative agenda to be taken forward over the medium term; *and*

- to develop links between UK and USA professionals, managers and others who have a commitment to address ethnic health issues.

The conference was addressed by the Secretary of State for Health; Ms Tessa Jowell MP, Minister of State for Public Health; Mr Paul Boateng MP, Parliamentary Under Secretary of State for Health in the House of Commons; and Mr Kevin Thurm, Deputy Secretary of the US Department of Health and Human Services. Papers of collaboration on black and minority health issues were signed by both countries and a forward plan for future work is being agreed by both countries. The key areas under consideration are development of the voluntary sector, and improving access to health services by black and minority ethnic groups.

The key thrust of the ministerial speeches was to address inequalities in health in relation to black and minority ethnic groups, and to recognise the diversity between the various black and minority ethnic groups. The proceedings of the conference, which was attended by some 150 delegates, will be published in 1998.

Ethnic diversity in England and Wales: an analysis by health authorities based on the 1991 Census[1] was published by the National Institute for Ethnic Studies in Health and Social Policy in October. This report highlights social inequalities among black ethnic minority groups in comparison to the white population in areas such as housing, overcrowding and employment.

DH continues to develop research into inequalities in health, and a catalogue of projects funded by the Department will be published during 1998.

Reference

1.   National Institute for Ethnic Studies in Health and Social Policy. *Ethnic diversity in England and Wales: an analysis by health authorities based on the 1991 Census.* London: National Institute for Ethnic Studies in Health and Social Policy, 1997.

(j)   Health in the workplace

The special chapter on health in the workplace in the Report for 1994[1] set out the background to the development of occupational health practice in the UK; described the main occupational health hazards and illnesses; and identified some future developments. It emphasised the importance of risk assessment and pointed to the role that occupational health professionals can play to improve health at work.

The Health and Safety Executive (HSE) has continued to build on the success of its 'Good health is good business' campaign, with a focus on dermatitis and occupational cancers during 1997. The development of the new Government health strategy[2] identified the workplace as a key setting. The HSE contributed to this initiative and continued its own work to develop a strategy on occupational health, which will help to inform decisions about future priorities.

Following publication in December of the Public Accounts Committee report *Health and safety in NHS acute hospital trusts in England*[3] the NHS Executive worked with the HSE to secure improvements in health and safety in the NHS. More than 80% of NHS Trusts and health authorities are now involved in the 'Health at Work in the NHS' project and representatives of primary care have been consulted about extending the project into general practice and community care settings.

During the year the Intra-Agency Network Group on Mental Health in the Workplace produced *Mental wellbeing in the workplace*[4], a resource pack for managers. The HSE published guidance on assessment and management of violence to staff in health services[5] in December, and prepared other information on glutaraldehyde[6], manual handling[7], and guidance for health-care employees on regulations about the reporting of injuries[8] for publication in early 1998. A distance-learning package for GPs about occupational health was also prepared.

References

1. Department of Health. *On the State of the Public Health: the annual report of the Chief Medical Officer of the Department of Health for the year 1994.* London: HMSO, 1995; 7, 88-127.
2. Department of Health. *Our Healthier Nation: a contract for health.* London: Stationery Office (in press) (Cm. 3852).
3. Committee of Public Accounts. *Health and safety in NHS acute hospital Trusts in England: second report.* London: HMSO, 1997.
4. Doherty N, Tyson S. *Mental wellbeing in the workplace: a resource pack for managers' training and development.* Sudbury (Suffolk): HSE Books (in press).
5. Health and Safety Executive. *Violence and aggression to staff in the health services: guidance on assessment and management.* Sudbury (Suffolk): HSE Books, 1997.
6. Health and Safety Executive. *Glutaraldehyde and you.* Sudbury (Suffolk): HSE Books (in press).
7. Health and Safety Executive. *Manual handling in the health service.* Sudbury (Suffolk): HSE Books (in press).
8. Health and Safety Executive. *Reporting of Injuries Diseases and Dangerous Occurrences Regulations (RIDDOR) 1995: guidance for employees in the healthcare sector.* Sudbury (Suffolk): HSE Books (in press).

(k)   Health of people in later life

DH continues to improve services for older people to promote their independent life in the community; to prevent inappropriate admission to hospital, residential or nursing home care; and, wherever practicable, to facilitate their return home after a stay in hospital.

Challenges identified in monitoring the implementation of guidance on NHS responsibilities for meeting continuing health care needs, issued in February 1995[1], are being addressed through a programme of development, as set out in the circular *Better services for vulnerable people*[2] issued to health and social services authorities in October. The three main areas on which DH is working with local health and social services authorities are the development of:

- joint investment plans in continuing care and mental health, to improve joint working between health and social services;

- a range of recuperation and rehabilitation services for older people, to give them the time and opportunity to recover from hospital episodes or to stay at home for longer; *and*

- a national framework for multidisciplinary assessment of older people in acute and community health care settings, undertaken jointly by health and social services, to provide the most appropriate care to the right people at the right time.

In November, the Secretary of State for Health announced that HAS 2000 (formerly the Health Advisory Service) would be commissioned to investigate the care provided for elderly people in hospital.

In November, *Eating matters*[3], a resource pack produced with DH funding to promote good practice in the dietary care of patients, was published.

References

1. Department of Health. *NHS responsibilities for meeting continuing health care needs.* Leeds: Department of Health, 1995 (Health Service Guidelines: HSG(95)8, Local Authority Circular: LAC(95)5).
2. Department of Health. *Better services for vulnerable people.* London: Department of Health, 1997 (Executive Letter: EL(97)62, Chief Inspector: CI(97)24).
3. Department of Health. *Eating matters: Chief Nursing Officer launches new guidance for good food in hospitals.* London: Department of Health, 1997 (Press Release: H97/355).

(l)   Mental health

Mental health continues to be a priority within the NHS[1], with increased emphasis on mental health promotion and preventive work across the Service at national and local levels. Mental health promotion activity has focused on reduction of the stigma attached to mental ill-health, reflected in positive and educational media coverage of mental health, and DH continues to work to increase employers' (including the NHS's) awareness of occupational mental health issues.

Data from GPs indicate that mental health problems are viewed by GPs as the second most common reason for a primary care consultation, often as a result of depression, anxiety, or alcohol or other substance misuse. Patients with severe mental illness may rely on support from primary rather than secondary care services.

The particular needs of young people with mental health problems are increasingly recognised, and the Department has continued to draw attention to these needs and has reviewed the provision of local services.

Services for people with severe mental illness continue to develop towards a comprehensive range of locally based facilities which focus upon individual need. The Independent Reference Group has done considerable work on the reprovision programmes of the remaining long-stay hospitals, and the major challenges presented by patients with co-existent severe mental illness and substance misuse have been highlighted[2].

In December, the National Confidential Inquiry into Homicides and Suicides by People with Mental Illness produced a progress report of work since it was relaunched with new data collection methods, which will inform future service developments.

Antisocial personality disorder is the focus of a major programme of work in services for mentally disordered offenders; research and training in forensic mental health services are also key areas.

References

1. Department of Health. *On the State of the Public Health: the annual report of the Chief Medical Officer of the Department of Health for the year 1995.* London: HMSO, 1996; 13-4, 95-126.
2. President of the Council's Office. *Tackling drugs to build a better Britain.* London: Stationery Office (in press).
3. National Confidential Inquiry into Suicides and Homicides by people with Mental Illness. *Progress report 1997.* London: Royal College of Psychiatrists, 1997.

(m)   Health of disabled people

The health of disabled people, highlighted in last year's Report[1], has high priority for health and social services alike, with emphasis on working through partnerships - increasingly involving disabled people and their carers and families - to meet national and local requirements (see page 180).

Reference

1. Department of Health. *On the State of the Public Health: the annual report of the Chief Medical Officer of the Department of Health for the year 1996.* London: Stationery Office, 1997; 20, 104-45.

CHAPTER 3

THE STRATEGY FOR HEALTH

(a)   Introduction

The Health of the Nation White Paper[1], which set out a strategy for health in England, was launched in July 1992 and would have reached its fifth anniversary during the year. However, following the May General Election the new Government appointed the first Minister of State for Public Health in England, Ms Tessa Jowell MP, and work to develop a new health strategy was put in hand. The new health strategy for England, *Our Healthier Nation*, is to be published as a Green Paper in early 1998[2], and will then be subject to three months' consultation, after which a White Paper will be published later in 1998.

The Minister of State for Public Health outlined the key features of the new strategy for health at a conference on 7 July[3]. It will recognise the impact on health of determinants such as poverty, unemployment, poor housing and a polluted environment; will be concerned with inequalities in health and informed by the outcomes of the Independent Inquiry into these inequalities chaired by Sir Donald Acheson, formerly Chief Medical Officer of the Department of Health (DH), and will be inclusive, taking in children and older people, schools and workplaces.

The new strategy will emphasise the need for partnerships and alliances to ensure concerted action to deliver better health. Central Government, local community organisations and individuals all have their parts to play in a successful strategy. The key to success will be joint working across organisational boundaries, and the Government has established a Cabinet sub-committee to oversee the health strategies in England, Scotland, Wales and Northern Ireland, and to ensure that key policies introduced by other Government Departments and Agencies take into account their likely impact on health.

The 'Our Healthier Nation' initiative will have a small number of national targets to be a focus for general action, complemented by local targets. The strategy for health will tie in with the implementation of the White Paper *The new NHS: modern, dependable*[4], in particular with the introduction of Health Action Zones and Health Improvement Programmes.

Data on the 27 Health of the Nation targets will continue to be monitored nationally, and they may in any case be adopted by health authorities as local targets should they match local health concerns. The independent interim review of the Health of the Nation initiative being conducted by Professor David Hunter, Professor of Health Policy and Management at the Nuffield Institute, and Dr Naomi Fulop, of the London School of Hygiene and Tropical Medicine, will report in 1998 in time to contribute to the development of the new health strategy White Paper, so that it can build on past experience.

References

1. Department of Health. *The Health of the Nation: a strategy for health in England.* London: HMSO, 1992 (Cm. 1986).
2. Department of Health. *Our Healthier Nation: a contract for health.* London: Stationery Office (in press) (Cm. 3852).
3. Department of Health. *Public health strategy launched to tackle root causes of ill-health.* London: Department of Health, 1997 (Press Release: H97/197).
4. Department of Health. *The new NHS: modern, dependable.* London: Stationery Office, 1997 (Cm. 3807).

(b)   Health of the Nation

The Health of the Nation White Paper[1] set 27 targets to improve health, most for the year 2000 but ranging in due dates from 1994 to 2010, with baselines mainly from 1990 but ranging from 1985 to 1992. Wherever possible, three-year average rates are used for monitoring purposes. The latest data are summarised below.

Targets A1 and A2: Coronary heart disease mortality rates

Mortality rates from coronary heart disease (CHD) in 1996 showed a continued downward trend. Over the five years since the 1989-91 baseline, CHD mortality in people aged under 65 years fell by an estimated 24%, after adjusting for the effects of changes in Office for National Statistics (ONS) coding and procedures in 1993. The CHD mortality rate for those aged 65-74 years fell by 17% over the same period.

Targets A3 and A4: Stroke mortality rates

Rates for stroke mortality show a mixed picture. The rate for those aged under 65 years remained virtually unchanged between 1995 and 1996, but fell by an estimated 10% over the five-year period since 1989-91, after adjusting for the 1993 coding changes. For those aged 65-74 years, the estimated fall has been 17% over the same period.

Targets A5/B6: Prevalence of cigarette smoking in adults

The prevalence of cigarette smoking by adults fell from 31% to 28% for men and from 28% to 27% for women between 1990 and 1996; the rate among women fluctuated during this period, falling to 25% in 1994 before rising to 27% in 1996 (see page 83)[2]. In view of the target of no more than 20% smoking prevalence for both sexes by the year 2000, the data indicate that the rate of decline would need to increase substantially compared with that between 1990 and 1996 to meet the target.

Target A6: Blood pressure

The 1996 Health Survey for England[3] will report that the mean systolic blood pressure among adults remained at 136 mmHg, compared with a baseline figure of 138 mmHg in 1991/92 and a target of 133 mmHg by the year 2005.

Target A7: Obesity

The 1996 Health Survey for England[3] will report that the percentage of 16-64-year-olds classified as obese showed an increase for both sexes, to 16% for men and 17% for women. These figures are higher than the baseline figures for 1986/87, and well above target levels of 6% and 8%, respectively, by the year 2005.

Targets A8 and A9: Consumption of total fats and saturated fatty acids

The percentage of energy derived from total fat and from saturated fatty acids fell further during 1996, continuing the slow but steady progress towards target levels shown in earlier years. Data from the 1996 National Food Survey[4] showed an average of 39.7% (total fat) and 15.4% (saturated fatty acids) as percentages of overall food energy intake.

Target A10: Prevalence of drinking in adults

Preliminary General Household Survey results for 1996, published in November 1997, showed no change in the percentage of men (28%) drinking more than 21 units of alcohol weekly between 1990 and 1996, whereas the percentage of women exceeding 14 units of alcohol weekly rose from 11% to 14%.

Target B1: Breast cancer mortality rate

Breast cancer remains the leading cause of death from cancer in England among women aged over 35 years. Death rates for breast cancer have fallen consistently since 1989-91 in the target age-group of 50-69 years by an estimated 13%,

97

adjusting for the change in coding in 1993. In 1994-96, the death rate from breast cancer for women in England aged 50-69 years was 81.3 per 100,000 population. Early detection by means of the national breast screening programme is a key element in tackling mortality from breast cancer, although it is still too early fully to assess the impact of the programme.

Target B2: Incidence of invasive cervical cancer

Incidence rates of invasive cervical cancer have fallen in each year since 1990. Provisional rates for 1991, 1992 and 1993[5] are all lower than the target figure of 12.8 cases per 100,000, with a fall of 26% between 1985-87 and 1991-93 (figures averaged over three years).

Target B3: Incidence of skin cancer

Although there have been occasional year-on-year falls in the incidence of malignant melanoma among men and women alike, the underlying upward trend has not yet been reversed. Incidence rates in 1993[5] for both sexes were at their highest point since the 1985-87 baseline, against a target to halt the year-on-year increase for all skin cancers by the year 2005.

Targets B4 and B5: Lung cancer mortality rates

Lung cancer mortality among men aged under 75 years continued to fall in 1996 and the rate for women remained virtually static, having fluctuated in earlier years. Over the five years since the start of the Health of the Nation initiative, the mortality rate for men fell by an estimated 17%, after adjusting for the effects of the 1993 coding changes, towards the target reduction of 30% by the year 2010; among women, however, the rate fell by only 3%, towards a target reduction of 15%.

Target B7: Smoking in pregnancy

Data from the five-yearly Infant Feeding Survey[6] in Great Britain showed a rise in the percentage of women giving up smoking in pregnancy from 24% in 1985 to 33% in 1995, apparently meeting the set target.

Target B8: Cigarette consumption

Provisional figures to mid-1997 show an average annual reduction of 2.6% in the total number of cigarettes released for home consumption over the six years from the 1989/90 baseline (including an estimate of European Union [EU] imports for the period following the establishment of the European single market on 1 January 1993) (see page 83).

Target B9: Smoking among 11-15-year-olds

This target was missed: the prevalence of smoking among 11-15-year-old children in 1994 was 12%, compared with a target level of 6%. Headline data for 1996, published in July 1997[7], showed a further slight rise in prevalence to 13% (11% for boys and 15% for girls).

Targets C1 and C3: Mental illness

A programme of work to reformulate the general mental health (C1) target on a quantified basis, and to develop proposals for national monitoring data, included development of the Health of the Nation Outcome Scale (HoNOS), launched in October 1996[8], and pilot work on the collection of data for suicide among mentally ill people (see page 172).

Target C2: Suicide and undetermined injury

The all-ages suicide rate showed a marked drop of 5% between 1995 and 1996 (although single-year changes can be volatile and should be treated with caution). Over the five years since 1989-91, a fall of 10% towards the target of 15% by the year 2000 was observed. Suicide rates among young men aged 15-29 years, which had been rising through the 1980s, have now stopped rising, and rates among people aged 75 years and over have fallen (figures for 1993 onwards have been recoded by the ONS so that they are now consistent with those for earlier years).

Target D1: Gonorrhoea, new cases

The target to reduce the rate of gonorrhoea by 1995 was already more than achieved in 1992 (46 new cases per 100,000 population, compared with a target of 53 per 100,000), and the rate fell to its lowest level in 1994 (37 new cases per 100,000). In 1995, however, the rate was 39 new cases per 100,000 population, still well below the target, but nevertheless representing a 5% year-on-year rise. Figures for 1996[9] show that the incidence rate increased further to 44 cases per 100,000, although this is still below the target level; these increases were evident among all age-groups for males, and the 16-24-years age-group in females.

Target D2: Drug misusers sharing equipment

National monitoring data that precisely follow on from the target baseline are not yet available, although progress has been made towards their collection (see page 81).

Target D3: Conceptions among girls aged under 16 years

Data on conceptions occurring in 1995 showed a further small increase of 3% compared with 1994, a rise similar to that between 1993 and 1994, bringing the national rate for 1995 to 8.5 conceptions per 1,000 females aged 13-15 years. Conception rates in this age-group had fallen in each of the previous three years, and it was hoped that the rising trend of the 1980s had been reversed. However, these increases are small in comparison with the earlier falls, and the overall fall in the rate since the 1989-91 baseline has been just under 14%.

Targets E1-E3: Accident mortality rates

Over the five years from 1989-91 to 1994-96, the reductions in death rates from accidents were: 34% among children aged under 15 years (target 33%), 25% among young people aged 15-24 years (target 25%) and 7% among people aged 65 years and over (target 33%). The target year is 2005 in all three cases.

Good progress has thus been made in both of the younger age-groups and, in both, target reductions for accidental deaths appear to have been reached. Among older people it would appear that progress towards the target is not yet sufficient for it to be met in the year 2005, and an increase of over 4% in the death rate between 1995 and 1996 is disappointing. However, in this age-group there are problems with comparability of data before and after 1993, so that the overall trend since the baseline was set cannot be confirmed, due to a change in coding practice - certain deaths from falls and fractures, previously coded to 'osteoporosis' as the underlying cause of death are now coded as 'accidental death'.

References

1. Department of Health. *The Health of the Nation: a strategy for health in England.* London: HMSO, 1992 (Cm. 1986).
2. Thomas M, Walker A, Wilmot A, Bennett N. *Living in Britain: results from the 1996 General Household Survey: an inter-Departmental survey carried out by the Office for National Statistics between April 1996 and March 1997.* London: Stationery Office (in press) (Series GHS; no. 27).
3. Prescott-Clarke P, Primatesta P, eds. *Health Survey for England 1996: a survey carried out on behalf of the Department of Health (vols 1 and 2).* London: Stationery Office (in press) (Series HS; no. 6).
4. Ministry of Agriculture, Fisheries and Food. *National food survey: annual report on food expenditure, consumption and nutrient intakes.* London: Stationery Office, 1997.
5. Office for National Statistics. *Incidence of and mortality from cancers of the lung, skin, breast and cervix: England.* London: Stationery Office, 1996 (Series MB1 96/2).
6. Foster K, Lader D, Cheesbrough S. *Infant feeding 1995: a survey of infant feeding practices in the United Kingdom.* London: Stationery Office, 1997.

7.   Jarvis L. *Smoking among secondary school children in 1996: England.* London: Stationery Office, 1997.

8.   Wing JK, Curtis RH, Beever AS. *HoNOS: Health of the Nation Outcome Scale: report on research and development July 1993-December 1995.* London: Royal College of Psychiatrists, 1996.

9.   Public Health Laboratory Service. Gonorrhoea. *Commun Dis Rep CDR Rev* 1997; **7(25)**:1.

(c)   Wider determinants of health

The Green Paper *Our Healthier Nation*, to be published in early 1998[1], will acknowledge that although the effects on health of an individual's age, sex, genetic make-up and lifestyle choices are indisputable, the circumstances under which they live, which may not be subject to choice, also have a major impact on their health (see page 14).

Low income is an important determinant of health in relation to being able, for example, to afford heating or protection from fire and accidents in the home, or to make lifestyle choices in relation to healthy food or taking exercise[2].

Joblessness has been linked to poor physical and mental health, and unemployed men and women are more likely to die from cancer, heart disease, accidents and suicide[3].

When social problems - such as poor housing, unemployment or low pay, fear of crime and isolation - are combined, people's health may suffer disproportionately. Social exclusion often involves not only social but also economic and psychological isolation, and its effects on health may be ameliorated by the provision of help and support to enable the socially excluded to participate in society, and thus improve their own economic and social circumstances.

The physical environment - such things as clean air and water and good quality housing - has a great bearing on health (see pages 108-40). For example, high levels of ozone in the air during Summer months is associated with increased hospital admissions for respiratory disorders[4,5]. Research indicates that the most significant risks from poor housing are associated with damp, which can contribute to diseases of the lungs and other parts of the respiratory system[6,7,8,9]; cramped living in poor conditions may lead to accidents, sleeplessness, stress and the more rapid spread of infections. Many deaths annually are due to cold conditions, as indicated by weekly death statistics (see Appendix Figure A.1); older people and the very young are particularly vulnerable to cold weather. There are many other environmental influences on health, including radon[10,11], noise pollution, global warming, ozone depletion and carbon monoxide in the home.

The quality of life in the local community and the extent to which people respect and support each other can also influence health: one study found that, compared with people with lots of social ties, the socially isolated were over six times more likely to die from a stroke and more than three times more likely to commit suicide[12].

References

1. Department of Health. *Our Healthier Nation: a contract for health.* London: Stationery Office (in press) (Cm. 3852).
2. Health Education Authority. *Health update 5: physical activity.* London: Health Education Authority, 1995.
3. Drever F, Whitehead M, eds. *Health inequalities: decennial supplement: Office for National Statistics.* London: Stationery Office, 1997 (Series DS; no. 15).
4. Stedman JR, Anderson HR, Atkinson RW, Maynard RL. Emergency hospital admissions for respiratory disorders attributable to summer time ozone episodes in Great Britain. *Thorax* 1997; **52:** 958-63.
5. Department of Health, Committee on the Medical Effects of Air Pollutants. *Quantification of the effects of air pollution on health in the United Kingdom.* London: Stationery Office (in press). Chair: Professor Stephen Holgate.
6. Sanders CH, Cornish JP. *Dampness: one week's complaints in five local authorities in England and Wales: a Building Research Establishments Report.* London: HMSO, 1982.
7. Department of the Environment. *English house condition survey.* London: HMSO, 1991.
8. Luczynska CM. Risk factors for indoor allergen exposure: health aspects of indoor air: Berzelius Symposium XXVIII. *Respir Med* 1994; **88:** 723-9.
9. Platt SD, Martin CJ, Hunt SM, Lewis CW. Damp housing, mould growth, and symptomatic health state. *BMJ* 1989; **298:** 1673-8.
10. Kendall GM. *Exposure to radon in UK dwellings.* Chilton (Oxon): National Radiological Protection Board, 1994 (NRPB-R272).
11. Central Office of Information. *Radon: a guide to reducing levels in your home.* London: Department of the Environment, 1996.
12. Kawachi I, Colditz GA, Ascherio A, et al. A prospective study of social networks in relation to total mortality and cardiovascular disease in men in the USA. *J Epidemiol Commun Health* 1996; **50:** 245-51.

(d)   Inequalities in health

Social class inequalities in death rates - as judged by the gradient in mortality between highest (I) and lowest (V) social classes - do not appear to have decreased over the past 40 years[1].

The Government recognises that the chances of good health vary not only between different social classes, but also between different regions, different genders and different ethnic groups, and has made a commitment to put plans in place to halt any further increases in inequalities in health[2,3,4], and to promote their reduction. The latest decennial supplement on health inequalities from the

ONS, published in September[5], gave further evidence of the involvement of socio-economic factors in ill-health and death, noting that "All sources show a marked socio-economic gradient in mortality and morbidity persisting into the 1990s". For example, in 1991-93, the national all-cause standardised mortality ratio (SMR) for men aged 20-64 years was almost three times higher among unskilled manual workers in social class V than among professional men in social class I. Moreover, half the deaths of men aged between 25 and 34 years were from accidents, suicide or homicide, which had strong social class gradients such that over 40% of deaths from these causes would have been prevented if all men in this age-group had had the same all-cause death rates as those in social classes I and II[5].

An analysis of national deaths data for 1991-93 to investigate whether the increased mortality risk observed in some migrant groups had more to do with their socio-economic circumstances, rather than some feature of migrant status as such, indicated that the social class of selected migrant groups could account for some but not all of the excess mortality observed. For example, for stroke, higher than average mortality was observed among men from the Caribbean, West/South Africa, the Indian sub-Continent and Ireland even after adjusting for social class[5].

The Government has accepted[2,3] that such differences are not just random variations, but the result of many complex factors that may often be outside individual control and which will require comprehensive solutions that embrace the whole of society. The new health strategy, and other initiatives, must address these concerns. Options recommended for a healthy lifestyle - such as eating well or taking exercise - may not be equally available to all; income will inevitably influence diet, the availability of local facilities will affect the opportunities to take exercise, and so on. Health promotion measures must take these factors into account and will require local partnerships and alliances between health authorities, local authorities, the voluntary sector and others (see page 14).

Responses to the forthcoming Green Paper *Our Healthier Nation*[3] will contribute to a White Paper on the new health strategy to be published next year, which will also be informed by an independent inquiry into inequalities in health which is being carried out at the request of Health Ministers by Sir Donald Acheson, formerly Chief Medical Officer of DH, in which he has reviewed the latest available information on inequalities of health from the ONS, DH and elsewhere, to summarise and to interpret the evidence about inequalities of health and expectation of life in England, and to identify trends. During the first half of 1998, Sir Donald will conduct an independent review in the light of this evidence to identify priority areas for future policy development that are most likely to offer opportunities to develop beneficial, cost-effective and affordable interventions to reduce health inequalities.

Access to health services is also a determinant of health, and the White Paper *The new NHS: modern, dependable*[4] includes fair access to health services in relation to need - irrespective of geography, class, ethnicity or gender - as one of the six main areas of its new national performance framework. Plans are under way to set up Health Action Zones in April 1998 to improve services in some of the most needy areas of the country.

For some people, poor health is just one of many problems that they face. In social exclusion, a combination of factors - such as unemployment, poverty and poor housing - all increase the chances of ill-health, which in turn lessens the chances of employment or developing new skills. Measures to combat social exclusion should also have a positive effect on health.

References

1. Department of Health. *Variations in health: what can the Department of Health and the NHS do?* London: Department of Health, 1995.
2. Department of Health. *Public health strategy launched to tackle root causes of ill-health.* London: Department of Health, 1997 (Press Release: H97/197).
3. Department of Health. *Our Healthier Nation: a contract for health.* London: Stationery Office (in press) (Cm. 3852).
4. Department of Health. *The new NHS: modern, dependable.* London: Stationery Office, 1997 (Cm. 3807).
5. Drever F, Whitehead M, eds. *Health inequalities: a decennial supplement: Office for National Statistics.* London: Stationery Office, 1997 (Series DS; no. 15).

(e)   Health alliances and healthy settings

The third annual Health Alliance Awards scheme culminated in a national awards ceremony in March, with 450 entrants nationwide - a 50% increase from 1996[1]. This increased interest was reflected across all eight NHS regions and in all the entrance categories. The regional and national prizes were sponsored by Johnson & Johnson. DH commissioned an evaluation of the scheme, which was favourable: a special edition of the *Target* newsletter[2] summarised all the projects which were national winners or runners-up.

The concept of alliances for health is now central to the new health improvement programmes to be established by each health authority in partnership with local authorities, local voluntary organisations, businesses and other interested bodies[3,4].

Healthy settings provide a helpful focus for health promotion activities and encourage imaginative approaches to population groups who might not otherwise be expressly addressed. The Health of the Nation initiative[5] identified seven different settings: schools, homes, hospitals, cities, the environment, workplaces and prisons. Given the overlap across settings - schools, hospitals and prisons are also workplaces, for instance - these covered the entire population. A range of different initiatives has been pursued during 1997 across these different settings, often as a result of cross-Government initiatives, in which DH worked closely with colleagues in other Departments: for example, in schools with the Department for Education and Employment (DfEE), and in prisons with the Prison Service Health Care Directorate of the Home Office (including the first year of the Prison Health Promotion Awards).

Other settings have encouraged work outside central Government: the network of health promoting hospitals, for instance, is now independent of the National Health Service (NHS) Executive; the Workplace Health Advisory Team has established alliances between small and medium-sized enterprises which will become self-supporting; work on healthy cities is carried out through the World Health Organization (WHO) 'Healthy Cities' project, co-ordinated by the 'Health For All Network (UK)' with support from DH.

The Green Paper *Our Healthier Nation*[4] will endorse the concept of healthy settings, particularly in schools and workplaces and with particular population groups (see page 14).

References

1. Department of Health. *On the State of the Public Health: the annual report of the Chief Medical Officer of the Department of Health for the year 1996.* London: Stationery Office, 1997; 100.
2. Department of Health. *Target* 1997; **24:** 1.
3. Department of Health. *The new NHS: modern, dependable.* London: Stationery Office, 1997 (Cm. 3807).
4   Department of Health. *Our Healthier Nation: a contract for health.* London: Stationery Office (in press) (Cm. 3852).
5. Department of Health. *The Health of the Nation: a strategy for health in England.* London: HMSO, 1992 (Cm. 1986).

(f)   Inter-Departmental co-operation

In the Health of the Nation initiative[1], DH and the NHS developed links to encourage colleagues in other Government Departments and Agencies to consider the wider health aspects of their own policy areas. The new Government's manifesto pledge to set targets for health, taking account of the effects of poverty, unemployment, poor housing and environmental pollution, and the appointment of a Minister of State for Public Health, reinforces the need to tackle health issues on a broad front. A new Cabinet sub-committee has been set up to oversee the development, implementation and monitoring of the Government's health strategy, and to co-ordinate the Government's policies on UK-wide issues that affect health; at its first meeting in July, it agreed to apply 'health impact assessments'[2] to appropriate Government policies. The development of the Green Paper *Our Healthier Nation*[2,3] has involved close work with a range of Departments that develop policies which may have an impact on health - particularly the Department of the Environment, Transport and the Regions (DETR), the DfEE, and the Health and Safety Executive (HSE).

DH continues to be closely involved in the DETR's National Cycling Forum, which oversees the progress of the national cycling strategy launched in July 1996. The Forum produced its first year report in December 1997[4], which set out progress towards the main aim of doubling (from 1996 levels) the prevalence of cycling by the year 2002, and doubling it again by the year 2012. The Department is also a member of the DETR's National Walking Working Group, which continues to work to set out a framework to encourage walking as a healthy alternative mode of transport. The Working Group, which comprises several Government Departments and local and national agencies with an interest in transport, will recommend a formal strategy in Summer 1998. DH has also been involved in the DETR'S proposed White Paper on Integrated Transport, due to be published in Summer 1998. The impacts of transport on public health are wide-ranging and include the health benefits that walking and cycling can provide within an integrated transport strategy; the impact of road traffic emissions on public health; the importance of accident prevention, particularly the need to ensure safe routes to schools, and the effects of transport strategies on social exclusion.

In September and October, DH organised two major inter-Departmental meetings to discuss new policy initiatives and to assess the efficiency of the current accident data collection systems, which included officials from the Department of Trade and Industry (DTI), the Home Office, the DETR, the ONS and the HSE. The DTI and DH subsequently agreed to develop a research proposal to assess national NHS accident and emergency data as part of a programme to improve data on accidents in home and leisure environments, currently held on DTI's home accident surveillance system; a draft specification was drawn up in November with a view to commission research in 1998.

In conjunction with the Home Office's 'Fire safety week', DH produced a special home safety leaflet, *Safe as houses*[5], which sets out simple precautions that can be taken to prevent accidents in the home, including fire safety, in September.

The Child Accident Prevention Trust continued to run its annual 'Child safety week' during June. In addition to contributions from individuals and industry, the event was co-ordinated and funded jointly by DH, the DfEE and the DETR.

DH and the HSE continued to collaborate on research into the attitudes and sun behaviour of outdoor workers, in relation to the Health Education Authority's 'Sun know how' campaign.

References

1. Department of Health. *The Health of the Nation: a strategy for health in England.* London: HMSO, 1992 (Cm. 1986).
2. Department of Health. *Public health strategy launched to tackle root causes of ill-health.* London: Department of Health, 1997 (Press Release: H97/197).
3. Department of Health. *Our Healthier Nation: a contract for health.* London: Stationery Office (in press) (Cm. 3852).
4. Department of the Environment, Transport and the Regions. *National Cycling Strategy: first year report.* London: Department of the Environment, Transport and the Regions, 1997.
5. Department of Health. *Safe as houses: handy tips to prevent accidents in your home.* London: Department of Health, 1997.

CHAPTER 4

ENVIRONMENT AND HEALTH

(a)   Introduction

Some of the interactions between the environment and health have been recognised for centuries - not for nothing is the weather a topic for conversation in this country, as the excess winter deaths shown in Appendix Figure A.1 testify; other factors are only now becoming apparent.

As noted in the Introduction, there has been a clear legislative link between health and the environment since the 1848 Public Health Act[1], which was followed by various pieces of legislation crucial to improve environmental health - for example, in respect of drinking water, sanitation and air pollution. In recent years there has been increasing awareness of other actual or potential environmental challenges to health - such as pollution linked to increased transport of people and goods[2], depletion of the ozone layer[3], and climate change[4]; the more subtle connections between environment and quality of life have also become more widely appreciated.

This chapter explores various aspects of the wider environment and its impact on health, including how climate change may affect some of these. Although nutrition, food supply and food contamination are linked with the environment (and of course health), these are covered in detail elsewhere (see Chapters 2 and 7); similarly, the occupational and educational environments may also have an impact on many people's health (see Chapters 2 and 3).

References

1.   *An Act for Promoting the Public Health 1848.* London: HMSO, 1848 (11 + 12 Vict. c. lxiii).
2.   British Medical Association. *Road transport and health.* London: British Medical Association, 1997.
3.   Department of the Environment, Transport and the Regions. *The potential effects of ozone depletion in the United Kingdom.* London: Stationery Office, 1996.
4.   McMichael AJ, Haines A. Global climate change: the potential effects on health. *BMJ* 1997; **315:** 805-9.

(b)   National and international issues

(i)   *Climate change and human health*

Human induced climate change

Human activities are increasing the atmospheric concentrations of 'greenhouse gases', such as carbon dioxide, methane and nitrous oxide, which tend to warm the atmosphere and are thought likely to lead to regional and global changes in climate[1]. The United Nations (UN) Inter-Governmental Panel on Climate Change (IPCC) projects an increase in global temperatures of about 1-3.5°C by the year 2100, and an associated increase in sea level of about 15-95 cm. Although there is uncertainty over the scale of these changes, there is confidence that such changes will occur. In its most recent report, the IPCC concluded that "The balance of evidence suggests a discernible human influence on the global climate"[1]; this conclusion is consistent with the rising trend in the observed global temperature record (see Figure 4.1). Potentially serious impacts of climate change could include an increase in temperature fluctuations, floods, droughts (with increased risk of widespread fires) and pest outbreaks, with longer-term effects on the composition, structure and function of ecosystems. Such environmental changes would inevitably affect agriculture, forestry, fisheries and water resources, with a profound potential impact on human health.

Figure 4.1: *Global average annual temperature anomalies by surface observations over land and sea, 1860-1997*

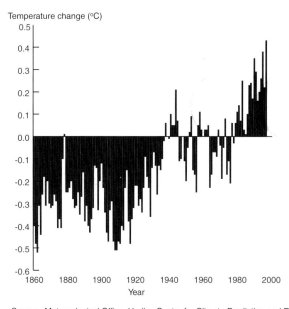

Source: Meteorological Office, Hadley Centre for Climate Prediction and Research

Global impacts of climate change on human health

The potential effects of climate change on human health globally (not restricted to the United Kingdom [UK]) could be serious and wide ranging. Direct impacts would include:

- deaths, illness and injury due to increased exposure to heat and ultraviolet radiation (UVR), although in some countries these might be offset by reductions in cold-related mortality and morbidity; *and*

- altered rates of death, illness and injury due to changes in the frequency or intensity of climate-related disasters (eg, droughts, floods and forest fires).

Indirect impacts on health would include:

- altered distribution and transmission of vector-borne infectious diseases;

- altered distribution and transmission of other communicable diseases, such as waterborne and foodborne infections, and some respiratory infections;

- effects upon agriculture and food production, particularly in tropical and subtropical regions (although beneficial effects may be seen in some temperate zones);

- effects on air quality via increased exposure to pollens, spores and certain air pollutants;

- potential consequences of a rise in sea level, leading to flooding, disrupted sanitation, soil and water salination, and altered breeding sites for infectious disease vectors; *and*

- impacts on health caused by demographic disruption and socio-economic factors arising from the effects of climate change on natural and managed ecosystems.

Among earlier possible effects would be increases in mortality in relation to heat waves and changes in the distribution of vector-borne infectious diseases (eg, malaria, leishmaniasis, dengue fever and tick-borne encephalitis); however, the potential public health consequences of a rise in sea levels and of regional changes in food production might not be apparent for several decades.

The potential effects of climate change on human health in the UK

In 1996[2], the Government's Climate Change Impact Review Group considered the potential effects of climate change on human health in the UK. Its conclusions were tentative and reflect limited data in respect of the UK. It is likely that climate change would lead to increased deaths in heatwaves and altered rates of infectious diseases and exposure to certain air pollutants. Possible impacts to human health in the UK include:

- an increase in deaths arising from heat stress during the summer, although these are likely to be outweighed by a reduction in winter deaths;

- an increase in diarrhoeal and dysenteric infections from foodborne and waterborne infectious agents, which are likely to spread more readily in warmer and wetter conditions;

- altered incidence and geographical distribution of vector-borne diseases, in which the life cycle and viability of both the vector and pathogen are responsive to climatic variation (malaria, for example, existed in the UK in Roman times, and was only effectively eradicated within the last half century). Moreover, climate change is likely to affect transmission of malaria and other infections in areas commonly visited by UK residents which are not currently thought of as sources of such infections;

- warmer summers and warmer, wetter winters would affect the proliferation of arthropod vectors (eg, ticks and mites), with implications for vector-borne diseases;

- a warmer climate is likely to amplify the biological effects of certain air pollutants; *and*

- an increase in the frequency or severity of hot summers may also increase the exposure of the population to UVR from the sun, irrespective of any changes related to stratospheric ozone depletion. In the short term, this could lead to increases in the incidence of sunburn and, in the long term, to an increase in skin cancer.

Preparing for climate change

Even though most developed countries have as a first step committed themselves to reducing their emissions of 'greenhouse gases' by 5.2% on 1990 levels by the period 2008-2012, these concentrations overall will continue to rise, such that some degree of climate change is likely, if not inevitable. The extent of such effects will depend on the efficacy of policies to reduce 'greenhouse gas' emissions; the impact of those effects will be influenced by the implementation of adaptation strategies to take account of climate change.

Historical analogues of anomalous climatic events provide opportunities to develop the understanding of the links between climate and human health and potential vulnerability to climate change. One study, *Economic impacts of the hot summer and unusually warm year of 1995*[3], whilst limited in scope, indicated that a move towards warmer conditions in the UK could lead to additional deaths during summer heatwaves but that these would be offset by decreases in winter mortality. A study of the 1976 heatwave[3] showed very similar results, despite the difference in the extent and timing of the heatwave; it also indicated that a change towards a warmer climate could lead to an increase in notified cases of food poisoning of 5-15%.

In view of these concerns, and the need for further data, the Government has established the UK Climate Impacts Programme at the University of Oxford to facilitate assessments of the impacts of climate change in relation to the UK. The programme offers guidance on research and aims to support local, regional and national studies, and provides opportunities for research on the impact of climate change on human health within a wider integrated programme - as many aspects relate to other social and environmental factors that will also change with the climate.

Concerns about the detection and attribution of the potential health impacts of climate change were reviewed in December 1997 at a workshop held by the World Health Organization (WHO), the UN Environment Programme (UNEP) and the Medical Research Council (MRC) on climate change and health monitoring. The workshop set priorities for research and monitoring and identified opportunities for collection of data and the integration of climate and health data - essential to identify important changes in disease incidence, health risk indicators or health status; to determine whether these changes are likely to be the result of local, regional or global environmental changes; and to develop counter-measures and to assess their effectiveness. The workshop concluded that the most important health indicators need to be established on a regional basis and that the public health infrastructure, including data collection and reporting, needed to be protected and strengthened. As a first step, the Department of the Environment, Transport and the Regions (DETR) is compiling a comprehensive set of indicators for the UK to track the impacts of climate change over time.

(ii)   Sustainable development

Sustainable development - a term increasingly used in recent years, particularly since the 'Earth Summit' held in Rio de Janeiro in June 1992[4] - recognises the need for technological development, but without environmental damage that might adversely affect the quality of life now, and for generations to come, and with the inclusion of all sectors of society.

The Government's broad approach to sustainable development recognises that it is not enough to focus on economic and environmental policies alone to achieve sustainable development. All groups in society must be included in the benefits of economic and environmental progress, which must take into account individual needs and aspirations as well as to ensure effective protection of the environment, prudent use of natural resources and maintenance of high and stable levels of economic growth and employment. Short-term solutions may give rise to long-term problems; interventions must be planned and carefully monitored; potential health gains must be weighed against possible health losses. Above all, there must be effective co-ordination between Government Departments and Agencies, and other bodies in the UK, and internationally.

The links between environment and health can be complex, but good air quality; safe, secure and good-quality housing; safe drinking water; access to open spaces; and the appropriate use of chemicals and hazardous substances are factors which influence human health.

The consultation paper *Opportunities for change*[5], on a new national sustainable development strategy, will address the links between health and environment issues within the overall theme of 'building sustainable communities'. It will consider how issues such as planning, transport, housing and construction, regeneration and health fit together within that framework. A new national strategy, based on the document and responses to it, will include indicators and targets to monitor progress, and will highlight the links between health, the living and working environment and the achievement of sustainable development, and will indicate how health policies can fit into an overall inter-Departmental framework for sustainable development.

(iii) 'Local Agenda 21'

Much can be, and is being, done to promote sustainable development locally. Since the Rio Earth Summit[4], British local authorities have been leading the way internationally in promoting 'Local Agenda 21' - a comprehensive action plan at the local level for sustainable development into the 21st Century. Many councils across the country have brought together business, voluntary and community sectors to identify what their local communities want and need, and then to co-ordinate delivery by means of local resources, taking account of local interests. Although this initiative was originally seen as primarily concentrating on environmental issues, many communities have included projects which have an impact on human health - such as the 'Safe routes to school' initiative, which encourages healthy transport to school by walking and cycling (and reduces traffic congestion), and projects to engage inner-city communities in improving their local environment and to produce fresh fruit and vegetables.

Almost 88% of local authorities are already committed to this work, and the Prime Minister has called on all to be involved by the end of this Century. To help them to achieve this, *Sustainable local communities for the 21st Century*[6], which contains guidance on why and how to put an effective local strategy in place and draws on the good practice that has already been established, will be published in January 1998. But no-one has all the answers, and communities will not become properly sustainable until local people are fully engaged in the initiative.

Implementation of a local strategy for sustainable development involves a number of elements. As well as managing and improving its own sustainability performance, the local authority has to integrate sustainability issues into all its policies and activities and ensure its employees and the local community understand what the concept means. It also has to consult and involve the community; to work in partnership with others; and to measure, monitor and report on progress and adapt policies accordingly.

Local health action plans should be a central element in such strategies. As a corporate strategy that brings together local authorities' environmental, economic and social objectives, 'Local Agenda 21' fits well with the aims of *Our Healthier Nation*[7] by tackling the environmental, economic and social factors that can influence health.

(iv)   National environmental health action plan

The Second European Ministerial Conference on Environment and Health, held in Helsinki in 1994, agreed the idea of an environment and health action plan for Europe (EHAPE)[8]. A principle feature of this was that environment and health Departments in individual countries would work together to prepare their own national environmental health action plans (NEHAPs). The UK NEHAP was the first of these to be published, in July 1996[9], after a public consultation exercise. It built on existing strategies for sustainable development, but concentrated on health implications and environmental policies in their widest sense. The UK's NEHAP follows the objectives of the EHAPE and a basic format agreed with other participating countries. The plan describes the institutional framework for action on environment and health, environmental hazards and means of control, the interaction between major economic sectors and enviromental health, and the UK's international contribution. The plan shows how the current provisions should deliver a steady improvement in environmental health, and ways in which they could be modified.

The agreed format means the plan covers five areas: institutional framework; environmental health management tools; specific environmental hazards; living and working environments; and economic sectors. A sixth area on international action was added, to reflect the UK's contribution in this area. In total, over 160 actions are listed, which form a checklist against which progress in improving environmental health in the UK can be measured. Three categories are identified, according to urgency:

- Group 1: The basic requirements for human health;

- Group 2: The prevention and control of medium and long-term health hazards; *and*

- Group 3: The promotion of well-being and mental health rather than the prevention of disease.

The wide range of actions covered include to:

- continue to review and amend the institutional framework and legislation to meet new requirements for improving environmental health;

- maintain and develop research initiatives to identify environmental health hazards and to evaluate associated risks to health;

- continue surveillance of food contamination and promote understanding and awareness of food hygiene;

- conduct research into links between noise and health; *and*

- take action to meet housing need, to improve the housing stock, to raise standards of housing management, to revitalise neighbourhoods, and to conduct housing surveys and research.

The Government gave a commitment in the report to review progress from time to time and report on the extent to which actions have been completed. The actions will be revised to take account of new knowledge and new policies.

To be effective, any NEHAP must be a useful tool relevant to current concerns, with effective joint working, and commitment, between all those involved in its implementation. The EHAPE also requires international co-operation, and the Third European Ministerial Conference on Environment and Health will be held in London in June 1999. Implementation of NEHAPs is one of the central themes of the conference, and the UK is leading a project to prepare guidance on NEHAP implementation to be considered at the conference. Government Departments and Agencies will be reviewing the UK NEHAP during 1998 to update it to reflect current concerns, new developments in policy and the need for greater integration between different policy areas.

The new public health strategy, *Our Healthier Nation*[7], will set goals to improve the overall health of the nation which recognise the effects that poor housing, poverty, unemployment and a polluted environment have upon health. It is increasingly recognised that responsibility for policies relevant to public health extends far wider than the immediate remit of the Department of Health (DH) alone, and work on the NEHAP, as well as on the 'Our Healthier Nation' initiative, serve to emphasise this. A number of environmental strategies relevant to health are under development or being reviewed, such as the national air quality, integrated transport and sustainable development strategies; and mechanisms are now put in place to take forward national environment and health policies across a broad front, but in a coherent manner, whilst taking account of local needs.

References

1. Houghton JT, Meirafilho LG, Callander BA, Harris N, Kattenberg A, Maskell K, eds. *Climate change 1995: the science of climate change.* Cambridge: Cambridge University Press, 1995.
2. United Kingdom Climate Change Impact Review Group. *Review of the potential effects of climate change in the UK.* London: HMSO, 1996.
3. Palutikof JP, Subak S, Agnew MD, eds. *Economic impacts of the hot summer and unusually warm year of 1995.* London: Department of the Environment, Transport and the Regions, 1997.
4. Department of Health. *On the State of the Public Health: the annual report of the Chief Medical Officer of the Department of Health for the year 1992.* London: HMSO, 1993; 171-2.
5. Department of the Environment, Transport and the Regions. *Opportunities for change: consultation paper on a revised UK strategy for sustainable development.* London: Department of the Environment, Transport and the Regions (in press).
6. Local Government Association. *Sustainable local communities for the 21st Century.* London: Local Government Association (in press).
7. Department of Health. *Our Healthier Nation: a contract for health.* London: Stationery Office (in press) (Cm. 3852).
8. Department of Health. *On the State of the Public Health: the annual report of the Chief Medical Officer of the Department of Health for the year 1994.* London: HMSO, 1995; 194-5.
9. Department of the Environment, Department of Health. *United Kingdom national environmental health action plan.* London: HMSO, 1996.

(c)   Lifestyle, environment and health

The concept of environmental health encompasses the workplace or classroom, home and leisure environments; each of these, in turn, has many components. In some instances it is possible to identify an individual environmental factor with a causal influence on health, and to modify it; in others the influences may be multifactorial and difficult to quantify. Moreover, some 'lifestyle' choices are made by an individual, but others are imposed - whether through the planning and structure of communities which limit individual choices, or as a knock-on effect of the choices of others. Three important factors that influence lifestyle and environment are housing and living conditions, transport and leisure activities.

(i)   *Housing*

A prime objective of Government interventions in housing over the years has been to promote public health. In general, with slum clearance and other initiatives, basic housing conditions have improved considerably over the past 50 years, such that people generally have more space, better services and live in homes in better physical condition, and hence are less likely to foster ill-health[1]. The number of homes without access to the most basic of amenities (an inside toilet, a wash handbasin, a bath or shower in an indoor bathroom, a kitchen sink and a supply of hot water) has now almost been eradicated (see Figure 4.2).

Nevertheless, a minority of houses pose health and safety risks:

- some 1.5 million households live in housing which is considered to be unfit for human habitation, generally because the dwelling is in a state of disrepair prejudicial to the health and safety of the occupant, or the conditions for the preparation and cooking of food are inadequate or unhygienic[1] (see Figure 4.3);

- some 100,000 dwellings are affected by concentrations of radon gas above the current action level[2];

- many homes pose a significant fire risk, particularly houses in multiple occupation[3]; *and*

- some half a million homes are overcrowded.

Figure 4.2: *Dwellings lacking basic amenities, England, 1971-91*

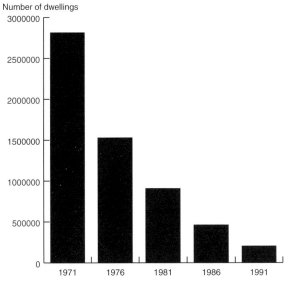

Number of dwellings

Source: DETR

117

Figure 4.3: *Reasons for unfitness of dwellings, England, 1991*

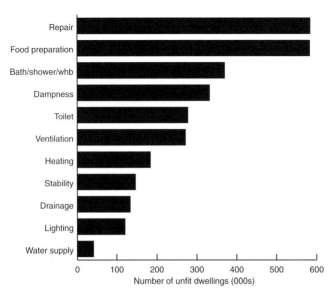

Note: whb = wash handbasin

Source: DETR

The most vulnerable members of society - defined in terms of income, families with small children and the elderly - are more likely to live in poor housing[1], and there are pockets of multiple deprivation and therefore social exclusion in some urban and, in more dispersed form, in some rural areas. Problems of housing and ill-health in these areas are interlinked with wider economic and social problems.

Many factors associated with the quality of housing have been shown to contribute to poor physical and mental health, although the relations are often complex and it may be difficult to establish or to quantify direct links, or to assess the influence of any one factor where several may interact. Poverty, unemployment, unhealthy lifestyles (eg, in relation to diet, cigarette smoking, alcohol consumption, drug misuse and lack of exercise) and limited access to medical services often go hand-in-hand with poor housing. It is therefore difficult to quantify benefits in terms of health gain that result directly from improvement in housing.

Nevertheless, in the UK, research indicates that the most significant health risks from poor housing appear to be associated with cold and damp[1]. As shown in Appendix Figure A.1, there are excess winter deaths - typically about 40,000 more deaths over January-March than the average rate for the other nine months of the year, although again other confounding factors abound, such as inadequate clothing and lack of exercise when outdoors, poorer diet and an increase in the incidence of infectious diseases such as influenza. International differences in

118

excess winter deaths indicate that the reasons behind the high UK increase in mortality rate may be more complex than the external temperature alone, and further work is needed to identify the causes. Housing and other environmental aspects are likely to be a major factor, particularly among elderly people, children and other vulnerable groups.

An important part of renovation and regeneration policies is directed towards tackling poor housing and recognising the health benefits that can arise from housing improvements. Policies seek to address the health risks that arise in relation to housing by tackling:

- housing in a physical sense: the structural aspects, including overall condition, design and layout, and the absence or condition of basic amenities and facilities;

- the indoor housing environment, such as air pollutants, radon, infestations and micro-organisms;

- the wider environment, in respect of the design and management of housing estates, access to shops and medical and other services and leisure facilities; *and*

- access to housing.

Key areas of current activity include:

- the 'Rough Sleepers' Initiative', to help homeless people off the streets in areas where there is a particular need;

- regulations to strengthen the safety net for homeless households;

- comprehensive building regulations which ensure that new buildings meet basic construction standards, including requirements for thermal insulation and ventilation;

- a review of the housing fitness standard, the statutory yardstick against which local authorities assess whether dwellings are fit for human habitation, to consider how it might cover more closely areas most likely to pose health and safety risks;

- a Government commitment to introduce a national licensing scheme for houses in multiple occupation, where some of the worst housing conditions may be found;

- the provision of advice and information so that householders can take action to limit their exposure to indoor pollutants such as dust mites, asbestos, carbon monoxide and radon;

- grant assistance to improve poor housing conditions targeted on the most vulnerable and, through disabled facilities grants, on those who need help with adaptations to facilitate full access into and around the home;

- the release of additional resources through the Government's Capital Receipts Initiative to help local authorities to meet priority housing and associated regeneration needs;

- grants under the Home Energy Efficiency Scheme to help elderly poor people and other low-income groups to keep their homes warmer and to use less fuel (in the seven years since this scheme started, over 2.5 million homes have been insulated at a cost of over £400 million); *and*

- regeneration programmes which provide resources to tackle the social, economic and environmental challenges posed by run-down urban and other areas, taking into account public health objectives and the needs and aspirations of local people.

Progress has been made over the years to tackle poor housing conditions, but more still needs to be done to improve people's health and their quality of life, as well as other goals. However, it is also important for research to establish more clearly the links between housing and health, and the most effective housing solutions to tackle health - taking into account other factors such as poverty, unemployment, education status and unhealthy lifestyles. Effective solutions call upon Government Departments and Agencies, local authorities, social services, health authorities and other local agencies to develop much closer working relations and to share existing knowledge and experience.

(ii)   Transport and health

Transport and health are linked in several respects, and not just in terms of stress caused to commuters stuck in a motorway traffic jam or a delayed train. Aspects of air pollution and lead outputs from fuel are discussed below, and aspects of access to transport has been considered above. As the British Medical Association's report, *Road transport and health*[4], pointed out, transport should not simply be a question of ease and convenience of access, but also of how that ease of access is met and whether the health of individuals is benefited or damaged.

DH has collaborated closely with the DETR on strategies that focus on the need to promote alternative and healthy modes of transport. The cycling strategy, launched in 1996[5], identified that 72% of all journeys are for fewer than five miles and 50% are for under two miles. The cycling strategy aims to double the number of journeys made by bicycle by the year 2002, compared with 1996 figures, and to double it again by the year 2012. The Department has drawn attention to the health benefits of cycling and is a key member of the National Cycling Forum, which monitors the progress of the strategy and published its annual report in December 1997[6]. As part of the Forum's commitment to healthy transport, a series of seminars for health promotion officers, health practitioners and local authority staff was organised for Spring 1998.

In parallel with this cycling initiative, the health gains from walking were also emphasised by the work of an inter-Departmental steering group to promote walking as a healthy and environmentally friendly mode of transport. The health benefits of a brisk walk of at least 30 minutes a day include the preservation of bone mineral density, protection against heart disease and stroke, and maintenance of the integrity of muscle function (which should protect against falls). A national strategy for walking, in co-operation with local and national agencies, is being developed.

Any policies to promote cycling and walking for health purposes must take into account any potential increased incidence of accidents, and accident prevention is a key feature in the Government's new health strategy[7], and DH, the DETR and the Department for Education and Employment (DfEE), as well as other Departments and Agencies and local authorities, have worked to co-ordinate an approach to safe alternatives to personal motorised transport.

(iii)   Leisure

Leisure pursuits play an important part in health promotion: increased physical exercise and reduction of stress are among the benefits. But it is also important to minimise any hazards associated with such activities, including microbiological hazards in the environment (see page 131).

The increased use of coastal and inland waters for a range of watersports raises new issues concerning water quality. Research indicates that the incidence of symptoms associated with water contact is related to the degree of contact and its duration, as well as to indicators of microbial pollution[8]. Water quality in designated bathing waters is governed by European Union (EU) Regulations. However, water contact now increasingly takes place outside these waters. High-contact water sports such as surfing and whitewater canoeing are likely to be associated with a higher incidence of symptoms, although these are often relatively mild and self-limiting. In recent years, there has been an increase in reports of algal blooms, in which increased water temperatures may play a part, and blooms of blue-green algae are of particular concern. In 1990, DH advised that "Illnesses, including skin rashes, eye irritation, vomiting, diarrhoea, fever and pain in muscles and joints have occurred in some recreational users of water who swallowed or swam through algal scum. There have been no reports of long-term effects or deaths in humans, but in some cases the illnesses were severe. Although algal scum is not always harmful it is a sensible precaution to avoid contact with the scum and the water close to it"[9].

Walking in the countryside is an important leisure pursuit for many people and schemes which promote access to the countryside deliver health benefits and improve the quality of life. But increased pressures on wildlife and landscape (already affected by agriculture, roads, industrial and housing development, and pollution) mean that Government, local authorities, landowners and the public need to work together to maintain and enhance the character of the countryside.

A risk of walking in woodland or long grass is that of tick bites, and climate change could increase this risk. Lyme disease caused by the spirochaete *Borrelia burgdorferi* occurs occasionally in the UK in regions where the tick vector, *Ixodes ricinus*, is prevalent - including places much used for leisure activities, such as the Lake District, the New Forest and Richmond Park. The tick's seasonal behaviour is temperature-dependent, with bimodal peaks in spring and autumn in warm regions and a unimodal pattern in colder regions. At present, only some 40 cases of Lyme disease are reported annually to the Public Health Laboratory Service (PHLS) Communicable Disease Surveillance Centre. A number of simple steps can be taken to prevent the disease, and in areas where ticks are known to be infected, simple advice sheets can be provided for residents and visitors.

Visits to open farms are another popular activity. The small risk of infection associated with such visits was highlighted in 1997 by several cases of verocytotoxin-producing *Escherichia coli* O157 (VTEC) infection, but it can be minimised by simple hygienic precautions[10,11,12,13].

References

1. Department of the Environment, Transport and the Regions. *English House Condition Survey 1996.* London: Department of the Environment, Transport and the Regions (in press).
2. National Radiological Protection Board. *Exposure to radon in UK dwellings.* London: HMSO, 1994 (Doc. NRPB R272).
3. Department of the Environment, Transport and the Regions. *Fire risks in homes: research report.* London: Department of the Environment, Transport and the Regions, 1997.
4. British Medical Association. *Road transport and health.* London: British Medical Association, 1997.

5.   Department of Transport. *National cycling strategy*. London: Department of Transport, 1996.

6.   National Cycling Forum. *National cycling strategy: first year report*. Department of the Environment, Transport and the Regions, 1997.

7.   Department of Health. *Our Healthier Nation: a contract for health*. London: Stationery Office (in press) (Cm. 3852).

8.   Department of the Environment. *Health effects of sea bathing (WMI 9021) - phase III: final report to the Department of the Environment*. Marlow (Bucks): WRc plc, 1994 (Report no. DOE 3412/2).

9.   National Rivers Authority. *Toxic blue-green algae: the report of the National Rivers Authority*. London: National Rivers Authority, 1990 (Water Quality Series; no. 2).

10. National Farmer's Union Professional Services Department. *Health and safety advice for farm open days*. London: National Farmers' Union, 1995.

11. Dawson A, Griffin R, Fleetwood A, Barrett NJ. Farm visits and zoonoses. *Commun Dis Rep CDR Rev* 1995; **5**: R81-6.

12. Health and Safety Executive. *School visits to farms*. London: Health and Safety Executive, 1989.

13. Department of Health. *Visits to farms*. London: Department of Health, 1997 (Professional Letter: PL/CEHO(97)6).

(d)   Environmental influences on health

Informed decisions about action to alter environmental factors to improve public health, and to understand which changes are likely to deliver the most effective outcomes, require an understanding of the links between individual environmental factors and effects on health, and of the complex interactions that underlie them. Some aspects are explored below.

(i)   *Air pollution*

Outdoor air pollution

Although air pollution has become, rightly, a topic of increasing public interest, it should be recognised that concentrations of several air pollutants have fallen dramatically in the UK during this Century. The Clean Air Acts of 1956[1] and 1968[2], and increased use of natural gas and electricity for domestic heating, led to a marked improvement in urban air quality. However, the extent of the anticipated improvement has been limited by the growth of traffic-generated air pollution, which is currently a major challenge.

Motor vehicles produce primary air pollutants directly - such as carbon monoxide, particulate matter and oxides of nitrogen; in addition, secondary air pollutants - such as ozone and more particulate matter - are generated by photochemical reactions in polluted air. This secondary production process takes time, and peak levels of ozone and secondary particles often occur far from the sources of primary pollutants. The photochemical nature of the production processes means that higher concentrations of secondary pollutants are generated in summer than in winter, with the possibility that climate change will increase the duration and peaks of these episodes[3]. Primary and secondary air pollutants alike all damage health.

Since 1990, DH and other Government Departments have reviewed the effects of air pollutants on health[4]; reports have been published on individual pollutants[5,6], related diseases[7], a national air quality strategy[8], and a handbook on air pollution and health[9]. Recent work has concentrated on estimating the extent of the effects of air pollution on health in the UK[10], the first time that such an attempt at quantification of the effects has been made; it provides a strong health basis for the need to improve air quality. The joint DETR/DH Expert Panel on Air Quality Standards (EPAQS) recommended a series of specifically health-based air quality standards which were incorporated into the national air quality strategy[8], which set out approaches to be taken to achieve objectives up to the year 2005; an accelerated review of the objectives is now under way.

Air pollutants damage health in a number of ways. Before 1990, it was generally accepted that there was a threshold of exposure for most air pollutants below which there would be no adverse health effects. More recently, epidemiological studies[11,12] indicate quantifiable effects of day-to-day variations in concentrations of common air pollutants - for example, particulate matter, ozone, nitrogen and sulphur dioxide, and possibly for carbon monoxide - such that effects on health can be predicted at even very low concentrations. This new evidence clearly may have implications for air quality objectives.

Although the health effects of air pollutants at low concentrations are proportionally small, they have the potential to affect many people, and the potential public health impact is large. To establish the strength of any causal link requires examination of a range of data and reassessment of previous theories. For example, recent studies[13,14] of the toxicological properties of small particles (less than 100 nm diameter) have produced results that would have seemed implausible just a few years ago; appreciation of a possible link between epidemiological studies and the work on ultrafine particles led Seaton and colleagues[15] to propose the 'ultrafine hypothesis' to explain the adverse effects of low mass concentrations of ambient particles, and studies of this hypothesis have been set up in the UK as part of the DH/DETR/MRC research initiative on air pollution.

Attention is now being focused on the common gaseous air pollutants - ozone, sulphur and nitrogen dioxide, and carbon monoxide - and the apparent lack of thresholds of effect. Here it is important to distinguish between the concepts of thresholds at individual and at population levels. For non-carcinogenic air pollutants, it is likely that for each individual there is a threshold of exposure which must be passed before effects occur, but at a population level there will be a considerable range of personal exposure and of personal sensitivity to air pollution. Even on a day when the recorded concentration of a pollutant may be very low, effects may be seen as a result of particular exposure of some sensitive individuals. It is hardly surprising that a population threshold does not easily emerge from such studies. Further research is needed, and the application of non-parametric statistical modelling techniques may yield more information about thresholds.

The effects of day-to-day variations in concentrations of air pollutants may be less important in public health terms than the much less studied effects of long-duration exposure. Two long-term studies[16,17], both from the United States of America (USA), indicate that long-term exposure to air pollution may lead to a reduction in average life expectancy. The size of this effect is being studied: preliminary calculations indicate that, if the findings are correct, the average reduction in life expectancy produced by current levels of air pollution in the UK would be of the order of months; in public health terms this is a significant effect.

The tightly focused research initiatives into air pollution, supported by DH, the DETR and the MRC, include novel epidemiological approaches, new chamber studies involving volunteers and advanced mechanistic studies. A review of what can be learnt from this research will be undertaken by the Committee on the Medical Effects of Air Pollutants in 1999/2000. UK research workers, together with DH and DETR officials, have been involved in the development of new air pollution directives in the EU and with the work of the WHO in updating the air quality guidelines for Europe and in the development of world air quality guidelines.

Indoor air pollution

Most people spend much of their day indoors - either at work, at school or at home - and therefore exposure to pollution and factors in the indoor environment may often be a major determinant of personal exposure to air pollution. Improved understanding of the links between health and outdoor air pollution has clear implications for the understanding of the health effects of indoor air pollution, but more work is needed to develop a fuller appreciation of this major determinant of exposure. A review of the health effects of certain indoor air pollutants by the MRC Institute for Environment and Health[18] contained several recommendations for research, and in July 1997 DH and the DETR launched a joint £1 million research programme focusing on indoor air pollution in the home, with emphasis on the need for a better assessment of personal exposure; the relation between the outdoor and indoor environment; the effects of indoor pollutants on sensitive individuals and sub-groups; the important toxicological interactions between environmental tobacco smoke, allergens and indoor air pollutants; and effects of damp in the home.

(ii)   Noise

The effects of noise on hearing in occupational settings are established[19]; the effects of environmental noise on other aspects of health are not, although it is a factor which causes concern and annoyance to many people. DH and the DETR held a workshop on the non-auditory effects of noise in May 1997, attended by international and national specialists. It concluded that: "a number of uncertainties remain about the non-auditory effects of noise; nonetheless, some conclusions have been reached. The evidence for effects of environmental noise on health is strongest for annoyance, sleep disturbance (onset and latency, awakening during the night and premature awakening in the morning, subjective sleep quality, mood next day), ischaemic heart disease, and performance in schoolchildren. The available data on other possible health consequences, such as low birthweight and psychiatric disorders are inconclusive"[20].

The conclusions also pointed to a need for further research to clarify the effects of environmental noise on non-auditory aspects of health, and for better characterisation of noise exposure and source, and better measurement of other health outcomes. It recommended longitudinal studies on susceptible groups (which might include changes in the siting of an airport, or intervention studies), investigation of possible chronic health effects, and identification of particularly sensitive individuals. In epidemiological studies, consideration should be given to confounding factors and effect modifiers in the association between noise and health. Publication of the report of the workshop in early 1998 will be followed by a joint call for research proposals over three years by DH and the DETR; a £600,000 research programme should be agreed later in 1998.

(iii)   Radiation in the environment

Radon

Radon, a natural radioactive gas produced in soil and rock, rises to the surface and disperses in the atmosphere; when it enters an enclosed space, such as a house, unusually high concentrations may be found. The areas in England with the highest concentrations of radon are Devon and Cornwall, and parts of Derbyshire, Northamptonshire and Somerset have moderately high levels[21]. Radon in the home is the main source of human exposure to ionising radiation; domestic exposure to radon may lead to lung cancer, although the risk of developing lung cancer from exposure to radon is ten times higher among smokers than non-smokers[22].

The DETR has a programme to identify homes with high radon concentrations in the most affected areas. Building regulations also specify that, in certain areas,

126

new houses must incorporate methods to stop radon ingress. Householders living in areas where radon concentrations might be high are able to obtain measurements and further advice. As part of the 'Our Healthier Nation' initiative[23] to reduce the number of deaths from cancer, local action in respect of radon concentrations in homes is being encouraged.

DH is supporting further research on dose and risk estimates from radon exposure for lung cancer and for other possible health effects, such as the induction of leukaemia and skin cancers, to reduce the uncertainties surrounding the possible effects of exposure to radon in the home. The Department is also funding research into public perceptions of radiation risks to discover why some sections of the public are less concerned about radon exposure than other aspects of potential radiation risk.

Electromagnetic fields

Electromagnetic fields (EMFs) such as those emitted by electrical equipment, electricity power lines, radio transmitter towers, mobile telephones and power generators have been the subject of public and media fears about potential adverse health effects. There is currently no clear causal link to provide a scientific basis for these fears[24], but the Department, along with many other agencies world wide, has supported research efforts to develop an understanding of what happens to human beings in these very low-intensity radiation fields. DH is also contributing to a five-year WHO international EMF project.

The Department has commissioned several studies into potential biological effects of EMFs, including investigations into potential influences of microwave radiation on learning ability and behaviour, and the biological responses of cells in an electromagnetic radiation field. In 1997, the Small Area Health Statistics Unit (SAHSU) investigated the incidence of leukaemia near 20 high-power television and radio transmitters in Great Britain, and found that living close to a transmitter was not associated with an increased risk of leukaemia[25] (see page 137).

Ultraviolet radiation

Excess exposure to the sun is associated with adverse health effects, particularly the development of skin cancer. The incidence of skin cancer in the UK has been rising over the last 30 years and exposure to UVR appears to play a major role: for non-melanoma skin cancers, cumulative life-time UVR exposure appears to be the most important causal factor, whilst for malignant melanoma intermittent high exposure to UVR and episodes of sunburn, especially in childhood, appears to have a major role[26]. The Health Education Authority's (HEA's) 'Sun know how' campaign, funded by DH, has emphasised the need to avoid sunburn, to cover up, to wear a hat, to avoid the mid-day sun, and to use a high-factor sunscreen. Although ozone depletion has been blamed for increases in skin cancer incidence, in the UK the unusual ozone patterns recorded here have occurred largely in the winter and spring when the sun is unlikely to cause sunburn. Although a reduction in ozone concentrations is likely to lead to an increased incidence of a number of effects such as sunburn, photo-ageing and skin cancer, it is not possible to attribute a causal relation at present, and prevention of excess exposure to UVR is the keystone to prevention of skin cancer. Measurements of solar UVR are made by the National Radiological Protection Board at several sites in the British Isles to assess exposure and to provide a baseline against which to compare future changes (see page 242).

Nuclear radiation

The Black Advisory Group was commissioned by the then Minister of Health in 1983 to investigate reports of a high incidence of leukaemia occurring in young people living in the village of Seascale, close to the Sellafield nuclear reprocessing plant. The Advisory Group confirmed that there was a higher incidence of leukaemia in young people resident in the area, but also concluded that the estimated radiation dose from the Sellafield discharges and other sources, received by the local population, could not account for the observed leukaemia incidence[27]. The uncertainties in the available data led the Advisory Group to make recommendations for further research and investigation. The Committee on Medical Aspects of Radiation in the Environment (COMARE) was established in November 1985 to assess and advise Government on the health effects of natural and man-made radiation in the environment, and to assess the adequacy of the available data and the need for further research.

A study in 1990[28] indicated that occupational exposure of fathers to radiation increased the risk of leukaemia and non-Hodgkin's lymphoma in their offspring. This study prompted the COMARE to recommend that studies should be set up to consider any possible effects on the health of the children of parents occupationally exposed to radiation.

A study published in November 1997[29] indicates that there is a higher incidence of leukaemia or non-Hodgkin's lymphoma (but not other cancers) among children whose fathers were radiation workers than in a control group of children living in the same part of the country whose fathers had a different occupation. It is not clear whether the findings in this study are due to chance or to a possible paternal link with the radiation work. However, the study found no relation with radiation dose. Further research is already under way.

The COMARE has published five reports on investigations into the incidence of cancer in children and young people living in the vicinity of several nuclear installations. The Committee has found no links between cancer incidence and the radioactive material released from these sites. It has considered several other hypotheses, including chemical and viral exposures and population mixing and other socio-economic effects. None of these hypotheses alone can account for any noted excess cancer incidence. The COMARE is continuing its investigations into this problem.

(iv) *Environmental chemicals*

DH advises other Government Departments on the health implications of chemicals in the environment in support of policy development and regulatory activity by those Departments. For many chemicals, including pesticides, the main route of exposure for the general population is food. Food safety issues are dealt with in Chapter 7. People may also be exposed to chemical pollutants in air, drinking water, soil or house dust. Although exposure to chemicals in the environment is usually low in comparison with exposures which might occur in an occupational setting, the level of public concern about this issue is high. The Department is funding a programme of work at the MRC Institute for Environment and Health (IEH) to establish priorities for public health responses to environmental chemical pollutants, including a review of environment and health problems as they arise and attempts to identify future concerns. In early 1998, the Department, together with the DETR, will set up a £900,000 research programme into the health effects of chemicals in the environment.

In terms of specific environmental chemical hazards, two areas of current concern include lead and endocrine disruptors.

Lead

Exposure to lead continues to decrease. The proportion of water supply zones in England and Wales that comply with the current standard for lead in drinking water increased from 78.9% in 1992 to 88.6% in 1997[30]. Further improvement is expected from additional modifications to water treatment processes. A revised EU directive on drinking water, including more stringent limits for lead, may be adopted in Autumn 1998. Nevertheless, as long as lead continues to be present in household plumbing, concentrations greater than the standard will occur at times in some consumers' water supply. The Drinking Water Inspectorate has published a public information leaflet on lead in drinking water[31], copies of which were sent to general practitioners in March 1997. Estimated dietary intakes of lead are lower than ever[32], reflecting changes in food processing and packaging (such as the greater use of welded rather than soldered cans), as well as reductions in environmental contamination (for instance, from the decreased use of leaded petrol).

Data on blood lead concentrations from the 1995 Health Survey for England were reported in March 1997 at a workshop at the IEH[33]. From 1984 to 1995, population blood lead levels fell by a factor of approximately three among adults, and by a factor of some 3.6-5 among schoolchildren[33,34]. Nevertheless, 3% of the sample exceeded a blood lead concentration of 0.5 µmol/l (10 µg/dl). Such concentrations do not cause clinical lead poisoning, but are associated with small decrements in intelligence quotient (IQ) in children, and small increases in blood pressure in adults. Evidence that even lower concentrations may also be harmful was presented at the workshop. Efforts to reduce lead exposure therefore continue.

Old leaded paint is a prominent cause of clinical lead poisoning, although such cases are now very rare. It also contributes to environmental exposure through dust and soil. The DETR will issue an updated public information leaflet on lead in paint in 1998.

Endocrine disruptors

Many[35], but by no means all[36], studies of trends in semen quality in many countries, including the UK[37], indicate that there has been a fall in sperm counts, perhaps for the past 50 years. Interpretation of these studies is not straightforward, and it is by no means clear whether the trend is real; moreover, there is no evidence that male fertility has fallen.

The explanation of any such trend in semen quality is not known, but there is considerable interest in the hypothesis that oestrogenic chemicals in food, consumer products and the environment may contribute to the incidence of this and other disorders of the male reproductive tract (such as testicular cancer, incomplete descent of the testis and hypospadias), and that exposures may have increased[38]. Scientific reviews[39,40] conclude that the evidence of a causal link is not persuasive, but that further research is needed. Government research in this area involves many agencies, including the DETR (which has taken on a co-ordinating role), DH, the Ministry of Agriculture, Fisheries and Food, the HSE, the Environment Agency, and the MRC. One important activity is the development, through the Organization for Economic Co-operation and Development (OECD), of harmonised test guidelines and a harmonised strategy for the screening and testing of endocrine-disrupting chemicals; the UK is playing a major role in this process. Other actions include:

130

- risk assessment of several relevant chemicals under the EU Existing Substances Directive;

- reviews, conferences and consultations commissioned through the IEH;

- participation in international discussions;

- identification and prioritisation of suspect chemicals; *and*

- research into exposures through food, food packaging, and the environment.

In Autumn 1997, DH, the DETR and the HSE issued a joint call for proposals for epidemiological studies to investigate trends in male reproductive health and the possible influences of occupational or environmental (or other) exposures to chemicals. This programme has a budget of £1.7 million, which includes a contribution of £350,000 from the European Chemical Industry Council.

(v) *Microbiological factors*

Foodborne and waterborne diseases for 1997 are described in detail on page 218. This section takes account of potential trends related to environmental factors.

Waterborne disease

The microbiological quality of mains water supplies in the UK is very high, and action is under way to improve the quality of the bathing waters around its shores. Climate change may affect this through reduced rainfall, rising sea levels and increased frequency and severity of extreme weather events such as floods and storms, but the major impact in the UK is likely to be on the quality of coastal waters - particularly an increase in microbial pollutants, which may increase pollution of shellfish and illness associated with recreational use of those waters.

Reduced rainfall and other factors may lead water suppliers to use source waters of poorer quality. Although conventional water treatment processes are able to deal with increased loads of micro-organisms sensitive to disinfectants, occasional, localised outbreaks of cryptosporidiosis do occur; if climate change occurs, organisms such as *Cryptosporidium*, which are resistant to disinfection, may pass through the treatment process in increased numbers. The risk of outbreaks of waterborne infections may also be increased by flooding following periods of drought.

Reduced rainfall may also lead to difficulties in maintaining a constant supply of mains water. Absence of water for hygienic purposes may be associated with an increased risk of infections transmitted by the faecal-oral route. Events during the 1995 drought indicated that interruptions to domestic water supplies were not acceptable as a means of controlling demand in periods of water shortage[41].

Climate change and pests

Warm winters are associated with increased numbers of rats, which are potential carriers of disease. They carry a number of organisms associated with food poisoning, including *Salmonella*, *Listeria* and *Yersinia enterocolitica*, as well as *Cryptosporidium*, but their role in transmitting disease via the food chain remains uncertain. The 1993 National Rodent Survey[42] showed that, whilst there had been an increase in rats in some domestic properties in comparison with earlier studies, the incidence of infestation in food premises had decreased; trends in infestation are being monitored through the five-yearly English House Conditions Survey.

Rats are also a reservoir for pathogens such as *Leptospira* and hantaviruses. Despite high levels of carriage in rats, human leptospirosis is uncommon in the UK. About half of the 40-60 cases reported by laboratories in England and Wales each year are due to *Leptospira icterohaemorrhagiae*, the species found in rats. As yet, few cases of human hantavirus disease have been reported in the UK but one study has shown evidence of infection in about 4-5% of UK rats[43].

Rats may be involved indirectly in the transmission of infection to humans. They may be a host for organisms such as *Toxoplasma* and *Coxiella burnetii*. Rat parasites, such as fleas, may also carry organisms capable of causing human disease (eg, *Yersinia pestis*), but these organisms are not currently present in the UK, and it is uncertain whether climate change is likely to influence this position.

Foodborne diseases

Most reported cases of food poisoning occur during the summer months when average temperatures tend to be higher, although there may also be more people returning from abroad with gastrointestinal infections at this time. The effect of possible future warmer summers on the projected numbers of reported cases of food poisoning has been examined by researchers at the University of East Anglia[44]. They have estimated increases of 2.3-7.6% per month by 2010 due to predicted temperature rises. Given that there is thought to be considerable under-reporting of food poisoning, the actual number of extra cases could be substantial.

A small increase in temperature can have a significant effect on the multiplication of foodborne bacteria such as *Salmonella* and *Escherichia coli*. Although *Campylobacter* is the most frequently reported gastrointestinal pathogen in England and Wales, most species are not known to multiply below temperatures of about 30°C. However, if climatic change leads to longer periods of higher temperatures, then there may be opportunities for *Campylobacter* to multiply outside animal hosts.

If pathogens are present in foods, then exposure to higher temperatures will increase opportunities for multiplication and cross-contamination to occur. Attention to good hygiene practice by all those who produce, prepare or store food will be of paramount importance if climatic change does lead to higher average temperatures in the UK.

Vector-borne diseases

Vector-borne diseases are particularly susceptible to changes in climate such as temperature, humidity and rainfall, and to ecological changes[45]. It is therefore likely that climate change and altered weather patterns would affect the distribution, intensity and seasonality of many vector-borne infectious diseases.

The commonest vector-borne disease world wide - malaria - is also the one most likely to change, and is also the one most studied in mathematical models of climatic change. Environmental changes affect the number, distribution, breeding pattern and behaviour of the vector (in this case anopheline mosquitoes), and the life-cycle of the malaria parasite. The extrinsic incubation of the parasite (the time between the vector ingesting infected blood and its being capable of transmitting infection), for instance, shortens dramatically at temperatures between 20°C and 27°C. Seasonal and year-on-year changes in transmission rates and geographical distribution of malaria already provide examples of the possible effects of more frequent extreme weather events such as droughts, storms and floods, or of a more sustained change in climate. In malarious countries, the lack of malaria at higher altitudes is a reflection of temperature: in Rwanda, in 1987, malaria was observed to have extended into higher altitudes, following record high temperatures and rainfall[46]. Based on such observations, in malarious areas a relatively small increase in minimum temperature is likely to facilitate the spread of malaria into large urban highland populations that are currently malaria free. The potential for malaria transmission would extend also into temperate zones, but the overall impact would depend on other factors such as population susceptibility and the ability to maintain environmental controls.

Of the other vector-borne diseases, those thought most likely to change are dengue fever - carried principally by the mosquito *Aedes aegypti* - and schistosomiasis, in which the vector is a snail[47]. Warmer temperatures affect the infectivity and development of the parasite within the snail; more importantly, water shortages increase the need for irrigation systems which have already been associated with an increased prevalence of schistosomiasis in some arid warm regions. Modelling has indicated an additional five million cases attributable to climate change by the year 2050[48].

Other diseases where changes are likely include lymphatic filariasis, onchocerciasis, African trypanosomiasis, and other arboviral diseases. Tick-borne diseases favour cooler temperatures: in the southern USA, the incidence of Rocky Mountain spotted fever could fall due to ticks' intolerance of high temperatures and diminished humidity[49].

(vi) *Biotechnology developments*

Biotechnology is broadly defined to include any technique that uses living organisms or parts of organisms to make or modify products, to improve plants or animals, or to develop micro-organisms for specific use. Commercial biotechnology consists of an ever-expanding range of inter-related techniques, procedures and processes for practical applications in health care, agriculture and industry, and although novel developments such as genetic modification and cloning attract most attention, it should not be forgotten that such well-established approaches as plant breeding, food fermentation and composting can also be labelled as 'biotechnology'.

The concept of sustainable development is based on the conviction that it should be possible to increase the basic standard of living of the world's growing population without unnecessarily depleting finite natural resources and further degrading the environment. Emerging biotechnologies, based on new scientific discoveries, offer novel approaches to strike a suitable balance between development needs and environmental conservation. The objectives of sustainable development could be fostered through the safe uses of biotechnology. Important contributions have been made in the use of biotechnology to combat major communicable diseases, to promote good health, and to improve programmes for treatment of and protection from major non-communicable diseases and to develop safety procedures. Use of DNA technology offers novel approaches towards the design and production of drugs, vaccines and diagnostic tools, as well as a powerful tool for the conservation, evaluation and use of genetic resources.

However, despite the enormous potential for benefit from novel uses of biotechnology, there must also be mechanisms in place to audit their effects, regulate their applications, and to ensure that new biotechnology techniques are safe and seen to be safe; they must also be seen to be ethical.

In March 1997, following earlier consultations on human and veterinary health care, agriculture and food, and environmental uses (including pollution clearance), a National Biotechnology Conference was held in response to a recommendation of the Government Panel on Sustainable Development that interested bodies should be brought together to draw up key principles to govern biotechnology and genetically modified organisms (GMOs). The background to the Panel's concern was that the current regulatory framework might not be adequate to take into account the wider issues of biotechnology that could have an impact on human health and environmental safety. The majority of concerns expressed at the conference related to the use of GMOs in food and agriculture rather than for health care purposes, although some themes - for example, the need for greater transparency and openness in decision-making and regulatory processes, a more clearly articulated set of underlying principles concerning the use of GMOs, and greater public consultation - apply to all sectors. A public consultation on the implications of biotechnology research will take place in late 1998.

References

1.   *The Clean Air Act 1956.* London: HMSO, 1956.
2.   *The Clean Air Act 1968.* London: HMSO, 1968.
3.   Department of the Environment, United Kingdom Photochemical Oxidants Review Group. *Ozone in the United Kingdom.* London: Department of the Environment, 1993.
4.   Department of Health. *On the State of the Public Health: the annual report of the Chief Medical Officer of the Department of Health for the year 1996.* London: Stationery Office, 1997; 24-6, 210-1.
5.   Department of Health, Advisory Group on the Medical Aspects of Air Pollution Episodes. *First report: ozone.* London: HMSO, 1991. Chair: Professor Stephen Holgate.
6.   Department of Health, Committee on the Medical Effects of Air Pollutants. *Non-biological particles and health.* London: HMSO, 1995. Chair: Professor Stephen Holgate.
7.   Department of Health, Committee on the Medical Effects of Air Pollutants. *Asthma and outdoor air pollution.* London: HMSO, 1995. Chair: Professor Stephen Holgate.
8.   Department of the Environment, Welsh Office, Scottish Office. *The United Kingdom national air quality strategy.* London: Stationery Office, 1997 (Cm. 3587).
9.   Department of Health, Committee on the Medical Effects of Air Pollutants. *Handbook on air pollution and health.* London: Stationery Office, 1997. Chair: Professor Stephen Holgate.
10. Department of Health, Committee on the Medical Effects of Air Pollutants. *The quantification of the effects of air pollution on health in the United Kingdom.* London: Stationery Office (in press). Chair: Professor Stephen Holgate.
11. Walters S, Griffiths RK, Ayres JG. Temporal association between admissions for asthma in Birmingham and ambient levels of sulphur dioxide and smoke. *Thorax* 1994; **49:** 133-40.
12. Katsouyani K, Touloumi G, Spix G, et al. Short-term effects of ambient sulphur dioxide and particulate matter on mortality in 12 European cities: results from time series data from the APHEA project. *BMJ* 1997; **314:** 1658-63.
13. Ferin J, Oberdörster G, Soderholm SC, Gebein R. Pulmonary tissue access of ultrafine particles. *J Aerosol Med* 1991; **4:** 57-8.

14. Peters A, Wichmann E, Tuck T, Heinrich J, Heyder J. Respiratory effects are associated with the number of ultrafine particles. *Am J Respir Crit Care Med* 1997; **155:** 1376-83.

15. Seaton A, MacNee W, Donaldson K, Godden D. Particulate air pollution and acute health effects. *Lancet* 1995; **345:** 176-8.

16. Dochery DW, Pope CA III, Xiu X, et al. An association between air pollution and mortality in six US cities. *N Engl J Med* 1993; **329:** 1753-9.

17. Pope CA III, Thun MJ, Namboodiri MM, et al. Particulate air pollution as a predictor of mortality in a prospective study of US adults. *Am J Respir Crit Care Med* 1995; **151:** 669-74.

18. Medical Research Council, Institute for Environment and Health. *Indoor air quality in the home.* Leicester: Institute for Environment and Health, 1996.

19. Department of Health. *On the State of the Public Health: the annual report of the Chief Medical Officer of the Department of Health for the year 1996.* London: HMSO, 1995; 110.

20. Institute for Environment and Health. *The non-auditory effects of noise.* Leicester: Institute for Environment and Health (in press) (Report no. R10).

21. National Radiological Protection Board. *Radon affected areas: England and Wales.* Chilton (Oxon): National Radiological Protection Board, 1996 (Doc. NRPB 7; no. 2).

22. National Academy of Sciences. *The health effects of exposure to indoor radon.* Washington DC: US National Academy of Sciences (in press).

23. Department of Health. *Our Healthier Nation: a contract for health.* London: Stationery Office (in press) (Cm. 3852).

24. National Radiological Protection Board. *Electromagnetic fields and the risk of cancer: report of an Advisory Group on Non-ionising Radiation.* Chilton (Oxon): National Radiological Protection Board, 1992 (Doc. NRPB 3; no. 1).

25. Dolk H, Elliott P, Shaddick G, Walls P, Thakrar B. Cancer incidence near radio and television transmitters in Great Britain: II: all high powered transmitters. *Am J Epidemiol* 1997; **145:** 10-7.

26. National Radiological Protection Board. *Board statement on effects of ultraviolet radiation on human health.* Chilton (Oxon): National Radiological Protection Board, 1995 (Doc. NRPB 6; no. 2).

27. Black D. *Investigation of the possible increased incidence of cancer in West Cumbria: a report of the Independent Advisory Committee.* London: HMSO, 1984. Chair: Sir Douglas Black.

28. Gardner MJ, Snee MP, Hall AJ, Powell CA, Downes S, Terrell JD. Results of case-control study of leukaemia and lymphoma among young people near Sellafield nuclear plant in West Cumbria. *BMJ* 1990; **300:** 423-9.

29. Draper GJ, Little MP, Sorahan T, et al. Cancer in the offspring of radiation workers: a record linkage study. *BMJ* 1997; **315:** 1181-8.

30. Department of the Environment, Transport and the Regions, Welsh Office. *Drinking water 1997: a report by the Chief Inspector, Drinking Water Inspectorate.* London: Stationery Office (in press).

31. Department of the Environment, Drinking Water Inspectorate, Welsh Office. *Lead in drinking water: have you got lead pipes?* London: Drinking Water Inspectorate, 1995.

32. Ministry of Agriculture, Fisheries and Food. *1994 Total Diet Study: metals and other elements.* London: Ministry of Agriculture, Fisheries and Food, 1997 (Food Surveillance Information Sheet no. 131).

33. Medical Research Council, Institute for Environment and Health. *Recent UK blood lead surveys.* Leicester: Institute for Environment and Health (in press).

34. Delves HT, Diaper SJ, Oppert S, et al. Blood lead concentrations in United Kingdom have fallen substantially since 1984. *BMJ* 1996; **313:** 883-4.

35. Carlsen E, Giwercmann A, Keiding N, Skakkebaek NE. Evidence for decreasing quality of semen during past 50 years. *BMJ* 1992; **305:** 609-13.

36. Berling S, Wölner-Hanssen P. No evidence of deteriorating semen quality among men in infertile relationships during the last decade: a study of males from Southern Sweden. *Human Reproduction* 1997; **12:** 1002-5.

37. Irvine S, Cawood E, Richardson D, MacDonald E, Aitken J. Evidence of deteriorating semen quality in the United Kingdom: birth cohort study in 577 men in Scotland over 11 years. *BMJ* 1996; **312**: 467-71.

38. Sharpe RM, Skakkebaek NE. Are oestrogens involved in falling sperm counts and disorders of the male reproductive tract? *Lancet* 1993; **341**: 1392-5.

39. Medical Research Council, Institute for Environment and Health. *Environmental oestrogens: consequences to human health and wildlife.* Leicester: Institute for Environment and Health, 1995.

40. Medical Research Council, Institute for Environment and Health. *European Commission workshop on the impact of endocrine disruptors on human health and wildlife: report of the proceedings of the workshop held on 2-4 December 1996, Weybridge, UK.* Leicester: Institute for Environment and Health, 1997.

41. Department of the Environment. *Water resources and supply: agenda for action.* London: Department of the Environment, 1996.

42. Meyer AN. National commensal rodent survey 1993. *Environ Health* 1995; **103**: 127.

43. Webster JP. Wild brown rats (*Rattus norvegicus*) as a zoonootic risk on farms in England and Wales. *Commun Dis Rep CDR Rev* 1996; **6**: R46-9.

44. Bentham G, Langford IH. Climate change and the incidence of food poisoning in England and Wales. *Int Biometeorol* 1995; **39**: 81-6.

45. Patz JA, Epstein PR, Burke TA, Balbus JM. Global climate change and emerging infectious disease. *JAMA* 1995; **275**: 217-23.

46. Loevinsohn M. Climatic warming and increased malaria incidence in Rwanda. *Lancet* 1994; **343**: 714-8.

47. World Health Organization. *Potential health effects of climatic change.* Geneva: World Health Organization, 1990.

48. Markens WJM. Modelling the effect of global warming on the prevalence of schistosomiasis. Bilthoven: RIVM, 1965 (GLOBO report series 10; report no. 461502010).

49. Haile DG. *Computer simulation of the effects of changes in weather patterns on vector-borne disease transmission.* In Smith JB, Tirpak DA, eds. *The potential effects of global climate change in the United States.* Washington DC: US Environmental Protection Agency, 1989 (Document 230-05-89-057).

(e)   Monitoring and surveillance of environmental indicators

An understanding of the implications of climate change and other environmental factors for human health requires the ability to identify changes in health and to determine whether such changes are linked to local or global environmental changes.

(i)   Clusters of disease and the Small Area Health Statistics Unit

Apparent clusters of disease can cause substantial public anxiety and generate considerable media interest; such clusters are often speculatively linked with a supposed local environmental hazard. Investigation of disease clusters is usually undertaken locally by district public health departments. At the national level, the SAHSU is funded by Government to investigate claims of unusual clusters of disease or ill-health, particularly in the vicinity of point sources of pollution from chemicals and/or radiation. The remit of the SAHSU also includes the need to build up reliable background information on the distribution of diseases among small areas so that specific clusters can be placed in proper context, and to develop small area statistical methodology. The SAHSU is based at the Imperial College School of Science, Technology and Medicine.

Three studies of general interest were published by the SAHSU during 1997. A study into a reported cluster of leukaemias and lymphomas near the Sutton Coldfield television and radio (TV/FM) transmitter confirmed that there was an excess of adult leukaemia within the vicinity of the transmitter in the period 1974-86, accompanied by a decline in risk with distance from the transmitter[1]. However, a further study of leukaemia incidence near 20 high-power TV/FM transmitters in Great Britain failed to confirm the pattern of findings seen at Sutton Coldfield and found no observed excess risk of leukaemia close to the transmitter sites when considered as a group[2] (see page 127).

The SAHSU also published a study of the incidence of angiosarcoma of the liver in Great Britain[3]. This cancer can be caused by occupational exposure to the chemical vinyl chloride, and the SAHSU looked in particular at possible 'neighbourhood' cases among residents living near vinyl chloride sites in view of the theoretical risk of possible low-level environmental hazard from the sites; no such non-occupational cases were found.

(ii)   Response to specific incidents

Over recent years there has been increasing concern, nationally and internationally, over health services' ability to respond effectively to the public health implications of chemical and other contamination incidents - whether accidental, through transport accidents or fires at industrial sites, or intentional, through terrorist activities.

In 1997, DH, together with the other UK Health Departments, established a national focus for work on the response to chemical incidents and the surveillance of the health effects of environmental chemicals at the University of Wales Institute, Cardiff[4]. During its first year, the Focus has supported the Health Departments in encouraging the development of a robust system for the immediate response to chemical incidents, the responsibility for which lies with individual health authorities; almost all health authorities have now established links with a specialist unit which can provide them with expert advice and support in the event of an incident. The Focus has also been involved with the revision of guidance for dealing with chemical incidents as part of major incident guidance in the National Health Service (NHS). This guidance emphasises the need for emergency planning, the importance of joint planning with other agencies (including the emergency services), and the role of health interests within integrated emergency management. During 1998, the Focus will implement a UK-wide surveillance system for acute chemical incidents, which will give a clearer indication of the number and type of such incidents to enable health authorities to make more informed decisions about resource allocation, and to improve the evidence base for future public health action. The national Focus will also consider the training needs of public health professionals in emergency planning, and the development of appropriate criteria for epidemiological follow-up of short-term and long-term health effects of chemical contamination incidents.

References

1. Dolk H, Shaddick G, Walls P, et al. Cancer incidence near radio and television transmitters in Great Britain: I: Sutton Coldfield transmitter. *Am J Epidemiol* 1997: **145**: 1-9.
2. Dolk H, Elliott P, Shaddick G, Walls P, Thakrar B. Cancer incidence near radio and television transmitters in Great Britain: II: all high power transmitters. *Am J Epidemiol* 1997; **145**: 10-7.
3. Elliott P, Kleinschmidt I. Angiosarcoma of the liver in Great Britain in proximity to vinyl chloride sites. *Occup Environ Med* 1997; **54**: 14-8.
4. Department of Health. National focus for work on response to chemical incidents and surveillance of health effects of environmental chemicals. *CMO's Update* 1997; **14**: 1.

(f)   The way ahead

The range and complexity of topics explored in this Chapter (and elsewhere in this Report) show the close and important links between public health, the environment and sustainable development. Attempts to forecast the impact of climate change on this complex network of linkages present methodological challenges; moreover, concern about potential future effects must not distract from addressing current challenges in environmental public health.

Continued and enhanced research into the links between environment and health will lead to a better understanding of which factors affect health, how they interact and the size of those effects. Risk assessments based on sound research will help to identify those environmental areas where action is most needed to improve health. Monitoring and surveillance of key indicators will enhance understanding of changes in public health which may be the result of changes within the environment, and help to audit the effectiveness of efforts to improve current environmental health problems. Some interventions may give benefits in both the short and the long term, such as action to reduce concentrations of air pollutants from motor vehicles (health benefits now, and reduced fossil fuel consumption, leading to more sustainable development and a reduction in 'greenhouse gases'), or improved energy efficiency of the housing stock (to reduce winter deaths and save in energy consumption, again with benefits in respect of sustainable development and the production of 'greenhouse gases'). But such interventions must not do more harm than good - for example, traffic calming schemes need careful consideration, where a potential decrease in accidents may be offset by an increase in noise and pollution.

Even of the known inter-relations between public health and environmental factors, many will be slow and difficult to change, and will need convincing evidence before ingrained habits or commercial interest will reflect a need for change. The resources and the will needed to maintain and to improve environmental health should not be underestimated, and can only be achieved by collaboration - individually, locally, nationally and internationally.

CHAPTER 5

HEALTH CARE

(a) **Role and function of the National Health Service in England**

(i) *Purpose*

The purpose of the National Health Service (NHS) is to secure through the resources available the greatest possible improvement in the physical and mental health of the population by: promoting health, preventing ill-health, diagnosing and treating disease and injury, and caring for those with long-term illness and disability. To achieve this purpose the NHS is required to:

- reduce the incidence of avoidable illness, disease and injury in the population;

- treat people with illness, disease or injury quickly, effectively and on the basis of need alone;

- enable people who are unable to perform essential activities of daily living, including those with chronic illness, disability or terminal illness, to live as full and normal lives as possible; *and*

- maximise the benefits to patients from the resources available to the NHS.

(ii) *Policies and strategies*

The Government is developing a new strategy for health and health care to enable the NHS to make progress towards meeting its objectives, including public health needs. This strategy will be based upon:

- a White Paper, which should be published in late 1998, taking into account responses to the Green Paper, *Our Healthier Nation*[1], to be published in early 1998 with proposals for concerted action across Government Departments and Agencies, and for the NHS to work in partnership with other organisations to improve health and reduce health inequalities. Work to develop and to deliver this public health strategy is supported by the Chief Medical Officer's project to strengthen the public health function, the review of inequalities in health chaired by Sir Donald Acheson, formerly Chief Medical Officer of the Department of Health (DH), and the Working Group on public health and primary care, and will be reinforced through the development of complementary strategies on key topics such as tobacco control, teenage conceptions and HIV/AIDS;

- the White Paper *The new NHS: modern, dependable*[2], published in December, which sets out the management and funding mechanisms through which the health strategy will be achieved;

- the Comprehensive Spending Review, launched in June 1997 to scrutinise expenditure across all Government Departments against the Government's objectives. Plans for expenditure in 1999/2000, and in later years, will be decided in the light of the results of this review which is due to be completed in 1998; *and*

- a Social Services White Paper, due to be published in Summer 1998, which will set out the objectives for social services and proposals for improved working at the interface between health and social care, building on the guidance on joint working in *Better services for vulnerable people*[3].

A number of key themes run through these major strategies which underpin the Government's policies for health and social care. These key themes, and some related actions, are to:

- *improve health and reduce inequalities:* health authorities have been charged with leading the development of health improvement programmes, which will set out the health needs of local people and what needs to be done to meet them. They will have local targets in priority areas to be identified in the Green Paper *Our Healthier Nation*[1] and will identify the contribution of partner agencies and NHS bodies to meeting them so that they will be developed and delivered by organisations responsible for local housing, education, employment and the environment, as well as those responsible for primary care, community and specialist services. The Government has also proposed new statutory duties on health authorities to improve the health of their local populations, as well as a duty of partnership on local authorities and other NHS bodies to ensure that this is achieved through appropriate joint working;

- *integrate services:* the White Paper *The new NHS: modern, dependable*[2] sets out a number of measures to integrate services more effectively. Primary and community care services are being brought together in new primary care groups, charged with the development of better relations with specialist services, and health authorities are required to agree joint investment plans with local authority social services. Local authority chief executives are to attend health authority board meetings, and further measures such as pooling budgets are being explored;

- *improve quality and responsiveness, and raise standards:* the aim here is to obtain better health outcomes as well as improving patients' experience of care. The White Paper *The new NHS: modern, dependable*[2] sets out local and national measures in which local 'clinical governance' arrangements are to be put in place to ensure that care is of the highest quality, to be backed up by a new statutory duty of quality for NHS Trusts; and new National Service Frameworks and a new National Institute of Clinical Excellence will be established to promote more effective and cost-effective clinical practice. A Commission for Health Improvement will be set up to support and oversee the quality of clinical governance and clinical services;

- *improve performance and efficiency:* a new national framework for assessing performance is being introduced to assess NHS performance in broader terms than the previous focus on efficiency. It will measure the NHS contribution to health improvement as well as the responsiveness and efficiency of services.

- *enable staff to make their maximum contribution*: a new human resources strategy for the NHS is being developed, with measures to ensure greater staff involvement; *and*

- *improve public confidence in the NHS:* the NHS, as a public service, must be more open and accountable to patients, and to the public, and shaped by their views.

Six areas, set out in the priorities and planning guidance for 1998/99[4], have been identified as priorities for the NHS over the medium term on the basis that they will require particular focus and attention by the Service as a whole over the next few years:

- *A:* To work towards the development of a primary care-led NHS, in which decisions about the purchasing and provision of health care are taken as close to patients as possible;

- *B:* In partnership with local authorities, general practitioners (GPs) and service providers, including the non-statutory sector, to review and maintain progress on the effective purchasing and provision of comprehensive mental health services to enable people with mental illness to receive effective care and treatment in the most appropriate setting in accordance with their needs;

- *C:* to improve the clinical and cost-effectiveness of services throughout the NHS and thereby secure the greatest health gain from the resources available, through supporting research and development and formulating decisions on the basis of appropriate evidence about clinical effectiveness;

- *D:* to give greater voice and influence to users of NHS services and their carers in their own care, the development and definition of standards set for NHS services locally and the development of NHS policy both locally and nationally;

- *E:* to ensure, in collaboration with local authorities and other organisations, that integrated services are in place to meet needs for continuing care for elderly, disabled, or vulnerable people and children which allow them, wherever practical, to be supported in the most appropriate available setting; *and*

- *F:* to develop NHS organisations as good employers with particular reference to workforce planning, education and training, employment policy and practice, the development of teamwork, reward systems, staff utilisation and staff welfare.

(iii)   Priority setting

The Government has made clear that the NHS should be available for all those who fall ill or who are injured, and that access to it will be based on need and not the ability to pay. It recognises that priority setting is a necessary part of decision-making in any health care system, and that priorities need to be set to give the best results for the population as a whole as well as meeting individual needs.

Nevertheless, there are unacceptable variations in access to some services and to the most effective treatments, and the Government has set out a range of measures to spread best practice, to promote clinical and cost-effectiveness and to ensure fairness. National consistency in access to services will be improved by the introduction of National Service Frameworks, and by the establishment of a National Institute for Clinical Excellence. Within these national arrangements and guidelines, clinicians and health authorities will decide the treatments and services required by patients and the population at local level.

(iv)   Research and development

The research and development strategy

Research and development (R&D) is a core function of the NHS and an integral part of the Department's responsibilities[5]. The R&D strategy comprises two complementary programmes: the Department's policy research programme and the NHS R&D programme. DH also promotes strong links with the scientific community, with research councils, charities and industry, and has established sound links with the European Union (EU). A national forum of research funders has provided an important means to establish closer working links between research interests in the NHS and elsewhere.

Policy-related research

The policy research programme provides a knowledge base for the development of strategic policy for health services, social services and public health.

Recent policy developments in relation to social care for children have been complemented by linked research designed to provide evidence to inform policy and practice development - eg, on residential care and delinquency. On social care for adults, the emphasis has been on longer-term research to evaluate community care arrangements and outcomes for users. Environmental health research has included studies on air pollution, skin cancer, hepatitis C and transmissible spongiform encephalopathies (TSEs)[6]. Health promotion research has focused on health inequalities, vaccine development, smoking, alcohol abuse, drug misuse, HIV/AIDS and nutrition.

On health service strategy, research has addressed policies on primary health care, prescribing, organisational and quality assurance, human resources, nursing and health economics. Strategies in relation to maternal and infant care, mental health, cancer, cardiovascular disease, and policies for disabled and elderly people are also being addressed, and studies to provide early evaluation of changes announced in the White Paper *The new NHS: modern, dependable*[2] are being put in place. Public health R&D is being documented and assessed to develop a co-ordinated approach to research in this area.

The NHS R&D Programme

The NHS R&D programme has a key role in the move to strengthen the scientific basis of health care. The programme aims to create a knowledge-based health service in which clinical, managerial and policy decisions are based on sound information from research. Work is under way to develop improved access to research findings across the NHS[7,8,9].

The national programme is being restructured to offer increased flexibility, better financial management and a more co-ordinated approach to determining needs and priorities for research. Two 'strands' of this new approach are in place - health technology assessment and service delivery and organisation; a third 'strand', new and emerging applications of technology, is in the early stages of development.

'Horizon scanning' for emerging clinical innovations and consultation with the NHS will inform priority setting across the new structure, and reviews of R&D needs in key areas will continue.

The new funding system for NHS R&D was introduced during 1997/98 and will be fully operational from 1998/99 onwards[10]. In the first bidding round to provide R&D support funding for NHS providers, some bidders received modest increases over their existing R&D allocations and a small number were successful in receiving R&D funding for the first time. During 1997/98, approximately £350 million were available to support R&D by NHS providers of care, and a further £75 million were available for R&D commissioned directly by the NHS Executive to meet NHS needs.

In May, the NHS Executive published *Responsibilities for patient care costs associated with research and development in the NHS*[11], which set out NHS support arrangements for externally funded non-commercial R&D, and the mutual obligations of the NHS and other research funders[12].

Since 1996, a Standing Advisory Group on consumer involvement in the NHS R&D programme, chaired by Ms Ruth Evans, Director of the National Consumer Council, has reported to the central R&D committee; its members have a wide range of backgrounds, including experience of involving consumers in health research. In early 1998, the Group will publish its first report, *Health research: what's in it for consumers?*[13], and it has also commissioned research to inform its work on consumer involvement in health research projects.

The National Working Group on R&D in primary care published its first report in November[14], which focuses on the need to develop a strategy to create and maintain an evidence base to underpin the work of primary care professionals as well as to deliver effective primary care services within the NHS. A number of recommendations have been made to achieve this, and DH will substantially increase its investment in primary care research over the next five years.

References

1. Department of Health. *Our Healthier Nation: a contract for health.* London: Stationery Office (in press) (Cm. 3852).
2. Department of Health. *The new NHS: modern, dependable.* London: Stationery Office, 1997 (Cm. 3807).
3. Department of Health. *Better services for vulnerable people.* London: Department of Health, 1997 (Executive Letter: EL(97)62, CI(97)24).
4. Department of Health. *Priorities and planning guidance for the NHS: 1998/99.* London: Department of Health, 1997 (Executive Letter: EL(97)39).
5. Department of Health. *Policy research programme: providing a knowledge base for health, public health and social care.* London: Department of Health, 1997.

6.   Department of Health. *Strategy for research and development relating to the human health aspects of transmissible spongiform encephalopathies.* London: Department of Health, 1996.

7.   Department of Health NHS Executive. *Report of the NHS health technology assessment programme 1996.* London: Department of Health, 1996.

8.   Department of Health Research and Development Task Force. *Supporting research and development in the NHS.* London: HMSO, 1994. Chair: Professor Anthony Culyer.

9.   Rook R. *Strategic framework for the use of the NHS R&D levy.* London: Department of Health, 1997.

10.   Rook R. *R&D support funding for NHS providers: an introduction.* London: Department of Health, 1997.

11.   Department of Health NHS Executive. *Responsibilities for meeting patient care costs associated with research and development in the NHS.* Leeds: Department of Health, 1997 (Health Service Guidelines HSG(97)32).

12.   Department of Health NHS Executive. *Statement of partnership for researchers, NHS providers and universities and charities.* Leeds: Department of Health, 1997 (Executive Letter: EL(97)77).

13.   Department of Health NHS Research and Development Directorate. *Health research: what's in it for consumers?: report of the Standing Advisory Group on Consumer Involvement in the NHS R&D Programme: 1996/97.* Leeds: Department of Health (in press). Chair: Ms Ruth Evans.

14.   Department of Health. *R&D in primary care: report of the National Working Group.* London: Department of Health, 1997.

(b)   Role of the NHS in maintaining public health

(i)   Public health and the NHS

Under the provisions of the White Paper, *The new NHS: modern, dependable*[1], health authorities will have a new statutory duty to improve the health of their local populations, which will take into account *Our Healthier Nation*[2], and other initiatives. To promote good health and prevent ill-health, the NHS will:

- hold hospitals, primary care and community health services, as well as health authorities, to account for their contribution to health promotion through performance management;

- ensure that everyone in the NHS accepts responsibility to promote good health and prevent ill-health;

- tackle inequalities by ensuring services reach areas of greatest need;

- ensure the right mix of local services;

- help to ensure that there is a wider understanding of what can be done to improve population health and how people and organisations can contribute;

- ensure that the many people with an interest in and contributions to make to further public health do so in a better co-ordinated manner; *and*

- address the need to ensure that there is adequate education, training, and personal and organisational development in relation to public health promotion.

Partnerships will be the key to deliver tangible benefits in public health and to tackle the determinants of ill-health. Joint working is key, not just for the NHS, but partnerships between all agencies. Health authorities must act in close partnership with other Government Departments and Agencies, local authorities and a range of other local organisations and communities to tackle the social, environmental and economic issues which affect people's health, and to develop effective joint planning and working mechanisms to bring together different parts of the NHS with other organisations in effective partnerships.

(ii)   Chief Medical Officer's project to strengthen the public health function

In June, the Chief Medical Officer was asked by Ministers to lead a project to consider the range of current public health activities at local, regional and national levels to ensure that a robust public health function was in place to deliver the Government's public health strategy. The first phase of the project was mainly to gather views from a wide range of people, mainly from outside the Department, on DH's and the NHS's public health function. A report of the findings, which takes account of these views, will be published in early 1998 for consultation and further debate.

The work of this project is linked directly to, and supports the implementation of, the White Paper *The new NHS: modern, dependable*[1], and the Green Paper *Our Healthier Nation*[2], and some of the issues raised during the course of the project will be taken forward through an integrated implementation programme rather than as a separate initiative.

Five main themes were identified during the first phase of the project - the need for a wider understanding of, better co-ordination of, an increase in the capacity and capabilities of, sustained development of, and for more effective joint working to enhance the public health function.

(iii)   Health care needs assessment

The second series of epidemiologically based health care needs assessments was published in January[3]. This series of assessments is part of a long-term programme for the production and dissemination of information to support commissioners of health care in their assessment of local health care needs. The first series, published in 1994[4], comprised reviews of 20 diseases, interventions and services selected for their importance - defined in terms of burden of disease (mortality, morbidity and cost), and the likely scope for changing patterns of commissioning of care - to purchasers of health care.

The eight health care needs assessments published in the second series were chosen after consultation on the most valuable potential topics: accident and emergency departments; child and adolescent mental health; low back pain; palliative and terminal care; dermatology; breast cancer; genito-urinary medicine services; and gynaecology. Additional chapters on elderly people; rehabilitation; and the health of black and ethnic minority groups are in preparation.

During the year, the process of updating the first series with current information and practice also started, along with work towards a third series of epidemiologically based health care needs assessments, which will take into account the key themes of the White Paper *The new NHS: modern, dependable*[1] to ensure their relevance to primary care commissioning.

(iv)   National Casemix Office and NHS Centre for Coding and Classification

National Casemix Office

The National Casemix Office has been set up to develop, maintain, issue and support patient grouping tools and classification methodologies for use in the NHS. Such health care resource and health benefit groupings (HRGs and HBGs) allow patient-based data to be aggregated in various ways to assist in analysis and management. Work during the year was concerned with:

- refinements of HRGs for inpatients and day cases;

- pilot projects of HRGs in mental health services and the care of elderly people;

- development of HRGs in outpatient and community services;

- pilot projects and continued development of HBGs to inform purchasing;

- review of the definition of 'episode of care' across acute and community services;

- provision of casemix-adjusted health service indicators, national HRG statistics and support for the production of HRG-based reference costs; *and*

- support of the implementation of casemix methods in the NHS through training courses, seminars, conferences and help-desk services.

NHS Centre for Coding and Classification

The NHS Centre for Coding and Classification (NHSCCC) continues to maintain and develop the Read Codes (a computerised thesaurus of health care terms), and also has responsibility to improve the quality of coded clinical data by support of the NHS standard classifications and by training in their use, and by facilitating coding standards. Work during the year included:

- support of the implementation of the new Read Codes version 3 by the establishment of partnerships with NHS organisations;

- facilitatation of the transition of users' data from earlier Read Code versions by the inclusion of all earlier versions in Read Codes version 3;

- development of term and code lists to support exchange of clinical messages;

- documentation of possible approaches for retrieval and analysis of clinical information from version 3 systems; *and*

- improvement of the quality of coded clinical data by development of a training programme for clinical coders.

(v)   *National Screening Committee*

The National Screening Committee was set up in July 1996 to advise UK Ministers and Departments of Health on the need for the introduction, review, modification or cessation of national population screening programmes. During the year, the Committee developed a framework for screening, to be published in its first report in Spring 1998[5]. As well as the specification of a population screening framework, in particular defining population screening and classifying programmes, and setting criteria to appraise the viability, effectiveness and appropriateness of a screening programme, the Committee defined a recommended format to process information on screening from systematic reviews and other research assessment programmes, and the recommendations of expert groups (a detailed questionnaire which requires information about all aspects of any proposal), and compiled the first inventory of over 300 screening programmes. Of these programmes, many are still at the research stage; although about 100 are currently used in clinical practice world wide. However, only three are nationally recognised in the UK and meet the Committee's stringent criteria for evidence of both effectiveness and quality - namely, breast and cervical screening among women, and neonatal bloodspot screening for phenylketonuria and hypothyroidism.

During the year, the Committee advised the Secretary of State for Health and other Health Ministers that there was no clear evidence that a national screening programme for prostatic cancer, with current techniques, would be of general benefit among men.

Workshops on colorectal cancer screening and child health surveillance (for hearing, vision, speech and language, and growth, among others) have been held to enable health care professionals to debate the clinical evidence, potential benefits and harm, and costs and clinical effectiveness. Several more workshops are planned for 1998. A sub-group was set up to consider population screening in pregnancy and after birth, and a conference on antenatal screening is planned for Spring 1998. Recommendations were also drawn up in relation to the introduction of screening for hepatitis B during pregnancy.

The subsequent work of the National Screening Committee will concentrate on development of screening policy, and improving quality. The efficacy and feasibility of screening for diseases such as *Chlamydia trachomatis*, cystic fibrosis, Down's syndrome, fragile X syndrome, haemoglobinopathies, ovarian cancer, and genetic testing for breast cancer will be explored over the next three years. In the light of the recommendations following formal reviews of the breast cancer screening programme at the Royal Devon and Exeter NHS Trust, and the cervical screening programme at the Kent and Canterbury Hospital, the Committee will draw up a strategic framework for the quality assurance of population screening programmes, which will review the management and monitoring arrangements of existing and future programmes, evaluate the clinical evidence for screening programmes and ensure that rigorous quality standards exist for the implementation of new and existing screening programmes. It will also set out arrangements to deal with those parts of the service which fail to meet agreed standards and targets.

The Committee will also review equality of access to screening and the need to ensure that the risks and benefits involved can be communicated to everyone in a clear and precise manner.

(vi)   Quality of service and effectiveness of care

Improvement of the clinical effectiveness of the services provided by the NHS is central to its purpose, and the NHS Executive is committed to ensure that the NHS increasingly adopts an evidence-based approach to decision-making. This approach has featured as a medium-term priority in the priorities and planning guidance for the NHS for five successive years[6,7,8,9,10], advising health authorities to ensure greater investment in interventions for which there is strong evidence on clinical effectiveness.

Assurance and improvement of the quality of care is a key theme of the White Paper *The new NHS: modern, dependable*[1], published on 9 December, which includes a number of specific proposals which set out a challenging but realistic agenda for quality improvement. These proposals include:

151

- a new statutory duty for NHS Trusts in respect of quality of care;

- the introduction of 'clinical governance' to provide a framework for continuous quality improvement in NHS Trusts and in primary care;

- a new, broader-based framework to assess and develop NHS performance, with a greater focus on service quality and outcomes by development of National Service Frameworks;

- a commitment to work with professional and regulatory bodies to strengthen the contribution which professional self-regulation and continuing professional development make to improvements in clinical outcomes and service quality; *and*

- the establishment of two new national bodies (the Commission for Health Improvement and a National Institute for Clinical Excellence) to help to drive and support the improvement of quality of service and effectiveness of care.

The Commission for Health Improvement would be established by Statute, with stated independence from Government, to support and guide the development of clinical governance nationally; to 'spot check' local clinical governance arrangements; and to offer targeted support to organisations facing serious clinical problems, either at their request or, where a problem is not effectively managed locally, at the direction of the Secretary of State for Health. The Commission may also carry out a series of systematic service reviews, and the terms of its establishment will be subject to consultation.

A new National Institute for Clinical Excellence will be established to give new coherence and prominence to information about clinical and cost-effectiveness by means of evidence-based clinical guidelines and effective clinical audit. This Institute will bring together the work of a number of professional organisations and other groups to work to a programme agreed by DH.

(vii)   Clinical and health outcomes

Existing health outcome indicators

Because of an increased volume of data, including trend data since 1985 for some indicators, the Public Health Common Data Set (PHCDS) for 1997 was published for the first time in compact disk read-only memory (CD-ROM) format in October[11]; it included an updated version of the set of Population Health Outcome Indicators[12]. Following a survey of the use of these indicators by health authorities[13], the Wessex Institute of Health Research and Development was commissioned by the Central Health Outcomes Unit (CHOU) to compile a series of case studies of local follow-up work. The CHOU has now received a report on these, which it hopes to publish during 1998.

Twenty six case studies from 18 health authorities cover topics such as coronary heart disease, stroke, diabetes mellitus, teenage conception and others. Each case study is a pragmatic account of why health authorities did the investigations, how they undertook the work, what happened as a result and any lessons learnt as a result. The studies show how national comparative data and initiatives prompt local investigations; the range of methods used; and examples of constraints with data quality, local health policy, health service delivery and access to health care. The studies also highlight concerns about definitions of indicators, inadequacies of current routine data, an inability to attribute local indicator values to local health care and the need for better indicators. Many of these concerns are already being addressed by the CHOU as part of its long-term outcomes development programme.

New outcome indicators

Nine of the ten working groups set up by the CHOU to develop new outcome indicators completed their work during the year[14]. Reports have now been received on asthma, stroke, diabetes mellitus, cataract, urinary incontinence, fractured proximal femur, myocardial infarction, breast cancer and severe mental illness. The tenth report, on normal pregnancy outcomes, is due during 1998. The whole set will then be published by the NHS Executive. Many of the indicators recommended require new data to be collected, and the feasibility of this process is now being tested by various researchers and clinicians.

Clinical indicators

A first set of 15 clinical indicators, reflecting aspects of clinical care that may raise questions about the quality of care for further investigation, was published as a consultation document[15]. It contained analyses of hospital-based death rates, complications following surgery, hospital readmissions, discharge home, adverse drug-related events and frequency of treatment, either for all admissions or for specific conditions as appropriate. The data were presented as age-standardised rates by type of admission (emergency/non-emergency) for NHS Trusts and health authorities, clustered into 'like' groups. The CHOU received just over 1,000 comments on the indicators. A select set of the indicators, revised in the light of consultation and based on the most recent data available, will be published during 1998.

Outcomes projects

The CHOU supports a number of projects which aim to develop the methods and information systems necessary to improve health outcomes assessment. One of the projects, Functional Assessment of Care Environments (FACE) completed its studies of validity and reliability and was made available for use by the NHS. FACE enables the collection of data on the health and social functioning of people with mental illness, learning disabilities and elderly people, plus the health and social care provided. It produces quantitative data for statistical purposes as a by-product of data collected for clinical care, and enables outcomes assessment from the perspectives of patients and carers as well as clinicians. Some 120 NHS providers of care have agreed to collect data for an outcomes project based on FACE.

(viii)   Regional epidemiological services for communicable disease

The contractual arrangement between the NHS Executive and the Public Health Laboratory Service (PHLS) for the provision of regional epidemiology services, which started on 1 April 1996, continued throughout the year. The planned recruitment of staff was completed, the functioning of each regional service unit was reviewed, and the establishment of regional databases for notifications of infectious diseases (with enhanced meningococcal surveillance) was completed.

During the year, regional directors of public health (RDsPH) asked regional epidemiologists to conduct a survey within their respective regions of local arrangements for communicable disease control, which was carried out between late June and mid-August. The results of this survey[16] revealed some shortcomings and steps have been taken where necessary to improve these local arrangements. Plans have been made for a survey of infection control in hospitals to be conducted during 1998.

References

1.   Department of Health. *The new NHS: modern, dependable.* London: Stationery Office, 1997 (Cm. 3807).
2.   Department of Health. *Our Healthier Nation: a contract for health.* London: Stationery Office (in press) (Cm. 3852).
3.   Stevens A, Raftery J, eds. *Health care needs assessment: the epidemiologically based needs assessment reviews: second series.* Oxford: Radcliffe Medical, 1997.
4.   Stevens A, Raftery J, eds. *Health care needs assessment: the epidemiologically based needs assessment reviews (vols I and II).* Oxford: Radcliffe Medical, 1994.
5.   National Screening Committee. *First report of the National Screening Committee.* Milton Keynes: National Screening Committee (in press).
6.   Department of Health. *Priorities and planning guidance for the NHS: 1994/95.* London: Department of Health, 1993 (Executive Letter: EL(93)54).
7.   Department of Health. *Priorities and planning guidance for the NHS: 1995/96.* London: Department of Health, 1994 (Executive Letter: EL(94)55).
8.   Department of Health. *Priorities and planning guidance for the NHS: 1996/97.* London: Department of Health, 1995 (Executive Letter: EL(95)68).
9.   Department of Health. *Priorities and planning guidance for the NHS:1997/98.* London: Department of Health, 1996 (Executive Letter: EL(96)45).
10.   Department of Health. *Priorities and planning guidance for the NHS: 1998/99.* London: Department of Health, 1997 (Executive Letter: EL(97)39).

11. Department of Health. *Public Health Common Data Set 1997: incorporating Health of the Nation indicators and population health outcome indicators: data definitions and user guide.* Guildford: National Institute of Epidemiology, University of Surrey, 1997.

12. Department of Health. *Population health outcome indicators for the NHS: 1993: England: a consultation document.* London: Department of Health, 1993.

13. McColl A, Ferris G, Roderick P, Gabbay J. *How do English DHAs use population health outcome assessments?: telephone survey report of DHAs in England.* Southampton: Wessex Institute for Health Research and Development, University of Southampton, 1996.

14. Department of Health. *On the State of the Public Health: the annual report of the Chief Medical Officer of the Department of Health for the year 1996.* London: Stationery Office, 1997; 157-9.

15. NHS Executive. *Clinical indicators for the NHS: 1994-95: a consultation document.* Leeds: NHS Executive, 1997.

16. Regional Services Division, Public Health Laboratory Service Communicable Disease Surveillance Centre. *A survey of the communicable disease control function in England.* London: Public Health Laboratory Service, 1997.

(c)   Primary health care

(i)   *Organisation of primary care*

The 1996 White Papers *Choice and opportunity*[1] and *Primary care: delivering the future*[2] set out various developments for primary health care services. The NHS (Primary Care) Act[3] foreshadowed in *Choice and opportunity*[1] was enacted on 21 March 1997. The principal objectives were to allow the establishment of different models for the delivery of primary care other than those seen in traditional GP surgeries, and to enhance the opportunities for delivery of a wider range of general medical services than was standard practice in primary care.

At the end of 1997, over 100 pilot projects under the Act (primary care act pilot schemes, or PCAPS) were due for consideration. Many of the proposals originated in existing general practices and community NHS Trusts, whilst some novel concepts were led by nurses working as primary care practitioners; a number of schemes involved the delivery of enhanced services to excluded populations, such as homeless people and travellers. The extra opportunities to adjust provision of services to meet locally sensitive needs proved particularly popular.

Section 36 of the NHS (Primary Care) Act[3] encourages and permits additional flexibility in the delivery of services in primary care paid for from the general allocation. Possible schemes under this section include programmes for local patient management schemes for particular diseases; enhanced standards of certain aspects of general medical service or of specific enhancement of services; additional improvement grants for premises; support for continuing professional development for all members of the primary care team; and additional work undertaken in nursing or residential homes or with drug misusers.

155

It has always been somewhat of a paradox that whilst all doctors after qualification are exposed to hospital practice in their training, often hospital doctors are not exposed to general practice. Changes made during debate of the NHS (Primary Care) Bill included provisions which would permit a wider range of GP practices than at present to provide training for pre-registration house officers, to allow those doctors who choose hospital specialties as a long-term goal to gain experience of working in the community at an early stage in their careers.

Development continued during the year of new features to deliver enhanced primary care through the General Medical Services (GMS) contract, including new opportunities for salaried employment for GPs, which should allow increased flexibility to GPs starting their careers, and enable practices better to fulfil the health needs of their registered populations. The financial system that supports practice premises development was revised; its goal is to fit the environment of general practice for the changing ways in which health care is delivered.

Towards the end of the year a further series of organisational changes was presaged in a further White Paper, *The new NHS: modern, dependable*[4]. For primary care, this paper promised new models of co-operation and organisation, with an emphasis on groupings of GPs and others serving natural communities through primary care groups. Responsibilities of these groups will include the commissioning of secondary services, and their constitution will reflect natural communities, seeking to integrate primary and community health services to work more closely with social services. They will promote the health of the local population, and will link to other initiatives in the White Paper such as clinical governance and enhanced quality assurance, so as to contribute to health authorities' local health improvement programmes.

(ii)   Development of emergency services in the community

The Chief Medical Officer's review of emergency services in the community, discussed in last year's Report[5], was published on 19 September[6] after a consultation period. The main initial action was to ask for tenders for emergency telephone helpline pilot schemes, which will start in early 1998 and be evaluated over the next two years to determine whether a national service would be cost-effective. The telephone helplines will be operated by the Two Shires Ambulance Service (in Milton Keynes), the Lancashire Ambulance Service (in Preston, Chorley and South Ribble), and the Northumbria Ambulance Service (in Northumberland, Newcastle and North Tyneside). If successful, immediate care advice lines could help to improve the accessibility of appropriate information to patients in the event of a perceived emergency, and help to ensure that appropriate resources are appropriately targeted to meeting patients' needs.

The spread of the co-operative movement for GP out-of-hours services continued. In May 1997, researchers at King's College London[7] identified 251 GP co-operatives compared with 130 the previous year. Supported by the development fund, out-of-hours services continued to develop quality criteria and standards during the year. A new national framework of standards was introduced via regulatory change and a letter to health authority management[8]. The framework covers the competence of doctors on duty, adequacy of service in relation to the population covered and the nature of the area, record-keeping, operational arrangements, communications, complaints, transport and the handling of clinical information to and from a patient's own doctor. Additionally, DH continued to work on schemes jointly with health authorities and the British Medical Association (BMA) through the doctor/patient partnership to reinforce the rights and responsibilities of patients in using primary care services.

(iii)   Health promotion in general practice

New arrangements came into force where the type of health promotion activity offered systematically by practices became subject to approval by a professional committee. Previous emphasis on data collection and banded payments ended. A research assessment on the success of the changes is taking place and should be completed in 1998.

(iv)   Review of continuing professional development

A review of continuing professional development in general practice was led by the Chief Medical Officer. The multidisciplinary team considered how general practice patient care might be better supported through improved alignment of continuing education, audit, research and the application of clinical effectiveness - together known as continuing professional development. The review team concluded that personal and practice professional development planning would better target learning needs and use resources more effectively. The report of the group was submitted by the CMO to Ministers in October, and should be published in Spring 1998.

(v)   Prescribing

NHS expenditure on drugs, dressings and appliances prescribed by GPs increased by 9% in 1996/97, reaching over £4,360 million (defined as net ingredient cost); this increase continues to be higher than the overall increase in NHS expenditure. Generic prescribing increased and averaged 60% in 1996/97. Further major increases in some drugs groups were seen - eg, lipid-lowering drugs (up 45% on a cost basis and up 40% by items prescribed); antipsychotic agents (up 42% and 6%, respectively); and drugs affecting bone metabolism (up 29% and 30%, respectively). The further 4% reduction in the frequency of antibacterial prescribing by GPs is of note in view of serious concerns in relation to antimicrobial resistance raised in this and earlier reports[9,10].

The review of prescribing, supply and administration of medicines, chaired by Dr June Crown, President of the Faculty of Public Health Medicine, started in March and consulted widely on current arrangements and on possible options for change. The Review team is due to submit two reports: on the supply and administration of medicines under group protocols by Spring 1998, and on all other aspects of the Review by Summer 1998.

Some health authorities set up pilot schemes of specific funding arrangements for some treatments - such as growth hormone and fertility drugs - to facilitate care for patients who might otherwise fall between the primary and secondary care sectors. The aim was to align clinical and budgetary responsibilities. Results so far indicate that patients do benefit from such revised arrangements, which foreshadowed the unification of budgets announced in the White Paper *The new NHS: modern, dependable*[4]. During the year, health authorities further developed area prescribing committees to aid prescribing decisions and an integrated approach to the use of medicines; these committees comprise representatives of health professions and managers from the primary, secondary and public health sectors.

The PRODIGY project of computer-aided prescribing decision-support for GPs during consultation underwent further pilot studies in a selected number of general practices across the country. Initial results show a positive influence in terms of following PRODIGY guidelines, and the software and knowledge base are being developed in line with feedback from users. A final report of the first phase, and an interim report of the second phase of the study, will be published in Spring 1998.

The nurse prescribing pilot scheme was successfully expanded to include a community NHS Trust in each of the seven health regions not previously involved.

During 1997 the Prescription Pricing Authority (PPA), in collaboration with the NHS Executive, piloted Electronic Prescribing Analysis and Cost (EPACT) data and installed it in all health authorities and Regional Offices. This system allows rapid access to, and more sophisticated analysis of, prescribing data held on the PPA's mainframe computers. The National Prescribing Centre started a two-year project to investigate the feasibility of providing equivalent analysis of hospital prescribing data, which could benefit professional training and clinical audit, as well as provide better data for performance and financial management.

A major issue in recent years has been the managed introduction of new drugs into the NHS in a way which secures equity of access for patients without distorting local health care priorities; some regions have set up local arrangements for guidance on their clinical and cost-effectiveness. As indicated in the White Paper *The new NHS: modern, dependable*[4], detailed proposals for a national system of appraisal of novel drugs and other new technology will be published in a consultative document in Spring 1998.

References

1. Department of Health, Scottish Office, Welsh Office. *Choice and opportunity: primary care: the future.* London: Stationery Office, 1996 (Cm. 3390).
2. Department of Health. *Primary care: delivering the future.* London: Stationery Office, 1996 (Cm. 3512).
3. *The National Health Service (Primary Care) Act 1997.* London: Stationery Office, 1997.
4. Department of Health. *The new NHS: modern, dependable.* London: Stationery Office, 1997 (Cm. 3807).
5. Department of Health. *On the State of the Public Health: the annual report of the Chief Medical Officer of the Department of Health for the year 1996.* London: Stationery Office, 1997; 161-2.
6. Department of Health NHS Executive. *Developing emergency services in the community (vols 1 and 2).* London: Department of Health, 1996. Chair: Sir Kenneth Calman.
7. Payne F, Jessop L, Dale J. *Second national survey of GP co-operatives: a report.* London: Department of General Practice and Primary Care, King's College London School of Medicine and Dentistry, 1997.
8. Department of Health, NHS Executive. *NHS (GMS) amendment regulations 1997: arrangements for the provision of deputies/health promotion.* Leeds: Department of Health, 1997 (Family Health Services Letter: FHSL(97)13).
9. Department of Health. *On the State of the Public Health: the annual report of the Chief Medical Officer of the Department of Health for the year 1995.* London: HMSO, 1996; 14-6, 176-7.
10. Department of Health. *On the State of the Public Health: the annual report of the Chief Medical Officer of the Department of Health for the year 1996.* London: Stationery Office, 1997; 13, 206-7.

(d)   Specialised clinical services

(i)   *Specialised services*

The National Specialist Commissioning Advisory Group (NSCAG), chaired by Mr Neil McKay, Regional Director of Trent Regional Office, has 14 members, representing purchasers of health care, the Joint Consultants Committee (JCC) of the BMA, and medical research. Its aim is to ensure that all NHS patients requiring treatment or investigation of a very specialised nature, or for a very uncommon condition, have access to the highest possible standard of care that can be delivered within available resources. The NSCAG therefore commissions centrally a small number of highly specialised services, including the former

Supra-Regional Services, and pays the service costs during evaluation of new treatments that are likely, if effective, to be centrally commissioned; it may also commission and issue purchaser guidelines for highly specialised services.

Three new established services were commissioned from 1 April 1997 (extra-corporeal membrane oxygenation for neonates and babies aged up to 6 months; the diagnosis and management of Gaucher's disease; and ocular oncology), and two were identified for further evaluation - small bowel transplantation, and anorectal reconstruction.

During 1997, 54 bids for designation and central commissioning were considered by the NSCAG. The Secretary of State for Health accepted recommendations from the NSCAG that the following services should be designated and centrally funded from 1 April 1998: severe personality disorder; inpatient psychiatry services for deaf children and adolescents; treatment of established intestinal failure; and gynaecological reconstruction.

An invitation to bid for designation and central commissioning as from 1 April 1999 was issued in May. By September, 19 bids had been received and are under consideration.

New arrangements for commissioning specialised services which fall outside the NSCAG's remit are promised in the White Paper *The new NHS: modern, dependable*[1]. The NHS Executive is to launch a wide consultation on such arrangements, with a view to issuing guidance in Autumn 1998.

(ii) Cancer

Work continued to implement the strategy to develop care services set in in *A policy framework for commissioning cancer services*[2], published in April 1995. To enhance progress already made locally, £10 million were made available in May to be used specifically for breast care services, to ensure that women with symptoms have rapid access to suitable diagnostic services and treatment.

Evidence-based guidance on the commissioning of services for individual cancer sites is being sequentially published to help commissioners and providers of care to identify aspects of cancer care which are most likely to make a difference to outcome. The second in this series, *Improving outcomes in colorectal cancer*[3], was published in November and guidance on lung and gynaecological cancers should be published during 1998.

A working group was established to advise on implementation of the Government's commitment to reduce waiting times for cancer treatment, and considered the feasibility of agreeing maximum intervals from referral by a GP to consultation with a specialist and the start of treatment.

The NHS Executive issued *Education and planning guidance*[4] to advise that education, development and workforce plans should adequately provide for delivery of cancer and palliative care services, and should consider staff education, training and support needs.

Breast and cervical screening continue to bring real benefits to women, despite local problems in the provision of such services that came to light. Shortcomings were identified in the accountability for quality assurance for both programmes, and responsibility and resources for quality assurance are accordingly being placed with NHS Regional Offices. In December, measures to improve quality standards in laboratories which read cervical smears were announced, including the need to apply for accreditation. Public confidence in screening is essential, and these changes will help to promote consistent high quality and dependability in breast and cervical cancer screening across the country.

(iii)   *National Confidential Enquiry into Perioperative Deaths*

The National Confidential Enquiry into Perioperative Deaths (NCEPOD) continued its work to raise professional and organisational standards of surgery and anaesthesia in this country, and published two reports during 1997. The first[5], covering the year 1994/95, contained key messages on the need for more effective communications between specialties and between staff in different grades, and on the transfer of patients with head injuries. The second, *Who operates when?*[6], was an audit of out-of-hours surgery in 1995/96; only 6.1% of all weekday operations occurred at night, and usually before midnight, but many of these operations were emergencies and may have been carried out without adequate supervision. The NCEPOD plans to repeat this study in five years' time.

(iv)   *Safety and Efficacy Register of New Interventional Procedures*

The Safety and Efficacy Register of New Interventional Procedures (SERNIP) works under the auspices of the Academy of Medical Royal Colleges and Faculties, with funding from DH. It is a voluntary system which allows novel interventional procedures to be introduced into the NHS in a controlled way. The SERNIP categorises each new procedure according to evidence about its safety and efficacy. In 1997, the SERNIP considered 67 procedures, of which 49 were categorised; 14 were considered safe and effective, whilst most of the others were thought to need further evaluation.

(v)   *Osteoporosis*

DH and the NHS continued to work towards the recommendations set out in the report of the Advisory Group on Osteoporosis[7]. The Department also began to develop a strategy for osteoporosis prevention and treatment, in consultation with clinicians and health care managers from all eight health regions. This strategy should target best practice in the prevention of fractures caused by osteoporosis, and set out priorities for action based on evidence about effective interventions.

The Department continued to work closely with the National Osteoporosis Society to promote public and professional awareness of osteoporosis. The Minister of State for Public Health, Ms Tessa Jowell MP, formally endorsed World Osteoporosis Day, on 24 June[8], and took part in the National Osteoporosis Society's 'Take your bones for a walk' campaign to promote the benefits of regular exercise in maintaining bone health.

(vi)   Transplantation

During the year, 2,293 cadaveric organ transplants were performed in England - very slightly more than in 1996. The number of donors year on year in the United Kingdom (UK) fell from 831 to 822, whilst the number of patients who might benefit by such interventions continued to rise and now stands at around 5,200. Demand for organs for transplantation continues to outstrip supply, in part a reflection of the success of the techniques, which means that a transplant is increasingly seen by clinicians as the treatment of choice. About one-quarter of potential donors are lost because relatives feel unable to consent to organ removal. However, research indicates that where a prior intention to donate organs in the event of death is known to relatives, few will refuse consent. The NHS Organ Donor Register, a permanent, computerised and confidential record of people who wish to donate their organs, which was established in 1994, is now available for local transplant co-ordinators to check at any time; by December 1997, over 4.65 million people had registered.

The Advisory Group on the Ethics of Xenotransplantation published its report, *Animal tissue into humans*[9], on 16 January. This report contained more than 60 detailed recommendations, including a recommendation that a national committee be established to supervise developments in xenotransplantation. In response, the Government launched a consultation exercise and announced the establishment of the United Kingdom Xenotransplantation Interim Regulatory Authority (UKXIRA). The UKXIRA, chaired by Lord Habgood of Calverton, met for the first time on 19 May, and a further three times during 1997. Its terms of reference are to advise the Secretaries of State for the UK Health Departments on the action necessary to regulate xenotransplantation, taking into account the principles outlined in *Animal tissue into humans*[9] and developments in xenotransplantation world wide.

(vii)   National renal review

Work continues to improve the level and quality of services for patients with end-stage renal failure, as recommended in the National Renal Review[10]. A survey which was carried out in 1996 (collecting data from 1995) showed a significant increase in access to treatment compared with 1992, associated with the opening of new satellite dialysis units. The results of this survey are due to be published in Autumn 1998. However, many renal units are under considerable pressure because of increased demand that arises partly from an enhanced ability to treat sicker patients.

The national renal registry, which was partly funded by the NHS Executive, completed its pilot phase in April 1997. It is now expanding to include more renal units. This computerised register of renal patients records outcomes and facilitates audit of the quality of care measured against standards agreed by the profession.

(viii)   Statins and coronary heart disease

A large increase in prescribing has been seen following the publication of two major trials of statins[11,12] that showed significant reductions in mortality from coronary heart disease (CHD) among people with raised cholesterol concentrations.   Expenditure on statins rose from £20 million in 1993 to over £113 million in 1997, and is expected to rise for some time. To advise doctors and health authorities how to address this change in prescribing practice, which has major implications for the NHS, a sub-group of the Standing Medical Advisory Committee (SMAC) considered the use of statins in people with known CHD and those at high risk of developing overt CHD.

The SMAC published a statement in August 1997[13], which was issued with the Sheffield table designed to help doctors to identify patients with a CHD risk of 3% or greater[14,15]. The statement defined the appropriate threshold for treatment as people with CHD or people with an annual CHD risk of 3% or greater whose level of risk could not be reduced by other means. The statement points out that drug treatment to lower blood cholesterol concentrations is one of a number of methods to reduce the risk of cardiovascular disease; other methods, such as lifestyle changes including smoking cessation and dietary modifications, should be tried before statins are prescribed. Most health authorities are drawing up their own guidelines to determine how this advice should be applied in the light of local priorities. Further advice, including an Effective Health Care Bulletin, will be published as more evidence becomes available.

(ix)   Adult intensive care

A number of policy initiatives in adult intensive care have followed the publication of guidelines on admission to and discharge from intensive-care units (ICUs) and high-dependency units (HDUs) in March 1996[16].

A national intensive care bed register brought together information from ICUs throughout the country from 1 December 1996. A doctor who needs to transfer a patient can now make a single telephone call at any time on any day to find the nearest suitable intensive-care bed.

A standardised national data set on intensive and high-dependency care activity has been collected from 1 October 1997 to support strategic decision-making by the NHS Executive, health authorities and NHS Trusts on the use, provision and distribution of ICU/HDU facilities, and will enable those who commission health care to place separate contracts for this type of care.

£5 million were made available to increase bed provision for Winter 1996-97, with a further £5 million supplemented by £15 million from health authorities for 1997/98, which ensured the availability of an additional 57 ICU beds and 104 HDU beds.

A forum on adult intensive care will take place early in 1998 to consider the future direction of policy.

(x)   Emergency care services

Winter 1996-97 again saw increased pressures on emergency services. Although demands varied across the country, a combination of a rise in the number of emergency admissions (up by a record 6.4% in the first quarter of 1997 compared with the same quarter the previous year), moderate levels of influenza, short periods of severely cold weather and shortages of staffing and acute hospital beds put the NHS under severe strain.

In preparation for the Winter of 1997-98, the Chief Executive of the NHS Executive and the Chief Inspector of the Social Services Inspectorate undertook joint visits to every health region to check on progress and to reinforce the message that better planning and joint working must be a priority. This programme was followed by a letter[17] from the Secretary of State for Health to all health authorities, NHS Trusts, leaders of councils and chairs of social services and housing departments to emphasise that:

- a first priority for the NHS is to make adequate provision for emergency care;

- hospitals (and their accident and emergency departments) must not close unilaterally to emergency admissions; *and*

- health authorities must share the risks faced by NHS Trusts in meeting unpredictable demand, and health authorities and NHS Trusts alike must be committed to improved co-operation with other NHS agencies and with social services departments.

164

The report of the Emergency Services Action Team (set up to work at local, regional and national levels)[18] included a check-list for action and a forward programme to enhance management of and planning for emergency pressures.

In October, an extra £269 million were made available to the NHS in England to help hospitals to cope with emergencies, to reduce delays in hospital discharges and to keep people out of hospital wherever possible, as well as generally to improve joint working across health and social services. This additional funding resulted in almost 1,500 new initiatives, and some £35 million of additional money was transferred to social services in respect of their contributions to improved joint agency working, particularly in relation to out-of-hours services and emergency cover arrangements.

(xi) Ambulance performance standards review

New performance standards were set in 1996 for ambulance services to be expected to reach 75% of life-threatening emergency (999) calls within eight minutes by the year 2001, with 90% as a long-term aim. Other 999 calls will continue to receive an ambulance response within 14 minutes (urban areas) or 19 minutes (rural areas), as at present. Ambulance services will be able safely to prioritise calls according to the patient's need by use of new control-room systems. Four ambulance services (in Berkshire, Derbyshire, Essex and the West Midlands) started to prioritise calls in April 1997, followed by a further five in October; the remainder will introduce such systems in April 1998 or shortly thereafter. Evaluation of the new standards in the first four services will include a study of the costs and benefits of raising the life-threatening 999 calls target from 75% to 90%, and will also explore alternative ways to deal with low-priority calls.

(xii) Palliative care

The *Policy framework for commissioning cancer services*[19], published in 1995 and subsequently endorsed and strengthened by this Government, includes palliative care as an integral part of the framework and of its implementation. The central philosophy is that there should be a consistent national approach to the provision of a uniformly high quality of service to patients with cancer wherever they live - an approach not just limited to cancer. In October 1996, the NHS Executive reminded commissioners of health care that they should ensure that palliative care is included in all services for those with cancer and other life-threatening diseases[20], advice which was repeated in June.

Palliative care has developed considerably over the last few years, with advances in pain and symptom control and in improving the overall quality of life for patients with cancer and life-threatening diseases. DH is committed to promote the benefits of these improvements in treatment and care for all patients. The NHS national R&D programme on cancer has funded a number of projects under the priority area 'What prevents terminally ill people from dying at home, if they so wish, and how can general practitioners and their teams access information to help them care more effectively for their patients at home?', which are now in progress. In December, the National Council for Hospices and Specialist Palliative Care Services published evidence-based guidelines on managing the last days of life in adults[21], which received funding from the NHS Executive.

The full spectrum of palliative care provision and support to meet the needs of terminally ill patients and their carers is being addressed from the point at which a patient's final illness is diagnosed, through to the carers' bereavement. This care and support is provided by a range of professionals in community, hospital and hospice settings.

(xiii) Diabetes mellitus

Diabetes mellitus affects up to 2.4% of the adult population. If not effectively managed, it can result in long-term complications including blindness, renal failure, lower limb amputation and cardiovascular disease. The international St Vincent Declaration, ratified in 1991[22], highlighted the scope to reduce complications resulting from diabetes and proposed a number of outcome targets.

The DH/British Diabetic Association (BDA) St Vincent Joint Task Force for Diabetes, which reported in 1995[23], made recommendations about good clinical and management practice. DH then set up a diabetes sub-group of the Clinical Outcomes Group (COG) to develop service guidance for the NHS, based on these recommendations. The sub-group's guidance, *Key features of a good diabetes service*[24], issued to the NHS in November, advises NHS managers of the key issues they need to consider, and if necessary act on locally, to provide a high-quality service to people with diabetes mellitus.

DH has also commissioned clinical guidelines on non-insulin-dependent diabetes mellitus, from a consortium of medical Royal Colleges and the BDA, and two Effective Health Care Bulletins on diabetes mellitus; these should be available by the end of 1999.

(xiv) Asthma

The 'Control your asthma' card, launched in October 1996[25,26], has been widely taken up by GP practices. Market research in Spring 1998 will evaluate the card and explore the scope for further ways to help patients to manage their own asthma treatment.

A major issue in asthma management is the phasing out of chlorofluorocarbons (CFCs), which damage the ozone layer, under the internationally agreed Montreal Protocol. CFCs have been used as propellants in almost all metered-dose inhalers (MDIs) for asthma and chronic obstructive pulmonary disease, and their phasing out requires the reformulation and relicensing of such MDIs. All MDI drugs with significant use will be reformulated over the next few years.

DH has been closely involved in the development of a draft UK strategy for the changeover to CFC-free MDIs, which fills out a draft European document and will be published for public consultation in 1998. The aim is to manage the transition with a minimum of disruption for patients and the NHS. DH is working with health professional organisations, patient bodies and the pharmaceutical industry to raise awareness of the change among professionals and the public alike. A range of information materials and services will be made available during 1998.

References

1. Department of Health. *The new NHS: modern, dependable.* London: Stationery Office, 1997 (Cm. 3807).
2. Department of Health, Welsh Office. *A policy framework for commissioning cancer services: a report by the Expert Advisory Group on Cancer to the Chief Medical Officers of England and Wales: guidance for purchasers and providers of care.* London: Department of Health, 1995.
3. Department of Health. *Improving outcomes in colorectal cancer: guidance on commissioning cancer services.* Leeds: Department of Health, 1997.
4. Department of Health NHS Executive. *Education and planning guidance.* Leeds: Department of Health, 1997 (Executive Letter: EL(97)58).
5. Gallimore SC, Hoile RW, Ingram GS, Sherry KM. *The report of the National Confidential Enquiry into Perioperative Deaths 1994/1995 (1 April 1994 to 31 March 1995).* London: National Confidential Enquiry into Perioperative Deaths, 1997.
6. Campling EA, Devlin HB, Hoile RW, Ingram GS, Lunn JN. *Who operates when? A report by the National Confidential Enquiry into Perioperative Deaths (1 April 1995 to 31 March 1996).* London: National Confidential Enquiry into Perioperative Deaths, 1997.
7. Department of Health. *Advisory Group on Osteoporosis: report.* London: Department of Health, 1994. Chair: Professor David Barlow.
8. Department of Health. *Tessa Jowell highlights protective measures against osteoporosis: Minister marks World Osteoporosis Day.* London: Department of Health, 1997 (Press Release: H97/144).
9. Advisory Group on the Ethics of Xenotransplantation. *Animal tissue into humans: a report by the Advisory Group on the ethics of xenotransplantation.* London: Stationery Office, 1997. Chair: Professor Ian Kennedy
10. Department of Health. *Report of the Health Care Strategy Unit: review of renal services: evidence for the review.* London: Department of Health, 1994.
11. Scandinavian Simvastatin Survival Study Group. Randomised trial of cholesterol lowering in 4,444 patients with coronary heart disease: the Scandinavian Simvastatin Survival Study (4S). *Lancet* 1994; **344:** 1383-9.
12. Shepherd J, Cobbe SM, Ford I, et al. Prevention of coronary heart disease with pravastatin in men with hypercholesterolemia: West of Scotland Coronary Prevention Study (WOSCOPS) Group. *N Engl J Med* 1995; **333:** 1301-7.

13.   Department of Health NHS Executive. *SMAC statement on use of statins.* Leeds: Department of Health, 1997 (Executive Letter: EL(97)41).

14.   Ramsey LE, Haq IU, Jackson PR, Yeo WW. The Sheffield table for primary prevention of coronary heart disease: corrected. *Lancet* 1996; **348**: 387-8, 1251.

15   Department of Health. Statins and coronary heart disease. *CMO's Update* 1997; **15**: 3.

16.   Department of Health NHS Executive. *Guidelines on admission to and discharge from intensive care and high dependency units.* London: Department of Health, 1996.

17.   Department of Health. *Managing winter 1997/98.* London: Department of Health, 1997.

18.   Department of Health NHS Executive. *Report to the Chief Executive on winter pressures.* London: Department of Health, 1997.

19.   Department of Health, Welsh Office. *A policy framework for commissioning cancer services: a report by the Expert Advisory Group on Cancer to the Chief Medical Officers of England and Wales: guidance for purchasers and providers of care.* London: Department of Health, 1995.

20.   Department of Health. *A policy framework for commissioning services: palliative care.* Leeds: Department of Health, 1996 (Executive Letter: EL(96)85).

21.   National Council for Hospices and Specialist Palliative Care Services. *Changing gear: guidelines for managing the last days of life in adults.* London: National Council for Hospices and Specialist Palliative Care Services, 1997.

22.   World Health Organization (Europe), International Diabetes Federation (Europe). Diabetes care and research in Europe: the St Vincent Declaration. *Diabet Med* 1990; **7**: 360.

23.   Department of Health, British Diabetic Association. *St Vincent Joint Task Force for Diabetes: the report: 1995.* London: Department of Health, 1995.

24.   Department of Health. *Key features of a good diabetes service.* London: Department of Health, 1997 (Health Service Guidelines: HSG(97)45).

25.   Department of Health. Asthma patient card. *CMO's Update* 1996; **12**: 6.

26.   Department of Health. *On the State of the Public Health: the annual report of the Chief Medical Officer of the Department of Health for the year 1996.* London: Stationery Office, 1997; 185.

(e)   Mental health

(i)   *Mental health promotion*

Mental health remains an issue surrounded by fear and misunderstanding. Stigma contributes greatly to the suffering of people with mental health problems, and inhibits people from seeking help for mental distress. While the social and economic costs of mental illness are high, public awareness of how to maintain and promote mental health is low. As part of DH's strategy to raise public awareness and understanding of mental health issues and to combat stigma, the Health Education Authority (HEA) co-ordinates the World Mental Health Day (WMHD) campaign. A guide to monitoring and evaluation, *Mental health promotion: a quality framework*[1], to support those working to promote mental health locally, was launched on 10 October. The WMHD campaign brings together over 50 national organisations; local participation has increased from 500 agencies in 1995 to nearly 6,000 in 1997. Initiatives are designed to meet the needs of different age-groups: 'Exam slam', produced in partnership with British Broadcasting Corporation (BBC) Radio 1, tackles coping with revision and examinations at schools; a joint project with the charity Mind targeted young people and engaged them in the debate around stigma through the use of controversial images; and materials produced in Mandarin, Vietnamese, Urdu, Bengali, Punjabi and Hindi addressed the concerns of different black and ethnic minority communities.

The HEA report *Making headlines*[2] noted widespread negative media coverage of mental health. The WMHD campaign helps to promote informed debate and to change media attitudes to its coverage of mental health issues. Over 1,300 events (in schools, workplaces, youth centres, shopping centres, hospitals, leisure centres, art galleries, places of worship and GP surgeries) helped to promote these aims.

(ii) Mental health in primary care

Mental health problems constitute a considerable part of the work of primary care. As diagnosed by a GP, mental health problems are one of the most common reasons for consultation[3], even though family doctors only tend to assign a psychiatric diagnosis to about half of those who present with them[4]. International[5] and UK studies[6] alike indicate that well-defined psychological problems are present in approximately one-quarter of consultations. The most common mental health diagnoses in primary care are depression, anxiety states, panic disorder, chronic fatigue and alcohol misuse. Of patients with schizophrenia, between 25-40% lose touch with secondary services and the GP is the health care professional most likely to remain in contact with them[7]. GPs also often prescribe medication recommended by specialist services for those with severe, enduring mental illness. Primary care services are therefore responsible for a significant proportion of the care for people with mental health problems, and DH continued to emphasise this area during the year.

The primary mental health care toolkit[8,9], published in January, is designed to be used by primary care teams within the context of their daily work and includes templates for assessment and management of common disorders; screening tools; guidance on the role of practice nurses; problem-solving and sources of self-help; audit; and resources. The Sainsbury Centre for Mental Health was commissioned to hold a conference on 'Innovations in primary mental health care' and to develop a database of programmes in primary mental health care to share examples of good practice. The training of primary care professionals in mental health skills is critical to the quality of care offered, and national audit of the mental health components of vocational training schemes for GPs has been started.

Mental health specialists continue to liaise closely with primary care colleagues in relation to the implications for primary mental health care following the White Paper *The new NHS: modern, dependable*[10], and the opportunities that it and new flexibilities in primary care may offer, with regional and national work to consider further the role of primary mental health care.

(iii)   Occupational mental health

Work continued during the year to increase employers' awareness of occupational mental health issues and to encourage further action. A three-year project in collaboration with occupational physicians to assess the risks associated with mental health in the workplace, to detect and manage mental health in the workplace and to influence organisational practice and company policy on mental health problems, commissioned by DH, started in late 1995. This project has analysed the training needs of occupational physicians and developed workshops to meet those needs, which will be promoted to training centres for occupational medicine. A series of 15 clinical updates, the 'ABC of mental health for occupational physicians', will be published between March and November 1998, followed by further work including case studies.

Work on occupational mental health is taken forward by alliances between DH and other Government Departments and Agencies (such as the Health and Safety Executive [HSE] and the HEA), human resource managers (through the Institute of Personnel and Development), the Faculty of Public Health Medicine, psychiatrists, psychologists, academic units and employers (such as the Confederation of British Industry [CBI] and the Small Business Federation) to ensure a wider understanding of occupational physicians' role in respect of mental health in the workplace. Strategies on mental health have been co-ordinated by the Mental Health at Work Inter-Agency Group, convened by DH, which also commissioned and oversaw production by Cranfield Business School of *Mental well-being in the workplace: an educational approach for managers*, an educational tool for managers to use in the identification and management of workplace stress, funded by the HSE.

Research continues into psychological symptoms among NHS staff; DH has supported the 'Health at work in the NHS project' and action to identify and manage the organisational causes of stress.

(iv)   Psychological treatment services

Following the publication in September 1996 of the NHS Executive's strategic review of psychotherapy services[11], a series of conferences was held to discuss the messages about good practice in the 'talking therapies', involving commissioners and providers of health care, employers and patient representatives, and to consider the implications for local services of the findings of the review. Despite some examples of very good practice and general evidence of progress, in many local areas there is some way to go to improve partnership and co-ordination in relation to 'talking therapy' services, and to increase their accessibility and effectiveness.

The NHS Executive also commissioned an independent review of funding for training in psychotherapy, circulated in January[12], which indicated a need for better information to be available for education and training consortia, which will ultimately take on responsibility for commissioning psychotherapy education and training at local level. Education and training planning guidance[13] was published in October to highlight issues in psychological treatment services, and further work is planned.

(v) Child and adolescent mental health

The Department continued initiatives to raise the profile of child and adolescent mental health and to ensure the development of services to reflect national planning and priorities guidance[14,15]. Regional offices of the NHS Executive, in conjunction with the Social Services Inspectorate, lead the implementation of national policy for a performance management framework, and a central forum was established for Regional Offices to report on progress in reviewing local child and adolescent mental health services (CAMHS), covering health, social services and educational aspects, in the light of wider Government initiatives to improve the health and well-being of young people.

The Health Select Committee of the House of Commons reported on CAMHS as part of its general examination of the health of children[16]. The Committee looked at the concept of mental health as it applies to children, outlined the types of mental health problems that children and young people suffer from and their prevalence rates, and looked at the problem of suicide among young people as well as the specific problems of antisocial behaviour and conduct and eating disorders; it also examined the provision of services for children and young people with mental health problems, and made recommendations how these could be improved.

In its response, published in November[17], the Government welcomed the Health Committee's report and its recognition of what had been achieved in recent years to raise the profile of child and adolescent mental health and to provide a sound basis for action to improve current provision of local services.

The Social Survey Division of the Office for National Statistics (ONS) was awarded a contract to undertake a national survey of the development and well-being of children and adolescents, which will provide data on the prevalence of

171

common child mental health problems, levels of impairment and service usage. Its findings are expected to be available in late 1999.

During the year two major studies (a wide-ranging inquiry into children's and young people's mental health by the Mental Health Foundation, and a comprehensive Audit Commission review) were started.

(vi)   *National Confidential Inquiry into Suicide and Homicide by People with Mental Illness*

The DH-funded National Confidential Inquiry into Suicide and Homicide by People with Mental Illness was established in 1992 (as the Confidential Inquiry into Homicides and Suicides by Mentally Ill People) to conduct a national audit of suicides and homicides by people who have a history of contact with mental health services; to make recommendations to Ministers on clinical practice and policy in mental health; and to identify training needs for mental health staff[18,19].

Under its current Director, Professor Louis Appleby, Professor of Adult Psychiatry at the University of Manchester, the Inquiry made progress during 1997 towards the establishment of new methods of data collection designed to produce a large and comprehensive sample of suicides and homicides for detailed study. A progress report published on 12 December 1997[20] set out the Inquiry's preliminary findings in the year from April 1996, when the new methods of data collection were established; a full report will be published in Spring 1999.

(vii)   *Specialised mental illness services*

DH remains committed to the provision of a range of services to those suffering from severe mental illness which are appropriate, easily available, of high quality, safe, and offer effective and accountable support by multidisciplinary teams working effectively together[4,21]. This comprehensive range of services should include hospital inpatient services, some of which require to be secure up to the level of the special hospitals; day hospital and other day-care provision; and crisis services, including accommodation, community mental health teams, specialist services, staffed residential provision and home-based support. Nationally, progress is being made towards implementation of this full range of services, although availability in some localities remains uneven; this process is monitored every Autumn in a formal review.

Responses to the Green Paper *Developing partnerships in mental health*[22] have contributed to planning of the provision of effective services, and with other initiatives[10,23] provide a context for the continued development of mental health services such that they become more integrated across primary and secondary care, and between health, social and housing services and other providers of care, including the independent sector.

The White Paper *The new NHS; modern, dependable*[10] offers an overall vision of integrated care, which is of central importance to mental health. The pivotal role of primary care in provision of and access to mental health care will be built upon, with a focus on staff training and development which should increasingly be multidisciplinary and serve to improve the morale and mutual support needed for effective team-working in mental health. Development of the assessment of outcomes will be enhanced by the new management framework, and there will be a focus on evidence-based interventions.

The Green Paper *Our Healthier Nation*[23] will acknowledge the major importance of mental health in relation to public health as a whole; suicide will represent an important focus. The all-age suicide (and undetermined deaths) rate fell by around 20% between 1982 and 1996, but there are striking variations in this trend related to age and gender: for example, the most dramatic falls in suicide rates are among women aged 45-84 years, whereas the rate for young men aged between 15-24 years rose during the 1980s. There also appears to be considerable variation between ethnic sub-groups, with particularly high rates among women of Indian and East African extraction. Further concerted action by Government, local authorities, the NHS, voluntary bodies, workplaces and individuals will be needed to reduce further the rate of suicide.

The independent reference group, set up in the Autumn of 1997 by Mr Paul Boateng MP, Parliamentary Under-Secretary of State for Health in the House of Commons, has an innovative role in the development of mental health services. Its first task has been to review the adequacy, in terms of service provision and of public confidence, of closure plans for the remaining long-stay mental health hospitals.

Severely mentally ill patients with co-existent substance misuse problems appear to be more resistant to treatment, to require longer periods of care, to provide more of a risk to the community and to be at high risk of relapse. A programme of work will therefore focus on these patients to seek out areas of good practice, to disseminate effective models of care and to encourage innovative work across providers of mental health services, substance misuse services, housing and social services agencies and other providers of care.

(viii) Services for mentally disordered offenders

In 1996, the High Security Psychiatric Services Commissioning Board (HSPSCB) established a research and development (R&D) Committee[24], which includes individuals who work in the high security psychiatric services as well as representatives from the prison service, probation and medium secure units, and various other relevant areas. One of the main objectives set by Ministers for the HSPSCB on its establishment was to develop a research strategy for forensic mental health, as well as research and development to underpin its commissioning strategy.

Much of the strategy of the R&D committee is based on the findings of the DH/Home Office *Review of health and social services by mentally disordered offenders and others requiring similar services*[25,26], which identified the need to develop the research infrastructure for training, and has been addressed by the establishment of networks, a bursary scheme, a fellowship scheme and tutoring facilities; a number of other initiatives are being considered. All these activities are multidisciplinary and multi-agency, and planned in consultation with the DH central R&D programme, with links to the Medical Research Council (MRC), the Economic and Social Research Council and other funding bodies in the UK, and has also established links with the EU.

A key policy area is that of antisocial personality disorder[27]: officials from the Home Office and DH are examining service provision in this area within the criminal justice system and the NHS; key areas of work include current service gaps, examples of good practice and advice to Ministers on future service development. This work draws on a number of other areas - including the overall HSPSCB strategy, which is under review by Ministers, a series of literature reviews due to report in Spring 1998 and general forensic mental health policy - and involves a wide range of services in the criminal justice system and the NHS. Personality disorder services are a major element of the HSPSCB R&D programme, and a conference in October identified key research priorities including the development of a framework of understanding personality disorders, the need for training of researchers in this area; and the need for further research, including randomised controlled trials and longitudinal cohort studies. The HSPSCB is providing funds to bring together 11 academic units across a range of disciplines and specialties to further these recommendations, and is also contributing to a number of national training projects into antisocial personality disorder.

A number of alleged incidents relating to pornography, drugs and paedophile activity at Ashworth High Security Hospital in early 1997 led to the establishment of a judicial inquiry into its Personality Disorder Unit; this inquiry is due to be completed by late 1998, and will report to the Secretary of State for Health and to the Home Secretary in early 1999.

(ix)   Mental health legislation

The Mental Health Act 1983[28] provides the framework for the detention of seriously mentally disordered patients in hospital. During 1997, this Act was amended to introduce a new sentencing power for the Courts by the Crime Sentences Act 1997[29], which introduced a direction which allows courts to impose a prison sentence combined with a hospital order. The new power came into force on 1 October. At present, this hospital direction is only available for offenders with a diagnosis of psychopathic disorder, but there are provisions for it to be extended to cover other categories of mental disorder.

During 1996/97, 203 patients were made subject to after-care under supervision (supervised discharge) under the Mental Health (Patients in the Community) Act 1995[30] The Department commissioned research into the use and impact of after-care under such supervision and guardianship, and an interim report is expected in Autumn 1998, with a final report in 1999. A three-year research project under way into decision-making and outcomes of Mental Health Review Tribunals should also report in 1999.

References

1. Gale E. *Mental health promotion: a quality framework.* London: Health Education Authority, 1997.
2. Gale E. *Making headlines: mental health and the national press.* London: Health Education Authority, 1997.
3. McCormick A, Fleming D, Charlton J. *Morbidity statistics from general practice: fourth national study: 1991-1992.* London: HMSO, 1995 (Series MB5; no. 3).
4. Department of Health. *On the State of the Public Health: the annual report of the Chief Medical Officer of the Department of Health for the year 1995.* London: HMSO, 1996; 13-4, 95-126.
5. Ustun T, Sartorius N, eds. *Mental illness in general health care: an international study.* Chichester: John Wiley, 1995.
6. Goldberg D, Blackwell B. Psychiatric illness in general practice. *BMJ* 1970; **2:** 439-43.
7. Kendrick T, Burns T, Freeling P, Sibbald B. Provision of care to general practice patients with disabling long-term mental illness. *Br J Gen Pract* 1994; **44:** 301-5.
8 Armstrong E, ed. *The primary mental health toolkit.* Wetherby (West Yorkshire): Department of Health, 1997.
9. Department of Health. Primary mental health toolkit. *CMO's Update* 1997; **15:** 4.
10. Department of Health. *The new NHS: modern, dependable.* London: Department of Health, 1997 (Cm. 3807).
11. Parry G, Richardson A. *NHS psychotherapy services in England: review of strategic policy.* London: NHS Executive, 1996.
12. Damon S. *Commissioning and funding of training in psychotherapies for the NHS in England.* London: Department of Health, 1997.
13. Department of Health. *Education and training: planning guidance.* Leeds: Department of Health, 1997 (Executive Letter: EL(97)58).
14. Department of Health. *NHS priorities and planning guidance: 1997/98.* Leeds: Department of Health, 1996 (Executive Letter: EL(96)45).
15. Department of Health, Department for Education and Employment. *Children's services planning: guidance.* London: Department of Health, Department for Education and Employment, 1996.
16. House of Commons Health Committee. *Child and adolescent mental health services: report from the Health Committee: Session 1996-97.* London: Stationery Office, 1997 (HC 26-I).

17. Department of Health. *Government response to the reports of the Health Committee on health services for children and young people: Session 1996-97.* London: Stationery Office, 1997 (Cm. 3793).

18. Department of Health. *On the State of the Public Health: the annual report of the Chief Medical Officer of the Department of Health for the year 1996.* London: Stationery Office, 1997; 174.

19. Steering Committee on the Confidential Inquiry into Homicides and Suicides by Mentally Ill People. *Report of the Confidential Inquiry into Homicides and Suicides by Mentally Ill People.* London: Royal College of Psychiatrists, 1996.

20. Appleby L. *National Confidential Inquiry into Suicide and Homicide by People with Mental Illness: progress report: 1997.* London: Department of Health, 1997.

21. Department of Health. *On the State of the Public Health: the annual report of the Chief Medical Officer of the Department of Health for the year 1996.* London: Stationery Office, 1997; 12-3, 170-80.

22. Department of Health. *Developing partnerships in mental health.* London: Stationery Office, 1996 (Cm. 3555).

23. Department of Health. *Our Healthier Nation: a contract for health.* London: Stationery Office (in press) (Cm. 3852).

24. Department of Health. *On the State of the Public Health: the annual report of the Chief Medical Officer of the Department of Health for the year 1996.* London: Stationery Office, 1997; 176-7.

25. Department of Health, Home Office. *Review of health and social services for mentally disordered offenders and others requiring similar services: final summary report.* London: HMSO, 1992 (Cm. 2088). Chair: Dr John Reed.

26. Department of Health, Home Office. *Review of health and social services for mentally disordered offenders and others requiring similar services: volume 4: the academic and research base: the reports of the academic development and research advisory groups.* London: HMSO, 1993. Chair: Dr John Reed.

27. Department of Health, Home Office. *Report of the Department of Health and Home Office Working Group on Psychopathic Disorders.* London: Department of Health, 1994. Chair: Dr John Reed.

28. *The Mental Health Act 1983.* London: HMSO, 1983.

29. *The Crime Sentences Act 1997.* London: Stationery Office, 1997.

30. *The Mental Health (Patients in the Community) Act 1995.* London: HMSO, 1995.

(f)   Maternity and child health services

(i)   *Implementation of 'Changing Childbirth'*

There has been continued progress towards implementation of the recommendations of the Expert Maternity Group's report, *Changing childbirth◊*, focusing on greater continuity and choice in maternity services.

During the year, the Changing Childbirth Implementation Team continued its programme of education and training initiatives. It organised, in partnership with the Royal College of Obstetricians and Gynaecologists' Clinical Audit Unit, two seminars on evaluation of maternity care and, in conjunction with the Institute of Health Sciences, a conference on critical skills appraisal, following on from a project on training for members of maternity service liaison committees. In July, the NHS Executive published *Learning together: professional education for maternity care*[2] as a reference source for the further development of multidisciplinary education. After a successful information campaign during 1996, work continued to enhance accessibility of the leaflet *How to get the best from maternity services*[3].

(ii)   Confidential Enquiry into Stillbirths and Deaths in Infancy

The Confidential Enquiry into Stillbirths and Deaths in Infancy's (CESDI's) annual report for 1995 was published in July[4]. This report made a number of observations about clinical and post-mortem practices, identified from the examination of cases for that year, which gave cause for concern. No consistent pattern was identified, but weaknesses appear to occur because of poor documentation and inadequate training. The report makes a number of recommendations, in particular that the medical and nursing Royal Colleges and other bodies responsible for teaching and accreditation should consider how levels of practical competence of professionals caring for women in labour and for newborn babies are achieved and maintained. It also emphasised the importance of a pathological examination and recommended that the availability of such services be audited. Despite the small numbers of births and deaths involved, the findings of the CESDI clearly indicate areas for improvement, and all the parties concerned are committed to the implementation of any recommended changes to clinical practice.

(iii)   Folic acid and the prevention of neural tube defects

The HEA's campaign to encourage mothers to increase their intake of folic acid around the time of conception to prevent neural tube defects continued throughout the year. Young people, especially those who may be at risk of an unplanned pregnancy, were particularly targeted via the media, pharmacies, a freephone advice line and food retailers. The folic acid 'flash' was agreed and is now used as a symbol on food packaging to indicate foods which are good sources of this vitamin. Spontaneous awareness among women of childbearing age of the benefit of taking folic acid rose from 9% in 1995 to 39% in 1997.

An expert group of the Committee on Medical Aspects of Food and Nutrition Policy (COMA) continued to review the health aspects of folic acid and its potential to prevent disease; a report is expected in 1999.

(iv)   Sudden infant death syndrome

The key messages to reduce the risk-factors which may lead to sudden infant death (cot death) are that:

 - babies should continue to be placed on their backs to sleep;

- cigarette smoking in pregnancy and around babies increases the risk of cot death;

- babies who become overheated are also in danger, and their bedrooms should be kept at an overnight temperature which is comfortable for a lightly clothed adult; *and*

- babies should sleep in such a way that their head does not become covered during the night, which can most easily be achieved by placing the baby to sleep with his or her feet near to the foot of the cot so that it is made difficult for them to move down the cot, and hence under their covers, during sleep.

Copies of the leaflet *Reduce the risk of cot death*[5], prepared with the assistance of the Foundation for the Study of Infant Deaths are still available. Since the launch in 1991 of the Department's campaign to reduce the number of cot deaths, the number of such deaths in infancy has halved in England and Wales from 1.4 per 1,000 live births in the post-natal period in 1991 to 0.65 in 1996 (1,008 deaths in 1991 to 424 deaths in 1996).

(v) Prophylaxis of vitamin K deficiency bleeding in infants

As discussed in recent Reports[6,7,8,9], by comparison with older children newborn babies are deficient in vitamin K, and in a small number - about 1 in 10,000 - this deficiency is associated with bleeding without warning, which can often lead to permanent disability or death. Understandably, it has been usual practice to give newborn babies prophylactic vitamin K, either orally or intramuscularly. During 1992, a possible association between vitamin K given intramuscularly and the development of cancer in childhood was reported[10,11,12]. The findings have been disputed, although concerns remain. These concerns have focused first on whether additional vitamin K in any form should be administered, and second on the most appropriate supplementation regimen.

It seems beyond dispute that vitamin K deficiency bleeding in newborn babies can be prevented by the administration of vitamin K. There should be clear benefits if additional vitamin K could be given safely to all newborn babies because there is insufficient vitamin K in breast milk to prevent vitamin deficiency bleeding in some babies, and additional amounts are needed to supplement their natural stores of vitamin K throughout the period of exclusive breast-feeding; vitamin K is already added to formula milk.

Intramuscular vitamin K effectively prevents vitamin K deficiency bleeding in virtually all babies after a single 1 mg dose given at birth. Oral doses of vitamin K are effective, but must be repeated to achieve equivalent effect to intramuscular usage; inadequate repeat oral supplementation will give less protection.

In view of continued debate on these issues, an expert group was convened in Autumn 1997 to consider all the evidence and to formulate advice, with the support of DH, the Medicines Control Agency (MCA) and the Committee on Safety of Medicines (CSM); the group is expected to report in 1998.

(vi) Retinopathy of prematurity

The multidisciplinary research project set up to assess and improve the care of infants with retinopathy of prematurity (ROP) continues[13,14]. The first phase of the project, a management survey of current screening policies and practices is complete and the data have been coded and analysed. Results showed some well organised and efficient local screening procedures, but also found some units where organisational challenges needed to be addressed. The survey continues to highlight areas for potential improvement of services and, by inquiring about the availability of printed information for parents and about record-keeping, has prompted several new local initiatives. A series of ROP roadshows continued to increase awareness of screening and management of pre-term babies, the natural history of the disease and counselling for parents of babies at risk of, and suffering from, ROP. Attendance by health professionals involved in ROP management has been very encouraging, and educational programmes will continue.

(vii) Paediatric intensive care

The report *Paediatric intensive care: a framework for the future*[15], from the National Co-ordinating Group set up in June 1996 to draw up a policy framework for paediatric intensive care, was published in July 1997. It noted the strengths of paediatric intensive care, which provides a high level of service to critically ill children. The Group's aim was to build upon these strengths and to produce a clear policy framework for the future.

Despite its strengths, the Group found that the key features of the current paediatric intensive care service showed that it had developed in an unplanned way and was provided in a wide range of settings apart from designated paediatric intensive care beds, which was not considered to be conducive to the best outcome for children under treatment. Specialist services to transport critically ill children to the nearest paediatric intensive care centre were still relatively few, and often not provided on a continuous basis. The report also indicated that there was a shortfall of clinicians and nurses with paediatric intensive care skills, and recommended greater overview through clinical audit and the designation of 'lead centres' for service provision; organisational structures were proposed, together with a set of standards to be implemented and a timescale for their implementation.

The Group's report, together with an accompanying report on nursing standards, education and workforce planning, *A bridge to the future: report of the Chief Nursing Officer's Taskforce*[16], was well received and implementation of the underlying recommendations is under way to ensure the best available service for the intensive care needs of individual children.

References

1. Department of Health Expert Maternity Group. *Changing childbirth: part 1: report of the Expert Maternity Group.* London: HMSO, 1993. Chair: Baroness Cumberlege.
2. Department of Health NHS Executive. *Learning together: a professional education for maternity care.* London: Department of Health, 1997.
3. Department of Health, Changing Childbirth Implementation Team, National Childbirth Trust. *How to get the best from maternity services.* London: Department of Health, 1996.
4. Confidential Enquiry into Stillbirths and Deaths in Infancy. *4th annual report: 1 January - 31 December 1995: concentrating on intrapartum related deaths 1994-95.* London: Maternal and Child Health Research Consortium, 1997.
5. Department of Health. *Reduce the risk of cot death: an easy guide.* London: Department of Health, 1996.
6. Department of Health. *On the State of the Public Health: the annual report of the Chief Medical Officer of the Department of Health for the year 1992.* London: HMSO, 1993; 130-1.
7. Department of Health. *On the State of the Public Health: the annual report of the Chief Medical Officer of the Department of Health for the year 1993.* London: HMSO, 1994; 132-3.
8. Department of Health. *On the State of the Public Health: the annual report of the Chief Medical Officer of the Department of Health for the year 1994.* London: HMSO, 1995; 148-9.
9. *Department of Health. On the State of the Public Health: the annual report of the Chief Medical Officer of the Department of Health for the year 1995.* London: HMSO, 1996; 182.
10. Golding J, Birmingham K, Greenwood R, Mott M. Childhood cancer, intramuscular vitamin K, and pethidine given during labour. *BMJ* 1992; **304:** 341-6.
11. Draper GJ, Stiller CA. Intramuscular vitamin K and childhood cancer. *BMJ* 1992; **305:** 709.
12. Hull D. Vitamin K and childhood cancer. The risk of haemorrhagic disease is certain; that of cancer is not. *BMJ* 1992; **305:** 326-7.
13. Department of Health. *On the State of the Public Health: the annual report of the Chief Medical Officer of the Department of Health for the year 1994.* London: HMSO, 1995; 149.
14. Department of Health. *On the State of the Public Health: the annual report of the Chief Medical Officer of the Department of Health for the year 1996.* London: Stationery Office, 1997; 182-3.
15. Department of Health NHS Executive, Health Services Directorate. *Paediatric intensive care: a framework for the future.* Leeds: Department of Health, 1997.
16. Department of Health NHS Executive. *A bridge to the future: report of the Chief Nursing Officer's Taskforce: nursing standards, education and workforce planning in paediatric intensive care.* Leeds: Department of Health, 1997.

(g)   Disability

(i)   General aspects of disability

Last year's Report[1] included a special chapter on the health of disabled people. The 1995 Health Survey for England[2], published in February 1997, provided

180

further data on the extent of self-reported disability based on questions recommended by the World Health Organization (WHO) to determine levels of disability[3]. Its findings indicated that 18% of males and females aged over 16 years who were living in private households had some degree of moderate or serious disability; 4% of men and 5% of women had a serious disability. The self-reported prevalence of disability increases with age: one-quarter of people were disabled by the age of 65 years; about 50% after 75 years-of-age; and three-quarters of people aged 85 years and older were disabled: these data equate to some 7.3 million people aged ten years and over who consider themselves to be disabled, of whom 47% are aged 65 years and over, 33% are aged 45-64 years and 20% aged 10-44 years.

Below the age of 55 years, the prevalence of self-reported disability is similar among men and women, but is higher for men among those aged 55-74 years who often report hearing disabilities, and higher among women aged 75 years and over who often report locomotor disabilities.

The 1995 Health Survey for England[3] classified disabilities into five broad types - locomotor, personal care, sight, hearing and communication. The most commonly reported cause of disability (34% of those with a disability) was disease of the musculoskeletal system and connective tissue, mainly cited as osteoarthritis, particularly among older people. Nearly one-quarter was caused by disease of the ear and mastoid process (chiefly causing deafness); 16% were caused by diseases of the circulatory system; 10% by respiratory diseases; and 8% by eye disorders. Serious disabilities were most likely to be caused by arthritis and rheumatism, diseases of the nervous system (particularly Parkinson's disease and multiple sclerosis) and circulatory disease (particularly stroke). People with moderate disabilities were more likely to report back and neck problems and deafness as causes of disability. Accidents are an important cause of disability among younger people, but are not considered to cause more than one-quarter of disabilities in any age- or sex-group.

(ii)   Types of disability

Physical disability

As well as trauma caused as a result of accident, almost any long-term, severe illness can cause disability. Demographic changes also mean an increasing number of older people survive with disability, where once they might have died.

Mobility

Although a number of advances in relation to mobility have allowed people with a range of disabilities to maintain or increase their independence as well as their quality of life[1], the General Household Survey was again asked to look at mobility in 1996[4], following its original survey in 1993[5]. From preliminary data for 1996, the number of people reporting mobility difficulties is similar to that in 1993[5], at 8%, but access to powered wheelchairs and the wheelchair voucher system has risen by 1%. Most of those with mobility difficulties (91%) regarded them as permanent rather than transitory.

In February 1996, schemes were announced for an additional £50 million to be made available to NHS wheelchair services in England over the following four years for the provision of electrically powered indoor/outdoor wheelchairs (EPIOCs) for severely disabled people who could benefit from them[6], and for the introduction of a voucher scheme to give users more choice over the types of manually operated chairs available to them[7]. EPIOC provision has now been implemented in all wheelchair services, and voucher schemes must be in place by 1 April 1998. Where services are unable to spend all their voucher allocation during 1997/98, Ministers have authorised these health authorities to transfer the shortfall to increase provision in mainstream wheelchairs and the powered chair service.

Falls

The need for rehabilitation and recuperation has been emphasised by *Better services for vulnerable people*[8] as well as by targets for accident prevention in the Health of the Nation initiative[9] and the forthcoming Green Paper, *Our Healthier Nation*[10].

A number of activities focused on falls among elderly people. The Community Care Development Programme has funded a study in the prevention of further falls among elderly people in Worthing, which is nearing completion, and the NHS Executive is supporting a multiprofessional clinical audit in falls guidance produced by physiotherapists and occupational therapists. The Public Health Directorate supported a three-day European conference on falls, particularly among elderly people.

Back pain

Following the Clinical Standards Advisory Group report on back pain in 1994[11], and subsequent guidelines produced by the Royal College of General Practitioners[12] and the physiotherapy, osteopathy and chiropractic professional bodies, DH supported an ONS survey on the prevalence of back pain. In summary, 40% of adults reported back pain in the previous year in 1996, and the overall figures, although similar to 1993, showed a slight rise in back pain among young adults (from 24% in 1993 to 30% in 1996 for young men and women alike). The differences between the two surveys in regard to treatment were negligible, with most people only spending about half a day lying down if their pain was severe. However, one-fifth were still being sent for X-ray (despite advice given in the guidelines[12]), although the proportion who visited their GP and received a sickness certificate appears to have dropped (although this change may be artifactual due to slightly different questions asked); preliminary data indicate that absences from work due to back pain were on average shorter[13], but future data are needed to determine trends.

Sensory disability

Visual impairment

Although 286,770 people in the UK are actually registered as blind or partially sighted with local authorities, the Royal National Institute for the Blind (RNIB) has estimated that 1.1 million people in the UK are eligible to be registered as blind or partially sighted[14]. Older people are more likely to have sight problems - 90% of people with a visual impairment are aged over 60 years, whilst only 8% of blind or partially sighted people were born with impaired vision.

People with hearing impairment

The Royal National Institute for Deaf People (RNID) estimates that 8.4 million adults in the UK have some form of hearing disability, whereas only 45,482 were registered as deaf and 125,939 registered as hard-of-hearing[15]; 75% of people with hearing impairments are aged over 60 years. The NHS Executive has commissioned a videotape for hospital trusts and other health care organisations about the needs of people who are deaf and hard-of-hearing when using hospital services, which is being made by a group of deaf film-makers and includes interviews with deaf and hard-of-hearing people as well as examples of good practice in the NHS and advice about solutions to some of the difficulties encountered by deaf people.

People with dual sensory impairment

Opinion regarding the possible number of deaf-blind people varies greatly. Some 250,000 people in the UK have both a visual and a hearing impairment of some degree, according to RNIB data, and the charities Deafblind UK and Sense estimate that some 23,000 people in the UK are deaf-blind. *Think dual sensory: good practice guidelines for older people with dual sensory loss*[16], published in July, set out guidelines for social and health care services in relation to older people for whom the normal ageing process is further complicated by dual sensory loss.

Learning disability

Following extensive consultation, *Signposts for success in commissioning and providing health services for people with learning disabilities* was prepared for publication in January 1998; a summary version will also be made available. It describes the services that people with learning disabilities (mental handicap) should expect from the NHS, and also refers to commissioning and service redevelopment; promotes the importance of positive attitudes and communication skills in staff and of meeting both the ordinary and special needs of this vulnerable group; describes good practice in primary care and general health services through health promotion, personal health records, routine health checks, responsiveness and flexibility; and the need for specialist services to be available as required - for example, to manage mental health needs, epilepsy, sensory impairments and physical disabilities. An audiotape and guidance, *The healthy way*, for people with learning disabilities themselves, will be issued at the same time, and four conferences will take place in 1998 to increase awareness of these publications and to promote good practice locally.

Mental disability

Disability as a result of mental illness was highlighted in last year's Report[1], and aspects of this are discussed elsewhere in this Report (see pages 94 and 168).

(iii)   Re-ablement

Re-ablement involves a wide range of services, some or all of which will be involved in the life of a disabled person at one stage of their lives or another. For people who have been disabled from birth, the process is not so much one of re-ablement, but of 'ablement' or enabling. Put simply, re-ablement or enabling is about removing or minimising the barriers encountered by disabled people. Such barriers may be physical or attitudinal - both, if they are not challenged, may effectively prevent disabled people from achieving their potential.

The joint initiative on the co-ordination of rehabilitation services for disabled people, funded by DH on behalf of the Inter-Departmental Group on Disability (IDGD), held four regional seminars during the year which drew together, at local level, representatives from social services, the NHS, the employment service, Training and Enterprise Councils, further education, the Benefits Agency, the voluntary sector, and users and carers. The aim of the initiative was to consider ways to improve communication and co-ordination of service planning and delivery between national and local agencies (statutory and non-statutory) concerned with the rehabilitation, education, training and employment of disabled people, and to encourage consultation between service users and agencies. A report, which will incorporate guidelines on good practice with local examples, is being prepared for publication in Summer 1998.

A programme of measures developed by the Department of Social Security, working closely in partnership with the Department for Education and Employment (DfEE) and other Government Departments, including DH, under the 'New deal' for disabled people has been designed to help people with a disability or long-term illness to find or to remain in work, and to help carers to balance their caring responsibilities with work or to take up work when those responsibilities come to an end. Part of this programme will test new ideas for helping people with a disability or long-term illness to move into work, and the process of commissioning such studies is now well under way. Plans for personal adviser pilot schemes in 12 areas, and changes in benefit structure to reduce disincentives to work, have also been announced.

Building on two conferences entitled *Patients disabled* - which were attended by hospital managers and staff, purchasers of care and disabled people - the NHS Executive is developing a good practice guide for the NHS, which will focus mainly on hospital services in relation to disabled people, although the guidance will be equally useful for other health care establishments.

Better services for vulnerable people[17], issued to health and social services authorities in October, sets out a development programme for a range of recuperation and rehabilitation services for older people to give them the time and opportunity to recover from hospital episodes or to stay at home for longer.

Much work continues to be done to promote awareness of and better services for disabled people. To underline its commitment to disabled people, the Government has announced that it will implement the remaining provisions of the Disability Discrimination Act 1995[18], concerned with access to goods and services for disabled people in the private and public sectors alike. A Ministerial Task Force to consult on how to implement civil rights for disabled people has been established; this Task Force will also make recommendations on the possible role and functions of a Disability Rights Commission.

The challenge of meeting the needs of disabled people will continue to be a priority for national and local agencies; progress will not be sustainable if some agencies act in isolation of others or of disabled people themselves. This emphasis on working through partnerships to achieve goals continues to be highlighted nationally across Government Departments and locally between different agencies, and involves disabled people and their carers and families.

References

1. Department of Health. *On the State of the Public Health: the annual report of the Chief Medical Officer of the Department of Health for the year 1996.* London: Stationery Office, 1997; 20, 104-45.
2. Prescott-Clarke P, Primatesta P, eds. *Health Survey for England 1995: a survey carried out on behalf of the Department of Health.* London: Stationery Office, 1997 (Series HS; no. 5).

3.   World Health Organization. *International classification of impairment, disabilities and handicaps.* Geneva: World Health Organization, 1980.

4.   Thomas M, Walker A, Wilmot A, Bennett N. *Living in Britain: results from the 1996 General Household Survey: an inter-Departmental survey carried out by the Office for National Statistics between April 1996 and March 1997.* London: Stationery Office (in press) (Series GHS; no. 27).

5.   Office of Population Censuses and Surveys. *Living in Britain: results from the 1993 General Household Survey.* London: HMSO, 1995 (Series GHS; no. 24).

6.   Department of Health NHS Executive. *Powered indoor/outdoor wheelchairs (EPIOCs) for severely disabled people.* Leeds: Department of Health, 1996 (Health Service Guidelines: HSG(96)34).

7.   Department of Health NHS Executive. *Wheelchair vouchers scheme.* Leeds: Department of Health, 1996 (Health Service Guidelines: HSG(96)53).

8.   Department of Health NHS Executive. *Better services for vulnerable people.* Leeds: Department of Health, 1997 (Executive Letter: EL(97)62).

9.   Department of Health. *The Health of the Nation: a strategy for health in England.* London: HMSO, 1992 (Cm. 1986).

10.   Department of Health. *Our Healthier Nation: a contract for health.* London: Stationery Office (in press) (Cm. 3852).

11.   Clinical Standards Advisory Group. *Back pain: report of a Clinical Standards Advisory Group Committee on back pain.* London: HMSO, 1994.

12.   Royal College of General Practitioners. *The management of acute low back pain.* London: Royal College of General Practitioners, 1996.

13.   Department of Health. *Health and personal social services statistics for England 1997.* London: Stationery Office (in press).

14.   Bruce I, McKennell A, Walker E, Royal National Institute for the Blind. *Blind and partially sighted adults in Britain: the RNIB survey.* London: HMSO, 1991.

15.   Davis A. *Institute of Hearing Research's report on hearing in adults.* London: Institute of Hearing Research, 1995.

16.   Department of Health NHS Executive. *Signposts for success in commissioning and providing health services for people with learning disabilities.* London: Department of Health (in press).

17.   Department of Health. *Better services for vulnerable people.* London: Department of Health, 1997 (Executive Letter: EL(97)62).

18.   *The Disability Discrimination Act 1995.* London; HMSO, 1995.

(h)   Complementary medicine

Work progressed further towards the implementation of the Osteopaths Act 1993[1] and the Chiropractors Act 1994[2]. The General Osteopathic Council was formally established on 14 January 1997; the statutory register of osteopaths is expected to open in May 1998. The designate General Chiropractic Council started preparatory work in January 1997 and, subject to progress, should be formally established in 1998.

Interest in the provision of complementary therapies within the NHS continued. The two-year pilot scheme of GP purchasing of osteopathy and chiropractic services, which started in July 1996, continued. The evaluation report of a pilot scheme, commissioned by DH from the Medical Care Research Unit at the University of Sheffield, is expected to be completed by Autumn 1998. The field work for a separate study on complementary therapy provision in primary care, commissioned by DH from the same Unit following earlier research, was completed at the end of 1997 and the report is expected to be published in Spring 1998.

References

1. *The Osteopaths Act 1993.* London: HMSO, 1993.
2. *The Chiropractors Act 1994.* London: HMSO, 1994.
3. Thomas K, Fall M, Parry G, Nicholl J. *National survey of access to complementary health care via general practice: final report to the Department of Health.* Sheffield: Medical Care Research Unit, University of Sheffield, 1995.

(i)   Prison health care

Noteworthy developments in prison health care were made during the year.

Training for prison doctors in the two-year Diploma in Prison medicine began in September 1996. The first ten doctors will complete the course in June 1998, and a further ten in 1999. Over this period, the course is being monitored by a committee drawn from members of the Royal Colleges of Physicians of London, General Practitioners and Psychiatrists, who have extended their role to advise the Prison Service on all aspects of training for prison doctors.

Prison governors were advised of the education of nurses necessary for compliance with the statutory post-registration education and practice requirements set by the UK Central Council for Nursing, Midwifery and Health Visiting. Training priorities have been in courses relating to substance misuse, HIV and AIDS, nursing degrees and diplomas, and National Vocational Qualifications (NVQs) for prison health care officers without nursing registration. Newly employed nurses are offered induction into working in a secure environment.

A new Health Promoting Prisons Awards Scheme was launched in 1996, reflecting the importance and viability of health promotion for the prison population. The first awards and certificates were presented to a total of 22 prisons in July 1997.

A provisional total of 750 mentally disordered prisoners were transferred to hospital under the provisions of Sections 47 and 48 of the Mental Health Act 1983[1], a similar figure to that in 1996. The ONS completed field work for a new study of the prevalence of mental disorder in prisons on behalf of DH. In Autumn 1997, the Health Advisory Committee for the Prison Service published the report of its review of the provision of mental health care in prisons[2], which included 16 recommendations to improve services.

A working group of officials from the Prison Service and DH was set up in November to review the organisation and delivery of health services for prisoners, in response to the report by the Chief Inspector of Prisons on prison health care, *Patient or prisoner?*[3] - which identified weaknesses in the present arrangements for the delivery of health care to prisoners, and argued that they could only be addressed by transferring the responsibility for prison health care from the Home Office and Prison Service to the NHS. The working group, chaired jointly by Dr Graham Winyard, Director of Health Services in the NHS, and Dr Michael Longfield, Director of Health Care of HM Prison Service, will report to Ministers with options and recommendations in Summer 1998, after consultation.

References

1. *The Mental Health Act 1983.* London: HMSO, 1983.
2. Health Advisory Committee for the Prison Service for England and Wales. *The provision of mental health care in prisons.* London: Stationery Office, 1997.
3. HM Inspectorate of Prisons for England and Wales. *Patient or prisoner?: a new strategy for health care in prisons.* London: Home Office, 1996.

CHAPTER 6

COMMUNICABLE DISEASES

(a)   HIV infection and AIDS

Health promotion strategy for HIV infection and AIDS

While combination antiretroviral drug therapy[1] has shown considerable clinical benefit during the year, health promotion based on current epidemiology remains the key to the control of the spread of HIV. Implementation of *HIV and AIDS health promotion: an evolving strategy*[2], published in November 1995, continued during 1997. While campaigns for the general public are still needed, greater emphasis is now placed on appropriate targeting of high-risk groups (ie, homosexual and bisexual men, people with links to high-prevalence countries, injecting drug users and partners of people from these groups). Health promotion for the general population and for homosexual and bisexual men continued during 1997. The integrated AIDS/Drugs Helpline also continued to play a valuable role. During the year, a health promotion programme for those who travel to or have links with high prevalence countries, particularly sub-Saharan Africa, was developed.

Epidemiology

AIDS

Surveillance of the epidemic is implemented through the voluntary confidential reporting systems run by the Public Health Laboratory Service (PHLS) AIDS Centre[3,4] and the Government's programme of unlinked anonymous HIV surveys[5].

Details of the AIDS cases reported in England are shown in Table 6.1 and Figure 6.1; 1,282 cases of AIDS were reported in 1997: these brought the cumulative total of AIDS cases reported since 1982 to 13,915, of whom 10,072 are known to have died.

The number of cases reported in 1997 was 26% lower than that reported in 1996, most probably due to the effect of combination antiretroviral drug therapies in delaying progression to a diagnosis of AIDS[6]. Monotherapy with antiretroviral drugs results in a loss of clinical benefit because of the development of virus resistance[7]. Combination therapy using two or more antiretroviral drugs aims further to reduce viral replication and so inhibit the development of resistance,

Table 6.1: *AIDS cases and known deaths by exposure category and year of report, England, 1982-31 December 1997*

(Numbers subject to revision as further data are received or duplicates identified)

How persons probably acquired the virus	Jan 1996-Dec 1996 Cases		Jan 1997-Dec 1997 Cases		Jan 1982-Dec 1997 Males		Females	
	Males	Females	Males	Females	Cases	Deaths	Cases	Deaths
Sexual intercourse:								
Between men	1075	-	703	-	9757	7365	-	-
Between men and women								
Exposure to 'high risk' partner*	4	32	7	17	45	30	158	113
Exposure abroad†	190	159	156	151	1014	584	797	431
Exposure in UK	7	18	5	12	81	62	87	60
Investigation continuing/closed‡	3	2	25	13	32	11	16	4
Injecting drug use (IDU)	79	30	47	22	430	291	183	124
IDU and sexual intercourse								
between men	35	-	20	-	250	180	-	-
Blood								
Blood factor								
(eg, treatment for haemophilia)	46	0	22	0	554	503	5	4
Blood/tissue transfer	7	3	6	4	47	31	72	55
Mother to infant	17	13	18	27	117	60	126	52
Other/undetermined/closed‡	17	2	21	6	124	98	20	14
Total	1480	259	1030	252	12451	9215	1464	857

*Partners exposed to HIV infection through sexual intercourse between men, IDU, blood factor treatment or blood/tissue transfer.

†Individuals from abroad and individuals from the UK who have lived or visited abroad, for whom there is no evidence of 'high risk' partners.

‡Closed = no further information available.

Source: CDSC, PHLS

Figure 6.1: *AIDS cases: total numbers and numbers where infection was probably acquired through sexual intercourse between men and women, England, to 31 December 1997*

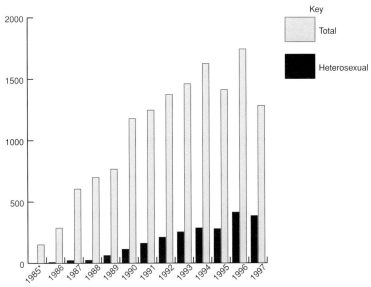

*1985 figure does not include previous years.

Source: CDSC, PHLS

Figure 6.2: *Incidence of AIDS cases diagnosed in Europe in 1996, adjusted for reporting delays: rates per million population*

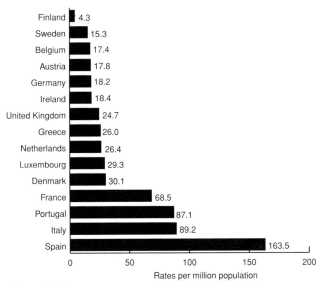

Source: WHO

191

thus delaying disease progression and reducing AIDS-related mortality. However, antiretroviral drugs whether alone or in combination are not a cure for HIV infection, and in the longer term it is possible that resistance to combinations of drugs currently in use will develop. It is therefore essential to maintain prevention efforts to control transmission of HIV infection.

Figure 6.2 compares the incidence rates of AIDS diagnoses per million population of the European Union (EU) Member States for 1996.

HIV infection

Table 6.2 and Figure 6.3 show details of the 2,334 newly diagnosed HIV infections in England, which brings the cumulative total since 1984 to 27,715. More than 2,000 new diagnoses have been reported annually since 1991; most were infections probably acquired as a result of sexual intercourse between men. Many factors influence the decision to be tested for HIV infection, and reported infections underestimate the true number of infections.

Unlinked anonymous surveillance

The fourth report from the Government's Unlinked Anonymous HIV Surveys Steering Group[5] for data to the end of 1996 was published in December. These

Figure 6.3: *HIV-antibody-positive people: total numbers and numbers where infection was probably acquired through sexual intercourse between men and women, England, by year of report to 31 December 1997*

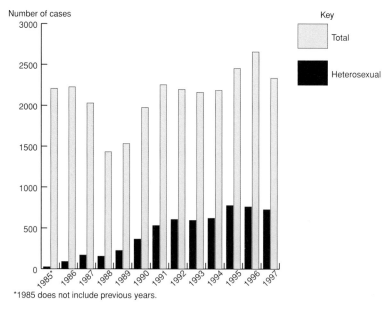

*1985 does not include previous years.

Source: CDSC, PHLS

192

Table 6.2: *HIV-infected persons by exposure category and date of report, England, 1984-31 December 1997*

(Numbers subject to revision as further data are received or duplicates identified)

How persons probably acquired the virus	Jan 1996-Dec 1996			Jan 1997-Dec 1997			Nov 1984-Dec 1997		
	Male	Female	NK	Male	Female	NK	Male	Female	NK
Sexual intercourse:									
Between men	1554	-	0	1254	-	0	17050	-	-
Between men and women									
Exposure to 'high risk' partner*	6	50	0	13	23	0	93	462	0
Exposure abroad†	268	337	3	206	283	2	2160	2248	11
Exposure in the UK	22	36	0	4	21	0	153	267	0
Investigation continuing/closed‡	18	21	0	83	88	4	125	130	4
Injecting drug use (IDU)	94	55	1	82	34	1	1359	628	4
IDU and sexual intercourse between men	46	0	0	18	-	-	450	-	-
Blood									
Blood factor	1	0	0	2	0	0	1152	10	0
Blood/tissue transfer	9	11	0	4	8	0	83	94	3
Mother to infant§	17	25	0	14	21	2	199	211	2
Other/undetermined/closed‡	60	18	2	111	51	5	634	146	37
Total	2095	553	6	1791	529	14	23458	4196	61

NK = Not known (sex not stated on report).

*Partner(s) exposed to HIV infection through sexual intercourse between men, with IDUs, or with those infected through blood factor treatment or blood/tissue transfer.

†Individuals from abroad, and individuals from the UK who have lived or visited abroad, for whom there is no evidence of 'high risk' partners.

‡Closed = no further information available.

§By date of report that established infected status of infant.

Source: CDSC, PHLS

Table 6.3: Prevalence of HIV-1 infection in the unlinked anonymous survey groups, England and Wales, 1996

Survey group	London and South-East England*				England and Wales outside South-East England				Prevalence ratio‡ London vs elsewhere
	Number tested	Number HIV-1 infected	% HIV-1 infected	Prevalence range (%)†	Number tested	Number HIV-1 infected	% HIV-1 infected	Prevalence range (%)†	
Males									
Genito-urinary medicine clinic attenders:									
Homo/bisexual§	4410	445	10	4.9, 17	1409	41	2.9	0.00, 4.8	3.5
Heterosexual§	13211	144	1.1	0.51, 2.3	17119	23	0.13	0.00, 0.29	8.1
Injecting drug users (IDUs) attending agencies#	552	7	1.3	1.1, 1.3	1884	5	0.27	0.00, 1.7	4.8
Hospital blood counts (sentinel group)	22261	158	0.71	0.21, 1.7	-	-	-	-	-
Females									
Genito-urinary medicine clinic attenders:									
Heterosexual§	18451	139	0.75	0.38, 1.1	16232	14	0.086	0.00, 0.18	8.7
IDUs attending agencies#	385	4	1.0	0.00, 1.6	552	5	0.91	0.00, 5.9	1.1
Pregnant women at delivery (infant dried blood spots)**	104666	200	0.19	0.00, 0.61	269633	43	0.016	0.00, 0.069	12.0
Pregnant women seeking terminations	7754	50	0.64	0.36, 1.5	-	-	-	-	-
Hospital blood counts (sentinel group)	45095	106	0.24	0.031, 0.50	-	-	-	-	-

* The injecting drug user (IDU) survey includes data from a few agencies in the South-East outside London; all other surveys present data for London.

† The range within a category is the lowest and highest rates recorded in individual genito-urinary medicine clinics (GUM survey), regions (IDU survey), districts (infant dried blood spot survey) or hospitals (termination of pregnancy, antenatal and hospital surveys).

‡ The ratio by which the prevalence of infection in London is greater than the prevalence in England and Wales outside South-East England.

§ Excluding known drug users.

\# Attending specialist centres for IDUs.

** Prevalence in South-East England outside London was 0.017% (13 of 77,773) in 1996. In Northern and Yorkshire Region data for pregnant women come from the antenatal survey.

Source: Unlinked Anonymous HIV Surveys

surveys supplement data from voluntary confidential testing and permit a more accurate picture of the epidemic. The surveys are established in a number of genito-urinary medicine (GUM) clinics, centres for injecting drug users (IDUs), London hospitals and antenatal clinics; screening of neonatal dried blood spots also takes place.

Results are summarised in Table 6.3 and show that, whilst prevalence is highest in London, HIV-1 infection is present in high-risk groups in every region surveyed. The prevalence in 1996 among homosexual/bisexual men attending GUM clinics was one in ten in London and the South East, compared with one in 34 elsewhere.

Prevalence among IDUs was about one in 80 for men and one in 100 for women in London and the South-East, and one in 380 for men and one in 110 for women elsewhere. There is little evidence of current substantial HIV transmission through injecting drug use, but about 18% of current IDUs report recent sharing of equipment, and these rates are higher among young injectors and women.

In London HIV-1 prevalence among pregnant women giving birth in 1996 was about one in 520 compared with one in 6,200 in the rest of England and Wales

Figure 6.4: *Trends in prevalence of HIV infection among women who give birth, by area of residence in Inner London, Outer London, and the rest of England, 1988-96*

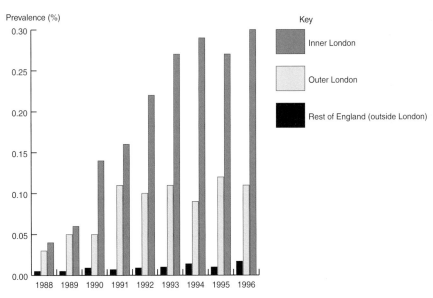

Source: Survey in North Thames and South Thames (West) co-ordinated by
Institute of Child Health, London; survey elsewhere co-ordinated by
PHLS AIDS Centre (commenced in 1990)

195

(see Figure 6.4). Comparison of data from the surveys with reported births to HIV-1-infected mothers indicate that in 1995-96 over 75% of these infections had not been clinically recognised, and consequently these women could not be offered interventions to reduce the risk of their baby being infected with HIV[5]. These interventions include the use of antiretroviral drugs during pregnancy, labour and, after birth, to the infant; avoidance of breast-feeding; and obstetric management measures. The risk of transmission from mother to baby can be reduced from one in six to one in 18 by the use of these interventions[8]. The Department of Health (DH) and others[9] recommend actively offering HIV testing to all pregnant women in higher prevalence areas so that the number of infected children born in the United Kingdom (UK) can be reduced. The Expert Advisory Group on AIDS set up a working group to produce a leaflet for pregnant women which provides information on which to base an informed decision about HIV testing. This leaflet will be tested for acceptability early in 1998. In addition, the Department is working with professional nursing and midwifery bodies to address training needs.

Post-exposure prophylaxis for occupational exposure

The risk of acquiring HIV infection after a needlestick injury is small, about three per 1,000 injuries. After a study in the United States of America (USA) which indicated that this risk could be reduced still further if zidovudine is taken prophylactically as soon as possible after occupational exposure[10], the Expert Advisory Group on AIDS considered the available evidence and issued guidelines in June[11]. Post-exposure prophylaxis (PEP) should be recommended to health care workers if they have been exposed to blood or other high-risk body fluids or tissues known or strongly suspected to be infected with HIV.

An improved surveillance system for occupational exposure was established at the Communicable Disease Surveillance Centre (CDSC) of the PHLS to monitor the uptake of and reaction to PEP for HIV, as well as any transmissions of HIV infection subsequent to such exposure.

HIV in blood donations

During 1997, 3.0 million blood donations in the UK were tested with anti-HIV-1+2 combined tests. Thirty-two donations (from 23 males and 9 females) were found to be anti-HIV-1 seropositive, or 1 in 95,000 (0.001%). The number of new donors tested was 317,094, of whom 22 were seropositive (1 in 14,413 or 0.007%). Again, no donations were found to be anti-HIV-2 seropositive during 1997.

Table 6.4 shows the number of donations tested in the UK between Autumn 1985 and the end of 1997, together with the number of donations confirmed as HIV

Table 6.4: *HIV in blood donations in the United Kingdom, October 1985 to December 1997*

Year	Donations tested (million)	Donations confirmed HIV-seropositive			
		Male	Female	Total	%
1985	0.6	13	0	13	0.002
1986	2.64	44	9	53	0.002
1987	2.59	18	5	23	0.0009
1988	2.64	18	5	23	0.0009
1989	2.74	25	12	37	0.001
1990	2.82	20*	12	32*	0.001
1991	2.95	23	8	31	0.001
1992	2.90	15	11	26	0.0009
1993	2.92	16	4	20	0.0007
1994	2.91	8	8	16	0.0005
1995	2.90	20	10	30	0.001
1996	2.91	13	9	22	0.0008
1997	3.04	23	9	32	0.001
Total	*34.56*	*256*	*102*	*358*	*0.001*

*Includes one anti-HIV-2-positive donation.

Source: PHLS, National Blood Authority

seropositive. The male:female ratio of seropositive donations in 1997 was 2.6 to 1, and was 2.7 to 1 for new donors.

HIV infection was diagnosed in a patient who had received many units of blood in the previous year and had no other risk-factors. Stored samples from the units given to the patient were investigated and none contained HIV antibodies but one contained HIV RNA, and the donor had subsequently developed HIV antibodies[12]. To reduce the risk of collecting blood from donors in the 'window period' before antibodies develop, individuals at an increased risk of HIV infection are advised not to donate blood. This case was the first documented incident of an HIV infectious donation entering the blood supply in England since anti-HIV testing of donations began in 1985.

References

1.	British HIV Association Guidelines Co-ordinating Committee. British HIV Association guidelines for antiretroviral treatment of HIV seropositive individuals. *Lancet* 1997; **349:** 1086-92.
2.	Department of Health. *HIV and AIDS health promotion: an evolving strategy.* London: Department of Health, 1995.
3.	Public Health Laboratory Service AIDS Centre. The surveillance of HIV-1 infection and AIDS in England and Wales. *Commun Disease Rep CDR Rev* 1991; **1:** R51-6.

4.   Waight PA, Rush AM, Miller E. Surveillance of HIV infection by voluntary testing in England. *Commun Dis Rep CDR Rev* 1992; **2:** R85-90.

5.   Department of Health. *Unlinked anonymous HIV prevalence monitoring programme: England and Wales: data to the end of 1996: summary report from the Unlinked Anonymous Surveys Steering Group.* London: Department of Health, 1997.

6.   Public Health Laboratory Service. Changes in the incidence of AIDS and in AIDS deaths: the effect of antiretroviral treatment. *Commun Dis Rep CDR Weekly* 1997; **7:** 381.

7.   Moyle GJ. Use of viral resistance patterns to antiretroviral drugs in optimising selection of drug combinations and sequences. *Drugs* 1996; **52:** 168-85.

8.   Connor EM, et al. Reduction of maternal-infant transmission of HIV-1 with zidovudine treatment. *N Engl J Med* 1994; **331:** 1173-80.

9.   Intercollegiate Working Party for Enhancing Voluntary Confidential HIV Testing in Pregnancy. *Reducing mother-to-child transmission of HIV infection in the UK.* London: Royal College of Paediatrics and Child Health (in press).

10.   Centers for Disease Control. Case-control study of HIV seroconversion in health-care workers after percutaneous exposure to HIV-infected blood: France, United Kingdom and United States: January 1988-August 1994. *MMWR* 1995; **44:** 929-33.

11.   Department of Health. *Guidelines on post-exposure prophylaxis for health care workers occupationally exposed to HIV.* London: Department of Health, 1997.

12.   Anonymous. *HIV infection transmitted through transfusion. Commun Dis Rep CDR Weekly* 1997; **7:** 137.

(b)   Other sexually transmitted infections

All figures for sexually transmitted infections (STIs) are derived from the KC60 reporting form for consultations in National Health Service (NHS) GUM clinics; cases diagnosed and managed elsewhere are not included. Responsibility for the collation and analysis of the data set was contracted to the PHLS CDSC in June 1997, and data for 1996 will be published in the *Communicable Disease Report (CDR) Review*[1].

The total number of new cases seen in GUM clinics in England in 1996 was 422,204 (see Table 6.5). Of these, approximately 23% were for wart virus infection, 18% for non-specific genital infection, 10% for uncomplicated chlamydial infection, 7% for herpes simplex virus (HSV) and 3% for gonorrhoea.

Total diagnoses of acute STIs rose by 7% between 1995 and 1996. The reasons for this increase are not clear, but the increased incidence is a reminder of the continuing need for information about sexual health and safer sex messages. The rises in diagnoses of uncomplicated gonorrhoea, uncomplicated chlamydial infection, the first attack of genital warts and genital herpes simplex were greatest among teenagers aged 16-19 years.

About 45% of acute STIs were reported in the Thames health regions. Regional distributions of different diagnoses varied considerably, but increased numbers of diagnoses were made in almost all regions. Around 20% of male diagnoses of

Table 6.5: *Sexually transmitted infections reported by NHS genito-urinary medicine clinics, England, in year ending 31 December 1996*

Condition	Males	Females	Persons
Total number of new cases seen	180828	241376	422204
All syphilis	763	442	1205
Infectious syphilis	*84*	*33*	*117*
All gonorrhoea	8939	5465	14404
Uncomplicated gonorrhoea	*7749*	*3902*	*11651*
Gonococcal ophthalmia neonatorum	*2*	*3*	*5*
Epidemiological treatment of suspected gonorrhoea	*1120*	*1346*	*2466*
Gonococcal complications	*68*	*214*	*282*
All *Chlamydia*	20257	24040	44297
Uncomplicated Chlamydia infection	*13694*	*18163*	*31857*
Complicated Chlamydia infection	*274*	*1007*	*1281*
Chlamydial ophthalmia neonatorum	*16*	*26*	*42*
Epidemiological treatment of suspected Chlamydia	*6273*	*4844*	*11117*
All Herpes simplex	11406	16090	27496
Anogenital Herpes simplex - first attack	*5641*	*9349*	*14990*
Anogenital Herpes simplex - recurrence	*5765*	*6741*	*12506*
All Wart virus infection	53116	44124	97240
Anogenital warts - first attack	*26636*	*27101*	*53737*
Anogenital warts - recurrence	*19673*	*11217*	*30890*
Anogenital warts - re-registered cases	*6807*	*5806*	*12613*
Chancroid/LGV/Donovanosis	52	27	79
Uncomplicated non-gonococcal/non-specific urethritis in males	45868	-	45868
Epidemiological treatment of NSGI	4312	16146	20458
Complicated non-gonococcal/non-specific infection	2189	7844	10033
Trichomoniasis	231	5302	5533
Anaerobic/bacterial vaginosis, male infection & other vaginosis/vaginitis/balanitis	13158	49524	62682
Anogenital candidiasis	7979	61732	69711
Scabies/pediculosis pubis	4257	1351	5608
Antigen-positive viral hepatitis B	445	195	640
Other viral hepatitis	880	354	1234
Other	6976	8740	15716

LGV = lymphogranuloma venereum; NSGI = non-specific genital infection.

Source: Form KC60

Table 6.6: *New cases of selected conditions reported by NHS genito-urinary medicine clinics by age (in years), England, 1996*

Condition	Sex	All ages	Under 16	16-19	20-24	25-34	35-44	45 and over	Not known
Infectious syphilis*	M	84	1	3	9	30	18	16	7
	F	33	0	3	4	10	9	5	2
Post-pubertal uncomplicated gonorrhoea	M	7749	26	869	2000	3526	947	309	72
	F	3902	126	1343	1243	922	179	53	36
Post-pubertal uncomplicated *Chlamydia*	M	13694	35	1326	4508	6055	1336	357	77
	F	18163	428	5508	6480	4646	764	165	172
Herpes simplex - first attack	M	5641	10	255	1222	2636	963	514	41
	F	9349	113	1572	2728	3282	1051	476	127
Wart virus infection - first attack	M	26636	83	1900	8828	11145	3066	1393	221
	F	27101	439	7056	9768	6785	1834	898	321

*Primary and secondary syphilis only.

Source: Form KC60

uncomplicated gonorrhoea were reported as homosexually acquired; in the North Thames region, at least 40% of new male cases of gonorrhoea were homosexually acquired, compared with 14% elsewhere.

In 1996, total reports of gonorrhoea rose by 17%, compared with 1995, to 14,404; the total number of diagnoses of uncomplicated chlamydial infection rose by 11% to 31,857 (an increase of 9% in men and 12% in women). Uncomplicated cases of non-specific genital infections rose by 4% from 63,593 in 1995 to 66,326 in 1996. There was a 10% fall in diagnoses of primary and secondary infectious syphilis (117 cases in 1996 compared with 130 in 1995).

First attacks of HSV infection rose slightly to 14,990 in 1996. First attacks of HSV declined in males by about 3% but first attacks rose by some 4% among females. Recurrence attacks rose by some 5% overall and accounted for 45% of all diagnoses of HSV infection during 1996. Total diagnoses of viral warts rose by about 6%, and recurrence attacks accounted for 32% of all reports of wart virus infection during 1996.

Other aspects of GUM clinic workload will be reported in the *Communicable Disease Report (CDR) Review*[1]; for example, 88,002 other conditions requiring treatment were identified and 138,144 individuals received pre-test discussion for HIV testing, of whom 84% underwent an HIV test.

Figure 6.5: *All gonorrhoea: number of new cases seen at NHS genito-urinary medicine clinics, England, 1980-96*

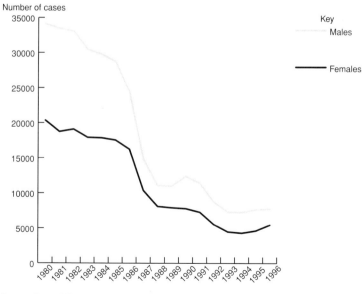

Source: Forms SBH60 and KC60

A high proportion of reports of STIs come from patients in younger age-groups (see Table 6.6).

Reference

1.   Simms I, Hughes G, Swan AV, Rogers PA, Catchpole M. New cases seen at genito-urinary
      medicine clinics: England: 1996. *Commun Dis Rep CDR Rev* (in press).

(c)   Chlamydia

Chlamydia trachomatis is the most common, curable sexually transmitted infection in England. Infections are often symptomless and consequently undiagnosed, but can have long-term consequences. Chlamydial infection is a well-established cause of pelvic inflammatory disease (PID) which can lead to infertility, ectopic pregnancy and chronic pain.

Symptomless disease will usually only be discovered by chance or by screening. Systematic screening for *Chlamydia* in the UK only takes place in GUM clinics, although evidence from other countries indicates health gains from wider screening. An Expert Advisory Group on *Chlamydia trachomatis* was established in November 1996 to help to identify the available options.

The Group's main conclusions, which will be published in Spring 1998[1], are that:

- good clinical practice requires testing of those with symptoms associated with chlamydial infection (eg, women with PID, men with non-specific urethritis, and infants with ophthalmia neonatorum and their parents), all attenders at GUM clinics and the partners of those infected, and all women seeking termination of pregnancy and the partners of those infected;

- evidence supports screening of symptomless, sexually active women aged under 25 years, especially teenagers, and also of symptom-free women aged over 25 years who have had a new sexual partner or have had two or more partners in a year; *and*

- opportunistic screening in settings where the risk of infection can be established before it is offered, such as in general practice and family planning clinics, would be a more appropriate option than a register-based call and recall procedure, which could not identify those who are sexually active and therefore at risk.

These screening proposals primarily concentrate on women because the consequences of infection are more severe for women than for men. It is expected that, after screening, positive cases would usually be referred to GUM clinics, which have the established protocols for partner notification necessary for the detection of symptomless cases among men.

Effective implementation of these proposals will require close collaboration between specialties to produce national guidelines and local protocols. The development of screening has been hampered by a lack of awareness of chlamydial infection and its long-term consequences, among health-care professionals and the general public alike, and education campaigns for both groups will be essential. Further research needs will also be identified.

The Group's report has been considered by the National Screening Committee and DH, and work on its recommendations will be taken forward during 1998.

Reference

1.   Department of Health Expert Advisory Group on *Chlamydia trachomatis. Chlamydia trachomatis: summary and conclusions of the Chief Medical Officer's Expert Advisory Group.* London: Department of Health (in press).

(d)   Immunisation

Immunisation coverage has remained at extremely high levels for all antigens (see Appendix Table A.9), although there has been a small but concerning decline in measles, mumps and rubella (MMR) vaccine coverage. Following publication of articles reporting purported associations between measles, measles vaccine and Crohn's disease, there has been considerable media interest in these putative associations, despite evidence to refute these theories (see page 13). Surveys of public attitudes on vaccine safety, carried out twice yearly on behalf of the Health Education Authority (HEA), indicate that parents' concerns have increased as a result of the suggested adverse effects. Despite the small decrease in reported coverage, measles notifications and reports of confirmed cases remain at extremely low levels, as do reports of other vaccine-preventable diseases.

In 1988, the World Health Assembly announced the objective of the global eradication of poliomyelitis by the year 2000. This will require every country to demonstrate that it has interrupted the transmission of wild virus poliomyelitis and has in place surveillance sufficiently sensitive to detect polio viruses should they be present. Since most poliovirus infections are inapparent, the virological surveillance is particularly challenging. An expert panel, chaired by Professor Alexander Campbell, Emeritus Professor of Child Health at the University of Aberdeen, has prepared a report that demonstrates the absence of polio from the UK, which has been accepted by the European Commission for Certification of Polio Elimination as sufficient evidence that wild virus transmission has indeed been interrupted in the UK.

(e)   Viral hepatitis

Data on viral hepatitis given below are obtained through the voluntary confidential reporting by laboratories of confirmed cases to the PHLS CDSC.

Hepatitis A

The incidence of hepatitis A infections fluctuates, the most recent peak being in 1990 when 7,248 cases were reported to the CDSC for England. Reports decreased in each of the six subsequent years with 1,024 reports received for 1996, but rose to 1,260 in 1997 (see Figure 6.6). This 23% increase, compared with 1996 figures, was due almost entirely to an increase of reports, from 588 to 871, among men. Most cases of hepatitis A infection seen in England are acquired in the UK and whilst most are sporadic, outbreaks do occur. However, a history of travel abroad in the six weeks before the onset of illness was recorded in 173 (14%) of cases reported to the CDSC in 1997; the Indian sub-Continent was the most frequently cited destination.

Hepatitis B

Reports of acute hepatitis B in England peaked in 1984 with 1,889 reports, and subsequently fell (see Figure 6.7). The CDSC received reports of 616 cases in 1997, a rise of 16% compared with 1996. Information about exposure risk was available in 368 (60%) cases; of these, 48% were likely to have acquired infection as a result of injecting drug misuse, 23% as a result of sexual intercourse between men and women, and 14% as a result of sexual intercourse between men. Much acute hepatitis B is subclinical, not diagnosed and hence not reported.

Hepatitis C

Hepatitis C rarely produces an acute symptomatic illness with jaundice, and hence few incident infections are diagnosed. Evidence of infection is detected by testing for antibodies to the virus (anti-HCV), although such tests do not distinguish between previous resolved, and established chronic, infection. Laboratory reports of the presence of antibodies to hepatitis C received by the CDSC for England increased from 27 in 1991 to 2,965 in 1997. This rise is consistent with the increasing frequency of testing over that period. In 1997, the prevalence of anti-HCV among new blood donors was 0.06%.

During the year, the Department commissioned a number of research projects, at a total cost of approximately £1 million, to study the prevalence, modes of transmission and natural history of hepatitis C. These included funding to set up

Figure 6.6: *Reports of hepatitis A to CDSC, England, 1980-97*

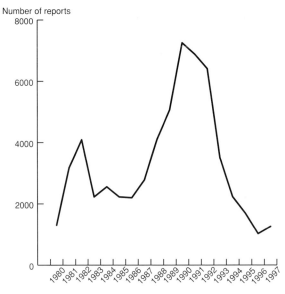

Number of reports

Source: PHLS, CDSC

Figure 6.7: *Reports of hepatitis B to CDSC (all reports and reports in injecting drug users), England, 1980-97*

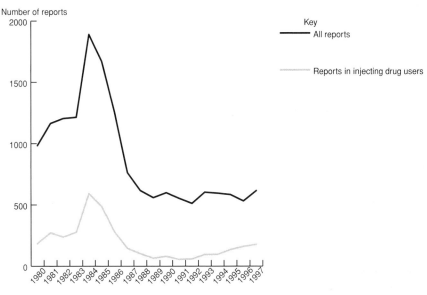

Number of reports

Key
— All reports

⋯ Reports in injecting drug users

Source: PHLS, CDSC

a national register of hepatitis C virus infections with known dates of acquisition to follow the natural history of hepatitis C infection and response to treatments. Testing also began of samples from the unlinked anonymous serosurveys of antenatal patients and GUM clinic attenders for anti-HCV to assess prevalence in these groups.

Hepatitis E

Hepatitis E is spread by the faecal-oral route, and large outbreaks have occurred in some endemic areas in association with faecally contaminated drinking water. The virus is not endemic in the UK. In 1997, the CDSC received reports of 19 cases for England; in the 11 for which information was available, all were associated with a history of recent travel to endemic areas, ten to the Indian sub-Continent and one to West Africa.

(f)   Influenza

Consultations to practices in the Royal College of General Practitioners' (RCGPs') Weekly Returns Service scheme for influenza and influenza-like illness, which had begun to increase towards the end of November 1996, reached a peak of 229 new consultations/100,000 population per week in the first week of January 1997; they had returned to baseline levels of below 50/100,000 population per week by early March. Isolates of influenza A (H_3N_2) viruses peaked at the same time. Although this rate of morbidity from influenza is only just above expected winter levels, a sharp rise in registered deaths from any cause - comparable in size to that seen during the last major influenza epidemic in 1989/90 - occurred in the first three weeks of 1997. The contribution of influenza to these deaths is unknown; only 274 deaths were attributed to influenza on the death certificate. The overall rise in mortality is likely to have been due to a combination of a sharp, very cold spell of weather towards the end of 1996, influenza and other co-circulating respiratory viruses.

The risk-groups recommended for influenza immunisation were unchanged for the 1997/98 influenza season. General practitioners (GPs) were reminded of the policy, and of the need to plan their influenza immunisation programmes, in August 1997[1]; the two DH leaflets on influenza were also re-issued[2,3]. A record 7.3 million doses of influenza vaccine were administered, a 16% increase from the 1996/97 season. However, preliminary data derived from the GP research database indicate that many in the recommended risk-groups, particularly among those under 65 years-of-age, remain unimmunised[4]. Further analyses of these data are awaited.

In March 1997, the UK Health Departments published their contingency plan for pandemic influenza[5]. This plan is primarily for central use, but provides a framework for the development of more detailed local plans. Health authorities were reminded of the need for their emergency plans to encompass the contingency of an influenza pandemic[6].

The pandemic plan describes a phased response, starting with the isolation from human beings of a 'new' influenza virus with a novel haemagglutinin and/or neuraminidase. In December 1997, an outbreak of illness due to an avian H_5N_1 influenza virus not previously known to infect man occurred in Hong Kong[7]. The UK plan was activated and an Influenza Advisory Committee convened. In the event, all the cases appeared to have been infected from chickens and no person-to-person transmission of infection was confirmed. The outbreak was controlled by a cull of all chickens in Hong Kong, and cleansing of chicken farms and markets before restocking. The UK Committee was subsequently stood down, although work continues internationally to develop an H_5 influenza vaccine for use should this virus, or a closely related variant, reappear.

References

1. Department of Health. Influenza immunisation. *CMO's Update* 1997; **15**:1.
2. Department of Health. *'Flu vaccination.* London: Department of Health, 1996.
3. Department of Health. *What should I do about 'flu?* London: Department of Health, 1996.
4. PHLS Communicable Disease Surveillance Centre. Uptake of influenza vaccine in high risk patients. *Commun Dis Rep CDR Rev 1997*; **45**: 401, 404.
5. UK Health Departments. *Multiphase contingency plan for pandemic influenza.* London: Department of Health, 1997.
6. Department of Health NHS Executive. *UK Health Departments' contingency plan for pandemic influenza: the influenza pandemic plan.* Leeds: Department of Health, 1997 (Executive Letter: EL(97)6).
7. Department of Health. *Avian (H_5N_1) influenza in Hong Kong.* London: Department of Health, 1997 (Professional Letter: PL(CMO)97/3).

(g)   Meningitis

Since 1995, there has been an increase in the incidence of meningococcal disease[1] which has continued into 1997. This increased incidence was associated with a shift in age distribution, with more cases being reported in older children and young adults, and an increase in the proportion of infections due to Group C meningococci. However, data for late 1997 indicate that the incidence has now started to fall (see Table 6.7). Among culture-confirmed infections, the proportion due to Group C meningococcal disease remained high (39%)[2], and clusters of Group C cases in schools and universities continued to be reported in the winter of 1997. Similar increases in meningococcal disease have been observed in recent years in Scotland[3], Canada[4] and the USA[5]. The increase in Canada was attributed to a new clone of Group C *Neisseria meningitidis*. Much

Table 6.7: *Meningococcal disease notifications and deaths reported to the Office for National Statistics (ONS), isolates referred to the Meningococcal Reference Unit (MRU), and estimated case fatality rates, England and Wales, 1989-97*

Year	Notifications to ONS	MRU reports	Deaths registered	Estimated crude case-fatality rate
1989	1362	1354	203	14.9
1990	1415	1500	169	11.9
1991	1390	1405	170	12.2
1992	1344	1301	162	12.0
1993	1451	1298	173	11.9
1994	1368	1129	149	10.9
1995	1847	1468	196	10.6
1996	2313	1495	235	10.2
1997	2660	1587	244	9.2

Source: ONS and MRU

of the recent increase in this country was attributable to serotype C2a infections and therefore probably represents the emergence of a new clone of Group C infection in England and Wales.

The total number of deaths was also higher than in recent years but the estimated crude case-fatality has continued to fall. This may be due to changes in clinical practice, such as fewer lumbar punctures being performed and the use of pre-admission antibiotics.

References

1. Ramsay M, Kaczmarski E, Rush M, Farrington P, White J. Changing patterns of case ascertainment and trends in meningococcal disease in England and Wales. *Commun Dis Rep CDR Rev* 1997; **4**: R49-54.
2. Kaczmarski EB. Meningococcal disease in England and Wales: 1995. *Commun Dis Rep CDR Rev* 1997: **4**: R55-9.
3. Fallon RJ. Meningococcal infection in Scotland. *J Med Microbiol* 1988; **26**: 161-87.
4. Whalen CM, Hockin JC, Ryan A, Ashton F. The changing epidemiology of invasive meningococcal disease in Canada, 1985 through 1992: emergence of a virulent clone of *Neisseria meningitidis*. *JAMA* 1995; **273**: 390-4.
5. Jackson LA, Schuchat A, Reeves MW, Wenger JD. Serogroup C meningococcal outbreaks in the United States: an emerging threat. *JAMA* 1995; **273**: 383-9.

(h)   Tuberculosis

Although there is continued concern about the failure to control tuberculosis in many parts of the world - particularly in Asia and Africa - notifications of cases of tuberculosis in England and Wales during 1997 remained fairly steady at 5,859 (provisional) compared with 5,654 in 1996 and 5,608 in 1995. Rates of drug-resistant disease remained low. There were 392 notified deaths.

Final results of the last five-yearly survey of tuberculosis notifications in England and Wales confirmed that, whilst the number of cases and the annual notification rate for previously untreated tuberculosis increased between 1988 and 1993, there were important differences between ethnic groups[1]. Among caucasians, the number of notifications fell and comprised 44% of all notifications, compared with 53% in 1988; however, the rate of decline in the notification rate seen between earlier surveys had slowed and was not seen in all age-groups. Total notifications among those from the Indian sub-Continent increased from 39% to 41%, and in 'other' ethnic groups increased from 8% to 14%. Forty-nine per cent of patients had been born abroad, with the highest rates among those who had recently arrived in the UK. Of adults aged 16-54 years with notified tuberculosis, 2.3% were estimated to be HIV-infected, although there was evidence of under-reporting.

The importance of early recognition of symptoms of tuberculosis in health-care workers was highlighted in a four-year prospective study from the West Midlands[2]. Doctors and nurses accounted for most cases of tuberculosis among hospital staff. All but one of the doctors had probably acquired their disease abroad, but all but one of the nurses had been born in the UK; their higher than expected incidence of tuberculosis raised the possibility that some of these infections had been occupationally acquired, and requires further monitoring.

The increasing problem of tuberculosis in cattle in the UK led to the Krebs review on bovine tuberculosis in cattle and badgers[3]. Currently, only 1-2% of isolates from human infection are identified as *Mycobacterium bovis;* these are mainly from older people and believed to represent reactivation of previous infection. Nonetheless, the Government accepted the recommendation that the risk to human beings should continue to be carefully monitored.

References

1.   Kumar D, Watson JM, Charlett A, Nicholas S, Darbyshire JH, on behalf of a PHLS/BTS/DH Collaborative Group. Tuberculosis in England and Wales in 1993: results of a national survey. *Thorax* 1997; **52:** 1060-7.
2.   Hill A, Burge A, Skinner C. Tuberculosis in National Health Service hospital staff in the West Midlands region of England, 1992-95. *Thorax* 1997; **52:** 994-7.
3.   Independent Scientific Review Group. *Bovine tuberculosis in cattle and badgers: report to the Rt Hon Dr Jack Cunningham MP.* London: Ministry of Agriculture, Fisheries and Food, 1997. Chair: Professor John Krebs.

(i)   Hospital-acquired infection

Interest in the prevention of hospital-acquired infection has increased further during the year, particularly in view of its role in reducing the spread of multiply antibiotic-resistant micro-organisms. In October, the House of Lords Committee on Science and Technology began an inquiry into microbial antibiotic resistance; this is referred to in more detail below, with other aspects of antibiotic-resistant infections including the production of new guidelines on methicillin-resistant *Staphylococcus aureus* (MRSA)[1].

The findings of a DH-funded study, *Hospital-acquired infection: surveillance, policies and practice*[2] were published in May. The study team and collaborators in the 19 study hospitals also produced consensus-based clinical guidelines[3], which provide a basis for the production of nationally accepted evidence-based clinical guidelines to allow hospitals to assess their own methods of prevention and control of hospital-acquired infection against a recognised standard. In July, DH issued an invitation to tender for production of these guidelines, planned for completion in the year 2000. As well as general principles for the prevention of infection, topics such as management of invasive devices, care of surgical wounds and patient isolation procedures will be addressed.

The new Nosocomial Infection National Surveillance Scheme, which also uses experience gained in the earlier project[2], allows hospitals to compare, on a confidential basis, their infection rates with those of others. This scheme has been well received and about 150 hospitals have so far been involved. Modules for hospital-acquired bacteraemia and surgical site infections became available during the year.

In the Autumn, the National Audit Office started an investigation into a number of aspects of hospital infection control, particularly in relation to compliance with existing guidance and the availability of hospital policies and procedures, which will continue during 1998.

References

1.   British Society for Antimicrobial Chemotherapy, Hospital Infection Society, Infection Control Nurses Association. Revised guidelines for the control of methicillin-resistant *Staphylococcus aureus* infection in hospitals. *J Hosp Infec* (in press).
2.   Charlett A, Cole N, Cookson B, et al. *Hospital-acquired infection: surveillance, policies and practice.* London: Public Health Laboratory Service, 1997.
3.   Cookson B, Glynn A, Taylor L, Ward V, Wilson J. *Preventing hospital-acquired infection: clinical guidelines: a supplement to hospital-acquired infection: surveillance, policies and practice.* Public Health Laboratory Service, 1997.

(j)   Antimicrobial-resistant infection

The emergence of resistance to antibiotics is to some extent an inevitable consequence of exposure to an antimicrobial agent; sensitive organisms are killed, leaving resistant ones free to flourish - be they infecting organisms or part of the normal commensal flora. Unfortunately, as we now know, resistance genes can then be transferred to other organisms[1].

Given the increasing prevalence of resistant organisms and the paucity of potential new agents for use in the immediate future, more concerted action is required to delay, if not reverse, the further development of resistance to antimicrobial agents in current use. Organisms of particular concern include *Staphylococci*, *Enterococci*, *Pneumococci*, *Salmonellae* and *Mycobacteria*. Among these, MRSA with reduced sensitivity to vancomycin, which renders them virtually untreatable, were reported from Japan during 1997[2].

Discussions on the control of antimicrobial resistance have mainly centred on the need to limit the use of antimicrobials, particularly where inappropriate; however, a truly strategic approach must consider human, veterinary and agricultural aspects of surveillance, antimicrobial use, infection control (to limit the need for antimicrobials as well as the spread of already resistant organisms), and research needs. International collaboration is essential.

In July, the House of Lords Select Committee on Science and Technology began a wide-ranging Inquiry into resistance to antibiotics and other antimicrobial agents; its report is expected in Spring 1998.

At the request of the Chief Medical Officer, the Standing Medical Advisory Committee established a sub-group chaired by Dr Diana Walford, Director of the PHLS, to examine antimicrobial resistance in relation to clinical prescribing practice and to make recommendations; its report is expected in Summer 1998.

The Advisory Committee on the Microbiological Safety of Food (ACMSF) working group on microbial resistance in relation to food safety continued its investigation into the role of food in the acquisition of antimicrobial-resistant organisms, and is expected to report during 1998.

DH continued to work with representatives from three professional organisations to revise the clinical guidelines on the control of MRSA.

Antimicrobial resistance is being given high priority in the programme of the World Health Organization's (WHO's) Emerging and other Communicable Diseases Surveillance and Control (EMC) Division.

211

References

1. Sanders CC, Sanders WE. Beta-lactam resistance in Gram negative bacteria: global trends and clinical impact. *Clin Infect Dis* 1992; **15**: 824-39.
2. Hiramatsu K, et al. Methicillin-resistant *Staphylococcus aureus* clinical strain with reduced vancomycin susceptibility. *J Antimicrob Chemother* 1997; **40**: 135-6.

(k)   New variant Creutzfeldt-Jakob disease and transmissible spongiform encephalopathies

In March 1996, the National Creutzfeldt-Jakob disease (CJD) Surveillance Unit, established in 1990 and funded by DH and the Scottish Office to monitor the incidence of CJD and to investigate its epidemiology[1], identified ten patients aged under 42 years who had a previously unrecognised form of CJD[2]. Now known as new variant CJD (nvCJD), this disease presents with unusual clinical features and shows a distinctive appearance in the brain tissues compared with classic CJD; all cases so far identified are in patients aged under 50 years. The independent expert Spongiform Encephalopathy Advisory Committee (SEAC) concluded that the most likely explanation was that these cases are linked to exposure to bovine spongiform encephalopathy (BSE) before the introduction of the specified bovine offals ban in 1989.

Further research published in October 1997[3,4] was considered by the SEAC, which concluded that it provided convincing evidence that the agent which causes nvCJD in human beings is the same as that which causes BSE in cattle. These findings do not, however, identify the means by which patients become infected.

There were three deaths attributed to nvCJD in 1995 and ten in 1996; during 1997 ten deaths from nvCJD have so far been identified, making a total of 23 cases of nvCJD, all of whom have died; in 22 of these, the diagnosis has been confirmed by the examination of brain tissue. Altogether, there were 74 deaths from definite or probable CJD and Gerstmann-Sträussler-Scheinker syndrome (GSS) during 1997. These figures remain provisional until the 1997 data are finalised (see Table 6.8).

It is still likely to be some years before sufficient data on the incidence of nvCJD are available to make soundly based assessments of the likely number of future cases, but a sub-group of the SEAC will keep all information on nvCJD under review so that any emerging trend in the incidence of the disease can be detected.

DH's overriding priority is the protection of public health and it continues to work with colleagues across Government Departments and Agencies and with

Table 6.8: *Deaths due to definite and probable cases of Creutzfeldt-Jakob disease (CJD) and Gerstmann-Sträussler-Scheinker syndrome (GSS), and referrals to the UK CJD Surveillance Unit, United Kingdom, 1985-97*

Year	Referrals	Creutzfeldt-Jakob disease				GSS	Total	Sporadic incidence/ million population*
		Sporadic	nvCJD	Iatrogenic	Familial			
1985	-	26	-	1	1	0	28	0.45
1986	-	26	-	0	0	0	26	0.45
1987	-	23	-	0	0	1	24	0.39
1988	-	22	-	1	1	0	24	0.38
1989	-	28	-	2	2	0	32	0.48
1990	53	28	-	5	0	0	33	0.48
1991	75	32	-	1	3	0	36	0.55
1992	96	44	-	2	4	1	51	0.75
1993	78	38	-	4	2	2	46	0.65
1994	116	51	-	1	4	3	59	0.87
1995	86	34	3	4	2	3	46	0.58
1996	134	41	10	4	2	4	61	0.70
1997†	157	55	10	6	3	0	74	0.94

nvCJD = new variant CJD (included from 1995).
*Based on UK population of 58.39 million.
†Provisional figures.

Note: These figures may differ from those published previously because the Unit is still identifying cases from previous years.

Source: UK CJD Surveillance Unit

scientific advisors to ensure that the public health implications of emerging findings on all transmissible spongiform encephalopathies (TSEs) are assessed and appropriate controls are put in place where necessary. Following the emergence of findings that infectivity had been detected in the dorsal root ganglia and provisionally in the bone-marrow of experimentally infected cattle, the Government introduced a ban of the sale of beef on the bone to consumers with effect from 16 December.

Despite a lack of epidemiological evidence to indicate a risk of transmission of classic CJD by blood or blood products, the Government has adopted a precautionary approach to the safety of blood and blood products following advice from the SEAC in October. DH has commissioned an assessment of the risks of nvCJD transmission through blood or blood products, which is due to be completed in Spring 1998.

Research remains a top priority, and DH works closely with the Medical Research Council (MRC) and other Government Departments and Agencies to commission studies into various aspects of nvCJD, BSE and other TSEs.

The National CJD Surveillance Unit was reviewed by a team of national and international experts in 1997, and DH will work with the Unit to implement the review's recommendations.

References

1. Department of Health. *On the State of the Public Health: the annual report of the Chief Medical Officer of the Department of Health for the year 1996.* London: Stationery Office, 1997; 3-4, 239-42.
2. Will RG, Ironside JW, Zeidler M, et al. A new variant of Creutzfeldt-Jakob disease in the UK. *Lancet* 1996; **347:** 921-5.
3. Bruce ME, Will RG, Ironside JW, et al. Transmissions to mice indicate that 'new variant' CJD is caused by the BSE agent. *Nature* 1997; **389:** 418-501.
4. Hill AF, Desbruslais M, Joiner S, et al. The same prion strain causes nvCJD and BSE. *Nature* 1997; **389:** 448-50.

(l)   Emerging and re-emerging infectious diseases

Several international initiatives demonstrated a growing will to collaborate to improve the surveillance, early warning and response to communicable disease incidents of international relevance, in which the WHO, through its new EMC Division, has a central role. In June, at Denver, Colorado, USA, the leaders of eight major nations undertook to promote development of a more effective global surveillance network, building on existing systems, and better co-ordination of international response to outbreaks, working especially with the WHO. The European Union-USA Task Force on Communicable Diseases continued to develop bilateral collaboration in surveillance and training, building on existing schemes and collaborating with the WHO. Through its EMC Division, the WHO continued its work to establish a system to monitor antimicrobial resistance at local, national and global levels.

Some of the more notable outbreaks in 1997 included Ebola haemorrhagic fever in Gabon at the beginning of the year; monkeypox in Zaire; typhoid fever resistant to the available first-line antibiotics in Tajikistan; meningococcal meningitis in West Africa; myocarditis, mainly in children, due to coxsackie B virus infection in Sarawak, Malaysia; Rift Valley fever in Kenya; dengue fever in Malaysia; and avian (H_5N_1) influenza in Hong Kong. The incidence of cholera showed further spread in Africa.

(m)   Travel-related and tropical diseases

Malaria

The PHLS Malaria Reference Laboratory reported 2,364 cases of malaria imported into the UK during 1997, compared with 2,500 in 1996 and 2,055 in 1995; there were 13 deaths. Falciparum malaria cases again increased (1,401 cases compared with 1,283 in 1996 and 1,113 in 1995); they were mainly contracted in East and West Africa. Cases of vivax malaria fell to 790, having been unusually high at 1,014 in 1996, and were mainly from Asia.

New guidelines for the prevention of malaria in travellers from the UK were published in September[1]. These acknowledge the difficulties doctors face in deciding which antimalarials to recommend, especially for visits to areas with highly resistant falciparum malaria. The issues are discussed in detail in a format that can be copied for patients; the variables that need to be taken into account for any individual traveller are also clearly listed.

The frequency of adverse reactions to chemoprophylaxis has to be balanced against the risk of severe malarial illness and death from falciparum malaria. The overall prevalence of adverse reactions, and of discontinuing chemoprophylaxis because of them, is comparable between the main regimens. The guidelines stress, however, that adverse reactions to mefloquine, if they do occur, are likely to be more distressing to the individual, and are more likely to interfere with the purpose for which travel was undertaken, than those to the main alternative, proguanil plus chloroquine. Greater caution is therefore recommended in the use of mefloquine unless there is a high risk of acquiring malaria that is highly resistant to chloroquine. In practice, this means that whilst mefloquine, unless contra-indicated in the individual, remains the preferred antimalarial for most of sub-Saharan Africa, it is reasonable to recommend proguanil plus chloroquine for short visits of two weeks or less to east African coastal resorts, and for visits to the Gambia between January and May, provided the traveller is aware of the increased risk of malaria. The country-by-country tables and text should be referred to for other destinations. More restricted use of antimalarials is recommended for Thailand, where highly resistant malaria occurs but transmission rates tend to be lower than those seen in sub-Saharan Africa.

Over 75% of adverse reactions to mefloquine are apparent by the third dose. The guidelines therefore recommend that people who are to use mefloquine start it, at least on the first occasion, two-and-a-half weeks before departure so that the third dose is taken early enough to make a change should an adverse reaction occur before leaving the UK.

The Department produced a malaria awareness leaflet particularly aimed at settled immigrants returning to visit family and friends abroad, and student back-packers[2]. The leaflet emphasises the four key elements of malaria prevention among travellers, namely to:

  - be aware of the risk;

  - take the recommended antimalarial tablets regularly;

  - prevent mosquito bites; *and*

  - remember that even with these precautions you could still catch malaria and should seek medical advice urgently should fever or 'flu-like symptoms develop.

The leaflets are available in Arabic, Bengali, Cantonese, Gujarati, Hindi, Portuguese, Punjabi, Somali, Spanish, Urdu and Vietnamese as well as in English.

Leprosy

Leprosy is uncommon in the UK; few health professionals therefore have experience of this disease, which requires highly specialised expertise in its diagnosis and treatment, and the long-term management of residual disabilities.

In August, DH and the Welsh Office issued an updated Memorandum on leprosy[3], replacing one previously issued in 1977. The Memorandum outlines the current epidemiology and management of leprosy. It also contains information on how to consult members of the Panel of Leprosy Opinion - a panel of experts who are available to advise about the diagnosis and management of patients with suspected or confirmed leprosy.

References

1. Bradley DJ, Warhurst DC. Guidelines for the prevention of malaria in travellers from the United Kingdom. *Commun Dis Rep CDR Rev* 1997; **7:** R137-52.
2. Department of Health. *Visiting Africa, Asia, South America? Think malaria.* London: Department of Health, 1997.
3. Department of Health, Welsh Office. *Memorandum on leprosy.* London: Department of Health, 1997.

CHAPTER 7

FOOD SAFETY

(a)   Introduction of the Food Standards Agency

During the year, the Government undertook work in preparation for the establishment of a Food Standards Agency. Professor Philip James, Director of the Rowett Research Institute, Aberdeen, had been commissioned by the Prime Minister, when leader of the Opposition, to write a report on the setting up of an independent Food Standards Agency in the United Kingdom (UK), which was published in May[1]. Public consultation on this report, which ended on 20 June, attracted over 600 responses, and showed widespread support for the general thrust of its proposals.

On 1 September, in preparation for the Agency's establishment, those parts of the Department of Health (DH) and the Ministry of Agriculture, Fisheries and Food (MAFF) with responsibility for issues in relation to food safety and standards were combined into an inter-Departmental group, the Joint Food Safety and Standards Group, reporting to both DH and MAFF ministers through the Group's head, Mr Geoffrey Podger. At the same time, the setting up of a new joint MAFF/DH Risk Communication Unit was announced to assist with strategic and practical aspects of communication to ensure that information about food safety and standards matters which may affect human health is presented clearly and comprehensively to the public. This initiative reflected developments within DH to look at more effective means to communicate the language of risk.

A White Paper to set out the Government's detailed proposals for the Food Standards Agency was drawn up in the light of the responses to the James Report, with a planned publication date early in 1998.

Reference

1.   James P. *Interim proposal for a Food Standards Agency.* London: Professor Philip James, 1997.

(b)   Foodborne and waterborne diseases

Foodborne diseases

Provisional figures from the Public Health Laboratory Service (PHLS) Communicable Disease Surveillance Centre (CDSC) show that there were 93,901 reported cases of food poisoning in England and Wales in 1997 (formally

Table 7.1: *Food poisoning: reports to the PHLS Communicable Disease Surveillance Centre, England and Wales, 1982-97*

Year	Total*
1982	14253
1983	17735
1984	20702
1985	19242
1986	23948
1987	29331
1988	39713
1989	52557
1990	52145
1991	52543
1992	63347
1993	68587
1994	81833
1995	82041
1996	83233
1997	93901**

* Statutorily notified to CDSC and ascertained by other means.
**Provisional.

Source: CDSC

notified and ascertained by other means) (see Table 7.1). This figure represents a rise of about 12.8% on the 1996 figure of 83,233.

The number of *Salmonella enteritidis* isolates increased in 1997 by 19% compared with 1996, of which *Salmonella enteritidis* phage type 4 (PT4) increased by 10.7%. Laboratory reports of *Salmonella typhimurium* fell by 19.9%, along with *Salmonella typhimurium* definitive type 104 (DT104), which fell by 26.4%. The number of cases of infection due to *Listeria monocytogenes* remained low, and an increase of 15.8% was seen in the number of *Campylobacter* isolates. The number of faecal isolations of verocytotoxin-producing *Escherichia coli* (VTEC) O157 showed a striking increase of 64.7% compared with 1996.

Campylobacter enteritis

Campylobacter remains the most commonly isolated bacterium associated with acute gastro-enteritis in human beings. There was a 15.8% increase in the number of laboratory-confirmed faecal isolates reported to the CDSC - provisionally 50,201 in 1997 compared with 43,337 in 1996.

Table 7.2: *Salmonella in human beings, England and Wales, January to December (inclusive), 1996 and 1997*

Serotype	1996		1997*	
	Total cases	Imported cases	Total cases	Imported cases
S. enteritidis				
Phage type 4	13127	752	1453	677
Other phage types	5129	745	7186	750
S. typhimurium				
Definitive type 104	3799	117	2796	122
Other definitive types	1743	239	1644	202
Other serotypes	4983	1153	4322	1070
Others untyped	202	30	N/A	N/A
Total	*28983*	*3036*	*30484*	*2821*

*1997 data provisional.

N/A = Not available; from 1997, figures quoted from the PHLS *Salmonella* data set are for isolates confirmed and typed by PHLS Laboratory of Enteric Pathogens (LEP).

Source: PHLS *Salmonella* Data Set

Salmonellosis

In 1997, the number of isolates of *Salmonella* from human beings in England and Wales recorded on the PHLS Salmonella Data Set was provisionally 30,484 compared with 28,983 in 1996 (see Table 7.2). *Salmonella enteritidis* PT4 continues to be the commonest phage type to cause human salmonellosis in England and Wales: in 1997, provisionally, there were 14,536 cases reported, compared with 13,127 in 1996. The second most prevalent *Salmonella* to cause human infection was *Salmonella typhimurium* DT104: in 1997, provisionally, there were 2,796 reported cases compared with 3,799 in 1996. About 96% of *Salmonella typhimurium* DT104 isolates are resistant to a number of antibiotics. The Advisory Committee on the Microbiological Safety of Food (ACMSF) has continued its work considering antibiotic-resistant micro-organisms in relation to food safety (see page 211).

Verocytotoxin-producing Escherichia coli (VTEC)

During 1997, there were provisionally 1,087 laboratory reports of faecal isolates of VTEC O157 in England and Wales, compared with 660 in 1996 - an increase of 64.7%. A PHLS case-control study has been funded by DH to identify and estimate the relative importance of risk-factors for the acquisition of infection with VTEC O157.

Listeria

Cases of human listeriosis in England and Wales continue to be reported at a low level: during 1997, there were provisionally 118 reported cases, compared with 115 in 1996.

Advisory Committee on the Microbiological Safety of Food (ACMSF)

The Committee's working group on foodborne viral infections has continued its work and should report in 1998. The ACMSF's working group on microbial antibiotic resistance in relation to the food chain has received evidence from relevant organisations and also hopes to complete its work in 1998. The ACMSF set up a sub-group to examine the results of a DH-funded survey of *Salmonella* contamination of eggs on retail sale in the UK to establish what conclusions could be drawn from the survey and to make recommendations for future work.

The Committee also considered two surveys on the microbiological status of raw cows' drinking milk on retail sale, one undertaken by the Agricultural and Development Advisory Service (ADAS) on behalf of DH, and the other by the PHLS. The Committee concluded that the sale of such milk in England, Wales and Northern Ireland should be banned.

Developments in food surveillance

The ACMSF has the responsibility to advise the Government on its microbiological food surveillance programme, and the Microbiological Food Surveillance Group (MFSG) co-ordinates relevant work undertaken by DH, other Government Departments, the PHLS and the Local Authorities' Co-ordinating body on Food and Trading Standards. The MFSG includes representatives from industry, retailers and research institutions; its food microbiological surveillance strategy and future work programme were endorsed by the ACMSF, and details published in the Food Safety Information Bulletin[1].

An Epidemiology of Foodborne Infections Group (EFIG) has also been established to collate and assess available information on animal and human infections, and to advise on the need for action where necessary.

The DH-funded study of Infectious Intestinal Disease (IID) in England continued in 1997, and a final report should be published during 1998.

A small focus group has continued its work to improve communications between and to co-ordinate the activities of DH, the MAFF and the PHLS in the area of food microbiology.

Waterborne diseases

Eight outbreaks of cryptosporidiosis were reported: four were probably associated with drinking water, including a large outbreak with 345 confirmed cases in North-West London and Hertfordshire. One other large outbreak was reported from North-West England but no common source was identified. An outbreak of *Campylobacter*, probably associated with a private water supply, was also reported.

Twelve outbreaks of gastro-enteritis associated with molluscan shellfish were reported. Small round structured viruses (SRSVs) were found in four of the eight outbreaks associated with oysters. Two outbreaks involved mussels, including one outbreak of diarrhoeic shellfish poisoning. Two, including one outbreak of *Salmonella enteritidis* PT19, involved cockles.

Reference

1. Microbiological Food Surveillance Group. Microbiological surveillance: the MFSG work programme. *Food Safety Information Bull* 1997; **90**: 3, 20-2.

(c)   Biotechnology and novel foods

A European Union (EU) Regulation[1] which came into force on 15 May introduced a statutory, pre-market clearance system for novel foods and novel food ingredients. Applications are made to the Member State in which the material will be marketed first for an initial assessment; the opinion of that Member State is then forwarded via the Commission to other Member States for review. The Advisory Committee on Novel Foods and Processes (ACNFP) will continue to provide expert advice on such applications in the UK. The Regulation allows for a 'fast track' procedure, with notification to the Commission for novel foods and food ingredients that can be demonstrated to the satisfaction of a recognised Authority to be substantially equivalent to conventional counterparts. The ACNFP has advised that this route should only be applicable to derived products that have undergone a high degree of processing and which have been shown not to contain intact novel DNA or protein.

In 1997, the Committee recommended approval of processed products derived from a genetically modified (GM) tomato variety and food products derived from a herbicide-tolerant GM maize, which had been submitted before the introduction of the EU Regulation.

Reference

1. Council of the European Communities. Regulation (EC) no. 258/97 of the European Parliament and of the Council of 27 January 1997 concerning novel foods and novel food ingredients. *Off J Eur Commun* 1997; **L43**: 1-6. (97/258/EC).

(d) Toxicological safety

The Committee on Toxicity of Chemicals in Food, Consumer Products and the Environment (COT) continued to advise the Department and other Government bodies on aspects of toxicological safety.

The Committee reviewed the toxicology of the polychlorinated biphenyls (PCBs) and agreed that certain congeners could be treated as analogues of the polychlorinated dibenzo-*p*-dioxins (PCDDs)[1]. Risks associated with the consumption of PCBs and PCDDs found in breast milk, diet samples and fish oils were considered; although these concentrations gave some cause for concern, the Committee noted that exposure during infancy would be for limited periods only and measurements showed that levels of these compounds in the diet appear to be falling.

After discussions with the dietary supplements industry, the Committee undertook a second review of the toxicity of vitamin B6. The Committee concluded that the lowest dose reported to have adverse effects in human beings was 50 mg daily[2].

Contamination of some samples of currants, raisins and sultanas with ochratoxin A, a mycotoxin which is carcinogenic in animals, led the Committee to advise that efforts should be made to reduce the concentrations of this contaminant to the lowest achievable levels[3].

The two working groups on peanut allergy and food intolerance established in 1996[4] made progress throughout the year, and will report back to the COT, which is expected to publish reports on these subjects during 1998.

The Committee provided advice on the toxicological risks of a range of other contaminants in food and/or the environment[5].

References

1. Committee on Toxicity of Chemicals in Food, Consumer Products and the Environment. *Statement on the health hazards of polychlorinated biphenyls*. London: Department of Health, 1997.
2. Committee on Toxicity of Chemicals in Food, Consumer Products and the Environment. *Statement on Vitamin B6 (pyridoxine) toxicity*. London: Department of Health, 1997.
3. Committee on Toxicity of Chemicals in Food, Consumer Products and the Environment. *Statement on ochratoxin A in dried vine fruits*. London: Department of Health, 1997.

4. Department of Health. *On the State of the Public Health: the annual report of the Chief Medical Officer of the Department of Health for the year 1996.* London: Stationery Office, 1997; 217-9.

5. Department of Health. *Annual report of the Committees on Toxicity, Mutagenicity, Carcinogenicity of Chemicals in Food, Consumer Products and the Environment: 1997.* London: Stationery Office (in press).

(e)   Pesticides

In March, the Advisory Committee on Pesticides (ACP) published the results of a survey of organophosphorus and carbamate residues in a range of individual fruits and vegetables[1]. Most residue levels fell well below the recommended maximum residue levels, but a small number of home-grown and imported individual apples and peaches had higher residue levels than is desirable. There is a wide margin of safety, a minimum of 10-fold, built into the acceptable levels set for pesticide residues. The findings of this survey reduce this margin of safety but were judged unlikely to cause adverse effects.

The UK is the first country to conduct a large-scale programme to monitor insecticide residues in individual fruits and vegetables to test the reliability of the bulk sampling methods used internationally. The findings indicate a need to examine further some international standards, and action is being taken to seek a review of such standards through the international food standards body, the Codex Alimentarius Commission.

The ACP had been asked to review the standards applied when approving pesticides for non-commercial use during 1996. The Committee completed its review and submitted a recommendation to Ministers in 1997 that a slightly more flexible approach could be applied to pesticide products for the home or garden, with greater emphasis on risk assessment and risk management. Ministers considered the ACP's recommendations but decided that no amendment to the present arrangements for such pesticides was needed.

The results of a survey of organochlorine residues in human fat samples were published during 1997 in the report of the Working Party on Pesticide Residues[2]. The results showed a continued fall in the levels of these pesticides - as illustrated by the residues of the pesticide dieldrin, which have shown a steady decline from a mean of 0.26 mg/kg reported in 1963-64 to a mean of 0.02 mg/kg found in 1995-97[2]. The levels of p,p'- dichlorodiphenyldichloroethylene (DDE), a metabolite of dichlorodiphenyltrichloroethane (DDT), have also shown a similar decrease. These organochlorine pesticides are no longer permitted for use in the UK.

References

1. Advisory Committee on Pesticides. *Unit to unit variation of pesticide residues in fruit and vegetables.* London: Advisory Committee on Pesticides, 1997.
2. Ministry of Agriculture, Fisheries and Food, Health and Safety Executive. *Annual report of the Working Party on Pesticide Residues: 1996: supplement to the Pesticides Register 1997.* London: Ministry of Agriculture, Fisheries and Food, 1997.

(f)   Veterinary products

Organophosphorus sheep dips

The Medical and Scientific Panel of the Veterinary Products Committee (VPC) met twice during 1997 and evaluated recent research in relation to organophosphorus (OP) sheep dips. DH continued to contribute to the funding of epidemiological research by the Institute of Occupational Medicine in Edinburgh and the Institute of Neurological Sciences in Glasgow into the health of sheep dippers.

The Working Group established by the Presidents of the Royal Colleges of Physicians and Psychiatrists to study the management of people who attribute ill-health to exposure to OP sheep dip met several times during 1997 and took evidence from those affected and other interested parties. It is anticipated that the Working Group's report will be completed during 1998.

Other veterinary products

UK health and agriculture Ministers are responsible for the authorisation of veterinary medicines. DH officials provided advice on human safety concerns associated with veterinary medicines, and attended meetings of the VPC and the VPC's Appraisal Panel for Human Suspected Adverse Reactions to Veterinary Medicines and the Advisory Group on Veterinary Residues. The Committees on Toxicity, Carcinogenicity and Mutagenicity of Chemicals in Food, Consumer Products and the Environment (COT, COC and COM) gave detailed advice on the toxicology of dipyrone and thiabendazole, which are used as veterinary medicines.

Toxicological advice was given to the EU's Committee on Veterinary Medicinal Products on consumer safety aspects of the setting of statutory European maximum residue limits (MRLs) for pharmacologically active substances used in veterinary products.

DH provided toxicological advice to the MAFF Food Contaminants Division with regard to human safety aspects of applications for approval of animal feeds and feed additives.

CHAPTER 8

EDUCATION, TRAINING AND STAFFING

(a)   Junior doctors' hours

Action to reduce junior doctors' hours continued, with the view to create better training opportunities and to improve patient care. By September, over 80%, or 23,808 posts, complied in full with all the hours targets originally set in 1991 in the 'New Deal' for junior doctors[1]. However, some posts, mainly at house officer and senior house officer (SHO) grades in acute specialties, still need further action to reduce work intensity and to maintain shorter working hours.

Until March, a central budget helped to provide extra doctors and non-medical staff and to promote local projects; subsequently, further money has remained available for the advisory and performance monitoring role of regional task forces, including the accreditation of successful National Health Service (NHS) Trusts, and NHS Trusts themselves have also continued to fund posts locally.

Activity to reduce junior doctors' hours has promoted organisational change to develop new working patterns, better team-working and cross-cover, effective skill-mix initiatives, (which may involve extended nursing roles), more daytime surgery and other service improvements.

Increased out-of-hours payments remained available during 1997 in cases where junior doctors' work intensity was too high for their contracted working pattern. Such payments have helped to promote local action to resolve difficulties by changing working practices. Actual hours of work are now monitored more accurately and regional task forces routinely involve junior doctors in the validation of these figures.

The provision of reasonable living and working conditions is a priority in the Government's developing human resources strategy. In December, the Department wrote to NHS Trusts to highlight the importance of high standards of on-call accommodation and out-of-hours catering as part of the training environment for junior doctors[2].

References

1.   Department of Health. *Hours of working of doctors in training: the new deal.* London: Department of Health, 1991 (Executive Letter: EL(91)82).
2.   Department of Health NHS Executive. *Managing human resources in the NHS.* Leeds: Department of Health, 1997 (Executive Letter: EL(97)73).

(b)   Advisory Group on Medical and Dental Education, Training and Staffing, the Specialty Workforce Advisory Group and the Medical Workforce Standing Advisory Committee

The structure of the Advisory Group on Medical and Dental Education, Training and Staffing (AGMETS) was changed in June to provide a more strategic focus and to enhance its relevance to the needs of the NHS. The overall aim of the Group is to bring together representatives of the professions and their regulatory bodies, academic and research communities, higher education, the NHS Executive, the Welsh Office, and NHS and patients' interests groups to help to shape the future strategic direction of medical and dental education, training and workforce policies, and to advise the Secretaries of State for Health and for Wales accordingly.

The new AGMETS structure has three main elements:

- a broadly based forum, which meets once or twice per year to seek consensus on strategic priorities for the following year and to review progress;

- a smaller working group, which includes representatives of the key interests, and meets quarterly to take forward priorities highlighted by the forum; *and*

- a series of sub-groups to undertake detailed work on specific issues.

The Specialty (formerly Specialist) Workforce Advisory Group (SWAG) is a sub-group of AGMETS, with a remit to assess future consultant demand and to advise Ministers on the required number of higher specialist trainees. For 1999/2000, the Group will also assess the need for general practitioners (GPs) and consider the balance between primary and secondary health care to ensure that the distribution of the medical workforce best reflects service needs. The SWAG recommended an increase of 850 trainees for 1997/98[1]: of these, 250 were new training placements funded by an additional £4.5 million in the Medical and Dental Education Levy, and 600 were made available by conversion of SHO or visiting registrar posts to specialist registrar (SpR) posts. Extra funds were targeted at specialties in which the demand for consultants had particularly increased, including some oncology and psychiatry specialties. The SWAG published its annual report for 1996/97[2] in November.

The third report of the Medical Workforce Standing Advisory Committee (MWSAC)[3] considered the future balance of medical workforce supply and demand in the United Kingdom (UK). Its main recommendation was for the annual intake to UK medical schools to increase by 1,000, a 20% increase over the target of 4,970 for the year 2000, together with a range of measures to improve the recruitment and retention of doctors. The Government will announce its decisions on all of the MWSAC's recommendations during 1998 in the light of the Comprehensive Spending Review.

References

1.   Department of Health NHS Executive. *Specialist Workforce Advisory Group recommendations: higher specialist training numbers: 1997/98.* Leeds: Department of Health, 1997 (Executive Letter: EL(97)14).
2.   Department of Health Specialist Workforce Advisory Group. *Medium term medical workforce planning: Specialist Workforce Advisory Group (SWAG) annual report for 1996/97.* London: Department of Health, 1997.
3.   Department of Health Medical Workforce Standing Advisory Committee. *Planning the medical workforce: third report.* London: Department of Health, 1997.

(c)   Postgraduate medical training

Specialist registrar grade

The introduction of the new SpR grade was completed on 31 March, when the final group of 14 specialties completed transition into the new grade. Overall, over 12,000 higher specialist trainees in 53 different specialties entered the new structured training programmes between December 1995 and March 1997.

Full implementation of the reforms will require higher specialist trainees, in addition to acquiring effective clinical skills, to be able to respond to service changes and to develop a wider range of competencies, including team-working and communication skills. However, the pace at which such changes can be made will have to take account of the capacity of the NHS to absorb the impact of any changes within available resources. Progress to implement these reforms of higher specialist medical training are greatly dependent on the helpful co-operation of the medical Royal Colleges and Faculties, universities and postgraduate deans, and on the enthusiasm of individual consultants, trainees, supervisors, tutors and advisors.

Summative assessment for general practice

Legislation to come into force in January 1998[1] will make a summative assessment of vocational training for general medical practice compulsory for all doctors who wish to become GPs. This assessment of GP registrars at the conclusion of the general practice element of their vocational training will:

- assure the competence of those joining the profession;

- reassure the public and protect patients from doctors whose performance is inadequate;

- confirm to individual doctors that they have reached an agreed minimum standard of competence; *and*

- identify those doctors who are not yet ready for independent practice and would benefit from further training or alternative career options.

Continuing professional development and medical education

Initiatives on continuing professional development and medical education to ensure that practitioners keep pace with developments in medicine, and continue to refine and develop new skills and abilities, continued throughout the year, and a major European conference on continuing medical education is planned for March 1998.

Reference

1.   *The NHS (Vocational Training for General Medical Practice) Regulations 1997.* London: Stationery Office, 1997 (Statutory Instrument: SI 1997; no. 2817).

(d)   Equal opportunities

New training arrangements introduced with the launch of the SpR grade have led to increased use of flexible training opportunities, which are managed by postgraduate deans. Introduction of the National Training Number (NTN), which represents a personal 'passport' for specialist training, helps doctors to take up flexible training or a career break.

The number of women doctors increased at all levels in the workforce, underlining the need for NHS to adopt 'family friendly' employment policies, and to recognise the need to balance work and other responsibilities. A working group was set up to generate ideas from which a more integrated strategy for flexible working could be developed. A survey of higher specialist trainees was also commissioned, to assist the design of flexible posts at consultant level.

The NHS Equal Opportunities Unit continued to be represented on the British Medical Association's (BMA's) racial equality working party. The Unit also explored ways to promote equal opportunities for doctors with the General Medical Council (GMC).

In April, a draft quality framework for hospital and community health services medical and dental staffing was issued[1]. This compendium of guidelines for a workforce based on quality emphasised the need for good practice in equal opportunities by all health authorities, NHS Trusts, medical schools and postgraduate deaneries in all areas of potential discrimination, including race, sex and disability. Emphasis is laid upon the need for local policies and practice to be in line with best practice; for fair and open competition through objective assessment, selection and appointment procedures; and for the identification of blocks and barriers to appointment and to career progress.

The priorities and planning guidance for the NHS[2] called for all NHS employers to have specified goals for the 'Opportunity 2000' initiative[3] and the programme of action for ethnic minority staff[4], and statements of local good practice in the recruitment and retention of staff with disabilities[5].

References

1. Department of Health NHS Executive. *Quality framework for hospital and community health services (HCAS) medical and dental staffing.* Leeds: Department of Health, 1997 (Executive Letter: EL(97)25).
2. Department of Health NHS Executive. *NHS priorities and planning guidance:1998/99.* Leeds: Department of Health, 1997 (Executive Letter: EL(97)39).
3. Department of Health NHS Executive. *Opportunity 2000: women in the NHS.* Leeds: Department of Health, 1995 (Executive Letter: EL(95)126).
4. Department of Health NHS Executive. *Ethnic minority staff in the NHS: a programme of action.* Leeds: Department of Health, 1996 (Executive Letter: EL(96)4).
5. Department of Health NHS Executive. *Employment of disabled people in the NHS: a guide to good practice.* Leeds: Department of Health, 1995 (Executive Letter: EL(95)143).

(e)   Retention of doctors

Estimates based on the 1991 Census indicate that the average working life in medical practice of male medical graduates in the UK is 30 years and of female doctors is 22 years. Equivalent figures based on the 1995 Labour Force Survey are 31.5 years for males and 22 years for females. From these figures, and a composite average of 27-28 years in medical practice, the MWSAC estimated an annual non-retention rate for all UK medical graduates (a composite of death, retirement and non-participation due, for example, to working overseas, a career break or a career move) at just over 3.5% annually[1].

Cohort studies by the UK Medical Careers Research Group indicate that, five years after qualification, some 5-9% of doctors (from cohorts who qualified in different years) were no longer in medical practice; and 9-17% were either not in practice or no longer practising in the UK. Equivalent figures some ten years or so after graduation appear to be broadly similar.

Reference

1. Department of Health Medical Workforce Standing Advisory Committee. *Planning the medical workforce: third report.* London: Department of Health, 1997.

(f) Undergraduate medical and dental education

Close co-operation between the NHS and universities is essential for the successful management of medical and dental education and research. Good progress continued to be made locally in the development of closer and more effective working relations in line with the recommendations of the fourth report of the Steering Group on Undergraduate Medical and Dental Education and Research[1]. Broader-based initiatives to enhance partnership between the NHS and universities include:

- closer working between the NHS Executive and the Higher Education Funding Council for England, including planning for a joint initiative to identify and disseminate good practice and to promote examples of good NHS/university partnership at local level;

- the development of closer working relations between the NHS Executive and the Council of Vice-Chancellors and Principals; *and*

- the establishment of an academic and research sub-group within the new AGMETS framework.

Reference

1. Department of Health Steering Group on Undergraduate Medical and Dental Education and Research. *Undergraduate medical and dental education and research: fourth report of the Steering Group.* Leeds: Department of Health, 1996.

(g) Maintaining medical excellence

In the two years since *Maintaining medical excellence*[1] was published, emphasising the need to ensure that the quality of medical practice is maintained at a high level, progress has been made to take forward its recommendations. In May, the Association of NHS Trust Medical Directors issued guidance to all medical directors to emphasise their responsibility to ensure that procedures were in place for doctors to report concerns about the conduct, performance or health of medical colleagues. In respect of the key recommendation that systems for mentoring should be introduced, the Standing Committee on Postgraduate Medical and Dental Education reviewed different approaches to mentoring, and hopes to report in early 1998.

A disciplinary resource pack was issued to all medical directors in September by the British Association of Medical Managers[2], which gave practical advice for dealing with problem doctors. The Central Consultants and Specialists Committee of the BMA and the NHS Confederation also worked together to agree a set of good practice principles to be applied to disciplinary procedures for senior hospital doctors, which should be issued during 1998.

The Medical (Professional Performance) Act 1995[3] was implemented in July 1997 to enable the GMC to take effective action in cases where a doctor's poor performance cannot be dealt with locally. Comprehensive guidance to support the new procedures was issued by the GMC in July[4], and the NHS Executive also published its own guidance on the role of the NHS in the GMC's performance procedures[5].

References

1. Department of Health. *Maintaining medical excellence: review of guidance on doctors' performance: final report.* Leeds: Department of Health, 1995.
2. British Association of Medical Managers. *When things go wrong: practical steps for dealing with the problem doctor.* Cheadle (Cheshire): British Association of Medical Managers, 1997.
3. *The Medical (Professional Performance) Act 1995.* London: HMSO, 1995.
4. General Medical Council. *The management of doctors with problems: referral of doctors to the GMC's fitness to practise procedures.* London: General Medical Council, 1997.
5. Department of Health NHS Executive. *The management of doctors with problems: guidance on the role of the NHS in the GMC's performance procedures and the rehabilitation of doctors.* Leeds: Department of Health, 1997.

(h)   Training developments for wider professional staff

The White Paper *The new NHS: modern, dependable*[1] highlighted integrated clinical care and quality, introduced the concept of clinical governance to underpin individual professionalism, and acknowledged the role of regional education and development groups and local education consortia to support the training and development needs of health care professionals.

The NHS Executive attaches great emphasis on continuing professional development and the need for health professionals to keep up-to-date with technological advances, novel and effective treatment methods and new approaches to service delivery, in line with the increasing emphasis on 'lifelong learning'.

The value of inter-agency and multidisciplinary team-working is increasingly recognised in respect of health and social care. The NHS Executive has promoted the development of multidisciplinary (shared learning) education[2], and continues to facilitate the development of team-based delivery of health care.

The proposed establishment of national training organisations in health and social care offers an additional opportunity for all sectors - public, independent and voluntary - and from all professional groups to work together.

Provision of public health is a fundamental part of pre-registration education, and local education consortia[3] are seeking to incorporate a strategic approach to health in education and development programmes and to assess training needs, in particular for the advanced specialist training of non-medical public health professionals including health promotion specialists.

In July, the NHS Executive Board established an education and workforce planning sub-committee to support and promote a more unified approach to professional education and workforce planning across the health service, with relevance to local and national priorities in health and social care.

Following an independent review of the Professions Supplementary to Medicine Act 1960[4], the Government will consult on proposals for new legislation, to provide public protection through the regulation of key groups of health professions. An independent review of the Nurses, Midwives and Health Visitors Act 1997[5] will report to the UK Health Departments in Summer 1998, with consultation before any proposals for new legislation.

The scientific and technical workforce in the NHS is heterogeneous and fragmented, and staff within it carry out a range of overlapping functions and duties. Career structures for scientists and technicians are sometimes unclear and their education or training needs ill-defined. The structure and function of this workforce are under review.

References

1. Department of Health. *The new NHS: modern, dependable.* London: Stationery Office, 1997 (Cm. 3807).
2. Department of Health. *Education and training planning guidance.* London: Department of Health, 1996 (Executive Letter: EL(96)46).
3. Department of Health. *Education and training planning guidance.* London: Department of Health, 1997 (Executive Letter: EL(97)58).
4. *The Professions Supplementary to Medicine Act 1960.* London: HMSO, 1960.
5. *The Nurses, Midwives and Health Visitors Act 1997.* London: Stationery Office, 1997.

CHAPTER 9

OTHER TOPICS OF INTEREST IN 1997

(a) Medicines Control Agency

(i) Role and performance

The Medicines Control Agency (MCA) is an Executive Agency which reports through its Chief Executive, Dr Keith Jones, to the Secretary of State for Health. Its primary objective is to safeguard public health by ensuring that all human medicines available in the United Kingdom (UK) meet appropriate standards of safety, quality and efficacy. Safety aspects encompass potential or actual harmful effects; quality relates to all aspects of drug development and manufacture; and efficacy is a measure of the beneficial effect a medicine has on patients.

This objective is achieved through a system of licensing and post-marketing surveillance. The MCA has an inspectorate that monitors standards of pharmaceutical manufacturers and wholesalers. The Agency also supports the work of the British Pharmacopoeia Commission in setting quality standards for drug substances. The MCA has responsibility for medicines control policy within the Department of Health (DH), plays a full role within the European Union (EU) and represents UK interests in respect of pharmaceutical regulatory matters in other international settings.

In an extremely busy and challenging year, the MCA's workload increased to the highest levels yet encountered, but almost all key licensing and safety targets were met, and often exceeded. As well as a record number of assessments of new active substances and legal reclassifications, there was important progress towards improved communication and provision of information about medicines.

(ii) Legal reclassification of medicinal products

The Prescription Only Medicine (POM) Order[1] was consolidated[2] and amended[3]. Beclomethasone dipropionate was reclassified to allow sale from pharmacies for the prevention of allergic rhinitis, as was cimetidine for prophylactic management of nocturnal heartburn. Pharmacists may supply ibuprofen and topical piroxicam to alleviate the pain of non-serious arthritic conditions, and a combination of hydrocortisone with clotrimazole for athlete's foot and candidal intertrigo.

To reduce the risk of overdose, aspirin and paracetamol will be added to the POM Order, with exemptions for pharmacy sale of packs of up to 32 non-effervescent tablets or capsules, in Autumn 1998. Aspirin and paracetamol will continue to be available on general sale, but with a pack size limited to 16 tablets or capsules[4].

The General Sale List (GSL) Order[5] was amended to add benzoyl peroxide for the treatment of spots and pimples on the face, dequalinium chloride for minor infections of the mouth and throat, loperamide hydrochloride for symptomatic treatment of acute diarrhoea, miconazole nitrate for treatment of athlete's foot, the laxative sodium picosulphate, and liquid paracetamol (in unit dose sachets) for children. A combination of menthyl valerate, quinine base and a higher dose of camphor was added to the GSL Order to allow general sale as an aid to smoking cessation.

(iii) Drug safety issues

Hormone replacement therapy and breast cancer

In October, a meta-analysis published in *The Lancet*[6] indicated an increase in the risk of being diagnosed with breast cancer in relation to the use of hormone replacement therapy (HRT), which disappeared within five years of stopping HRT. Overall, the results were not considered markedly to alter the balance of benefits and risks of HRT, but in view of the potential for concern amongst users of HRT, the Chairman of the Committee on Safety of Medicines (CSM) sent a message to health professionals through the Chief Medical Officer's Epinet electronic communication cascade system and a leaflet was provided which could be given to patients or used to explain the issues involved[7].

Terfenadine

Reports of serious cardiac adverse effects continued to be received despite steps taken in 1992 and 1994 to introduce safeguards in product information. In view of these reports, and concern about the increasing complexity of the precautionary measures required, the CSM advised that terfenadine should only be used under medical supervision, and following consultation it was restricted to prescription-only use. Doctors and pharmacists were informed of the consultation by letter[8], and of the final decision in *Current Problems in Pharmacovigilance*[9].

Troglitazone

Troglitazone, a novel anti-diabetic agent which acts by enhancing the action of insulin, was marketed in the United States of America (USA) and Japan from

March and in the UK from October. Reports of serious liver toxicity, some fatal, were first received from the USA and Japan in mid-October. Following the accumulation of further evidence from the USA and Japan, the manufacturers withdrew the drug from the UK market with effect from December[10].

Anorectics and valvular heart disease

In July, 24 cases of unusual cardiac valvular disease predominantly associated with use of the combination of fenfluramine and phentermine were reported in the USA[11]. Although primary pulmonary hypertension is well recognised to be associated with anorectic drugs, these cases were pathologically distinct, and subsequently over 100 cases of cardiac valvular disease associated with anorectics were reported. In another US survey, 30% of obese patients treated with fenfluramine or dexfenfluramine were found to have symptomless valvular heart abnormalities[12]. The manufacturers withdrew fenfluramine and dexfenfluramine from sale in September. In the UK, doctors and pharmacists were informed of this issue by the manufacturers and through the Epinet electronic cascade system[13], and in *Current Problems in Pharmacovigilance*[14].

(iv) Pharmaceutical developments in the European Union

On 30 July, the European Commission adopted a decision to ban the use of specified-risk materials (SRMs), which should, inter alia, safeguard against the risks of transmission of transmissible spongiform encephalopathies (TSEs) by medicinal products. These controls should be implemented from 1 April 1998.

The Directive on good clinical practice and clinical trials was referred to the Council of Ministers in Autumn 1997. It includes statements of principle supported by ten Guidelines, which are under development. The Directive will require research ethics committees to be brought within the scope of UK law, and seeks to harmonise some aspects of administrative and procedural practice in the conduct of clinical trials in the EU.

Negotiations are also under way on the Directive governing good manufacturing practice (GMP) in starting materials. The European Commission proposal for a Council Regulation on fees payable to the European Medicines Evaluation Agency (EMEA) will be taken forward under the UK Presidency of the EU during the first half of 1998.

References

1. The *Medicines (Products Other than Veterinary Drugs) (Prescription Only) Order 1983*. London: HMSO (Statutory Instrument: SI 1983; no. 1212).
2. *The Prescription Only Medicines (Human Use) Order 1997*. London: Stationery Office, 1997 (Statutory Instrument: SI 1997; no. 1830).

3.   *The Prescription Only Medicines (Human Use) Amendment Order 1997.* London: Stationery Office, 1997 (Statutory Instrument: SI 1997; no. 2044).

4.   *The Medicines (Sale or Supply) (Miscellaneous Provisions) Amendment (No. 2) Regulations 1997.* London: Stationery Office, 1997 (Statutory Instrument: SI 1997; no. 2045).

5.   *The Medicines (Products Other Than Veterinary Drugs) (General Sale List) Order 1984.* London: HMSO, 1984 (Statutory Instrument: SI 1984; no. 769).

6.   Collaborative Group on Hormonal factors in Breast Cancer. Breast cancer and hormone replacement therapy: collaborative re-analysis of data from 51 epidemiological studies of 52,705 women with breast cancer and 108,411 women without breast cancer. *Lancet* 1997; **350:** 1047-59.

7.   Department of Health. *HRT and breast cancer.* London: Department of Health, 1997 (Cascade Electronic Message: CEM/CMO(97)8).

8.   Committee on Safety of Medicines. *Terfenadine: proposed changes to prescription use.* London: Committee on Safety of Medicines, 1997.

9.   Committee on Safety of Medicines. Terfenadine. *Curr Probl Pharmacovigilance* 1997; **23:** 9.

10.   Committee on Safety of Medicines. Troglitazone *Curr Probl Pharmacovigilance* 1997; **23:** 13.

11.   Connolly H. Valvular heart disease associated with fenfluramine/phentermine *N Engl J Med* 1997: **337:** 581-8.

12.   Food and Drug Administration. FDA announces withdrawal of fenfluramine and dexfenfluramine. *HHS News* 1997 (15 September).

13.   Department of Health. *Withdrawal of fenfluramine ('Ponderax') and dexfenfluramine ('Adifax'): effects on heart valves.* London: Department of Health, 1997 (Cascade Electronic Message: CEM/CMO(97)7).

14.   Committee on Safety of Medicines. Withdrawal of fenfluramine and dexfenfluramine. *Curr Probl Pharmacovigilance* 1997; **23:** 13-4.

(b)   Medical Devices Agency

The Medical Devices Agency (MDA) is an Executive Agency of the Department which reports through its Chief Executive, Mr Alan Kent, to the Secretary of State for Health. The role of the Agency is to advise Ministers and to take all reasonable steps to safeguard public health by ensuring that all medical devices meet appropriate standards of safety, quality and performance and comply with the relevant European and UK legislation.

Developments in the European Union

The Agency has continued to represent the UK in negotiations to bring about a single European market in medical devices. Two European Directives have already been implemented:

- The Active Implantable Medical Devices Regulations 1992[1], covering all active implants, came into force on 1 January 1993; *and*

- The Medical Devices Regulations 1994[2], covering all other medical devices with the exception of in-vitro diagnostic devices, took effect from 1 January 1995. Manufacturers have until 13 June 1998 to comply with these Regulations.

Political agreement on a common position was finally reached on a third Directive to cover in-vitro diagnostic (IVD) medical devices at the Internal Market Council on 27 November, following two years of negotiations. The proposal to extend the Medical Devices Directive to include a restricted range of devices containing substances derived from human tissues has been removed from this Directive. In 1997, the Commission decided to ban the use of certain animal material (Specified Risk Material) as from 1 April 1998. This ban will affect some medical devices but, as currently drafted, excludes IVDs.

The MDA acts as the UK's Competent Authority in the implementation and monitoring of compliance with the European Medical Devices Directives, and set up a compliance unit in April. In addition to investigating all potential breaches of the Regulations drawn to the MDA's attention, this Unit has started a programme of inspections of manufacturers who place products on the market on a self-declaration basis.

The MDA continued to audit the independent certification organisations (known as Notified Bodies) which assess manufacturers' compliance against the requirements of the Regulations. Substantial improvements in compliance have been made, and the Agency has kept other Member States informed of lessons learnt in the UK. Additionally, 58 applications were received for products that required clinical investigation assessments before being placed on the market. A panel of external assessors set up to assist the Competent Authority in these assessments has continued to provide valuable advice.

Adverse Incident Reporting Centre/vigilance system

During 1997, 5,383 adverse incidents were reported to the MDA, of which 47 involved fatalities[3]; this represents a 30% increase on 1996.

The number of adverse incidents of CE-marked devices reported by manufacturers in line with their obligations under the Medical Devices Regulations increased from 128 in 1996 to 215 in 1997. As a result, the MDA sent out 31 reports to other European Competent Authorities to alert them to measures taken or contemplated to prevent recurrence, and received 28 reports from other Competent Authorities. Further substantial increases are expected next year with the end of the transition period.

As a result of adverse incident investigations, 16 Hazard Notices, 20 Safety Notices, four Pacemaker Technical Notes and four Device Bulletins were issued, the last providing guidance and information on more general medical device issues. Recent topics have included a major investigation into the effects of mobile telephones on medical devices[4], selection and use of infusion devices for ambulatory use[5], and the impact of the year 2000 (in respect of year coding in microchips used not only in computers but in other systems) on the function of certain medical devices[6]. The production and distribution of these safety warnings have been accelerated by the introduction of a number of measures, including a 'fast fax' system for Hazard Notices.

Evaluation programme

The evaluation programme, set up to provide impartial information on safety, performance and clinical experience, assessed nearly 200 new devices during the year, including pathology kits and instrumentation, diagnostic and monitoring devices, equipment used in surgery and intensive care, and equipment for people with disabilities. Assessments were made at specialist national evaluation centres, and 140 detailed reports were published[7].

References

1. *The Active Implantable Medical Devices Regulations 1992.* London: HMSO, 1992 (Statutory Instrument: SI 1992; no. 3146).
2. *The Medical Devices Regulations 1994.* London: HMSO, 1994 (Statutory Instrument: SI 1994; no. 3017).
3. Medical Devices Agency. *Adverse incident reports 1997.* London: Medical Devices Agency, 1997 (Device Bulletin: MDA DB 9701).
4. Medical Devices Agency. *Electromagnetic compatibility of medical devices with mobile communications.* London: Medical Devices Agency, 1997 (Device Bulletin: MDA DB 9702).
5. Medical Devices Agency. *Selection and use of infusion devices for ambulatory applications.* London: Medical Devices Agency, 1997 (Device Bulletin: MDA DB 9703).
6. Medical Devices Agency. *Medical devices and the year 2000.* London: Medical Devices Agency, 1997 (Device Bulletin: MDA DB 9704).
7. Medical Devices Agency. *Catalogue of evaluation reports.* London: Medical Devices Agency, 1997.

(c)   National Blood Authority

The National Blood Authority (NBA) is a Special Health Authority set up in April 1993 to manage the National Blood Service (NBS) in England. The Service comprises the Bio-Products Laboratory, the International Blood Group Reference Laboratory and the Blood Centres (which until April 1994 were managed by the then Regional Health Authorities).

As a result of concerns raised about potential effects on services provided to local hospitals of the NBA's plans to transfer bulk donation processing and testing from the Liverpool to the Manchester Blood Centre, the Secretary of State for Health set up a review of the services provided by the Merseyside Blood Centre. This review, carried out by Professor John Cash, President of the Royal College of Physicians of Edinburgh, produced an interim report in September, which recommended that the transfer continue as planned on safety grounds. The NBA subsequently decided not to proceed with the planned transfer of processing activities from Plymouth to Bristol. Professor Cash will deliver his final report, which is expected to have implications for the wider service, during 1998[1].

Increased evidence of a link between bovine spongiform encephalopathy (BSE) and new variant Creutzfeldt-Jakob disease (nvCJD) (see page 212) led to concerns about the theoretical risk of transmission of nvCJD through blood and blood products; during the year precautionary measures to reduce or remove that potential risk included collaboration in an independent assessment of the risks of human-to-human nvCJD transmission and preparation of a strategy to implement a programme of leucodepletion, should the risk assessment indicate that this is necessary.

The NBA has worked with DH to find ways to increase the number of regular donors to meet rising hospital demand for blood and blood products and to reduce the need for emergency appeals, with the launch of a major long-term publicity strategy. The emergence of the possible risk of nvCJD transmission also highlighted the need to ensure the efficient use of blood by clinicians, to develop alternative approaches to blood transfusion and to promote good transfusion practice.

Reference

1.   Cash J. *Independent review of proposals for the transfer of bulk blood processing and testing from Liverpool to Manchester.* London: Department of Health (in press).

(d)   National Biological Standards Board

The National Biological Standards Board (NBSB), a non-Departmental public body set up in 1976, has a statutory duty[1,2] to assure the quality of biological substances used in medicine.

The Board fulfils this function through its management of the National Institute for Biological Standards and Control (NIBSC). The NIBSC is a multidisciplinary scientific organisation which tests the quality, reliability and safety of biological medicines such as vaccines, products derived from human blood and those produced by biotechnology; develops the biological standards necessary for this testing; and carries out associated research. This work is relevant to various areas of preventive medicine, therapeutics and diagnostics. The Institute also monitors progress in emerging fields such as gene therapy and xenotransplantation and collaborates with other bodies to generate scientific guidance on quality and safety in these areas.

The Board and the Institute work within the Government's overall public health programme to:

  - respond to and advise on public health problems involving biological agents;

- address new developments in science and medicine; *and*

- take a leading role in developing the scientific basis for the control and standardisation of biological agents in Europe.

The NIBSC examines almost 2,000 batches of biological medicines annually, in addition to testing over 3,000 plasma pools for virological safety. The Institute is designated an Official Medicines Control Laboratory within the EU and is accredited to the internationally recognised quality standard EN45001 for testing biological substances.

The Institute is a World Health Organization (WHO) International Laboratory for Biological Standards and prepares and distributes the bulk of the world's international standards and reference materials. These activities are certified to the quality standard ISO9001.

The NBSB recently commissioned an independent, international scientific review of biological standardisation and control, chaired by Professor Sir Leslie Turnberg, formerly President of the Royal College of Physicians of London. This review, which stresses the growing importance of biological agents in medicine, will enable the NIBSC to review its own future scientific strategy and will have a major impact world wide[3].

References

1.   *The Biological Standards Act 1975.* London: HMSO, 1975.
2.   *The National Biological Standards Board (Functions) Order 1976.* London: HMSO, 1976 (Statutory Instrument: SI 1976; no. 917).
3.   World Health Organization. Biological standardisation and control: the scientific basis of standardisation and quality control/safety monitoring of biological substances used in medicine. Geneva: World Health Organization, 1997 (*WHO Tech Rep* WHO/BLG/97.1).

(e)   National Radiological Protection Board

The National Radiological Protection Board (NRPB) is a non-Departmental public body which reports to the Secretary of State for Health. The functions given to the Board[1,2] are:

- by means of research and otherwise, to advance the acquisition of knowledge about the protection of mankind from radiation hazards (for both ionising and non-ionising radiation); *and*

- to provide information and advice to persons (including Government Departments), with responsibilities in the UK in relation to the protection of the community as a whole or of particular sections of the community from radiation hazards.

It also provided that the Board should have the power:

- to provide technical services to persons concerned with radiation hazards; *and*

- to make charges for such services and for providing information and advice in appropriate circumstances.

The NRPB contributes to public health strategy[3,4] by a combination of formal advice, research, the publication of scientific reports and the provision of advice directly to health professionals and others involved with radiation work, as well as to the general public.

During the year, the Board published formal advice on a range of issues, which included intervention for recovery after accidents and the application of emergency reference levels of dose in emergency planning and response[5]; the relative biological effectiveness of neutrons for the induction of cancer[6]; chromosome 2 hypersensitivity and clonal development in murine radiation acute myeloid leukaemia[7]; carcinogenic response at low doses and dose rates[8]; and assessment of skin doses from exposure to ionising radiation[9]. Research projects included publication of an epidemiological study of record linkage between radiation workers and their children[10]; development of the practical application of a novel dosimetry model for the respiratory tract for assessment of the consequence of inhalation of radionuclides[11]; the calculation of doses to the embryo and fetus from intakes of radionuclides by the mother[12]; studies in support of EU research into various aspects of radionuclides in the environment; maintenance of the National Patient Dose database and the examination of doses in paediatric radiology[13]; examination of the protection against solar ultraviolet (UV) radiation provided by a range of clothing fabrics in support of the campaign to reduce the risk of skin cancer[14]; and measurements of exposure of children to electric and magnetic fields, radon and natural gamma radiation as part of the National Study of Childhood Cancer (to be published).

The NRPB provides administrative support for the Administration of Radioactive Substances Advisory Committee (ARSAC), supplements efforts in nuclear emergency exercises, participates with the Health Education Authority (HEA) in the programme to reduce skin cancer, and provides the secretariat for the Committee on Medical Aspects of Radiation in the Environment (COMARE), which assesses and advises Government on the health effects of natural and artificial radiation. Aspects under review by the COMARE include the geographical distribution of childhood malignancies in Great Britain, and epidemiological studies of radon in homes, of the children of radiation workers and of electromagnetic fields.

The NRPB itself has two advisory groups on which external experts serve and which contribute to the development of advice. Among the topics being tackled by the Advisory Group on Ionising Radiation are the heterogeneity of human response to radiation exposure; the epidemiology of second cancers following radiotherapy; the risk of radiation-induced leukaemia and solid cancers, and the reassessment of reference doses in diagnostic radiology. The Advisory Group on Non-ionising Radiation is to produce a comprehensive review of the dosimetry, biology and epidemiology of occupational and residential exposures to power frequency electromagnetic fields, and will also monitor information on the effects of UV radiation.

At the international level, the Board continued to strengthen the UK's representation on commissions and agencies that deal with matters of radiation protection - including the International Commission on Radiological Protection, the International Commission on Non-ionising Radiation Protection, the United Nations (UN) Scientific Committee on the Effects of Atomic Radiation and the WHO - and in particular contributed to the research and regulatory programme of the European Commission.

References

1.   *The Radiological Protection Act 1970.* London: HMSO, 1970.
2.   *Extensions of Functions Order 1974.* London: HMSO, 1974.
3.   Department of Health. *The Health of the Nation: a strategy for health in England.* London: HMSO, 1992 (Cm. 1986).
4.   Department of Health. *Our Healthier Nation: a contract for health.* London: Stationery Office (in press) (Cm. 3852).
5.   National Radiological Protection Board. *Intervention for recovery after accidents: application of emergency reference levels of dose in emergency planning and response: identification and investigation of abnormally high gamma dose rates.* Chilton (Oxon): National Radiological Protection Board, 1997 (Doc. NRPB 8; no. 1).
6.   National Radiological Protection Board. *Relative biological effectiveness of neutrons for stochastic effects.* Chilton (Oxon): National Radiological Protection Board, 1997 (Doc. NRPB 8; no. 2).
7.   Bouffler SD, Meijne EIM, Morris DJ, Papworth D. Chromosome 2 hypersensitivity and clonal development in murine radiation acute myeloid leukaemia. *Int J Radiat Biol* 1997; **72**: 181-9.
8.   Cox R. *Carcinogenic response at low doses and dose rates: fundamental issues and judgment.* In: Goodhead DT, ed. *Proceedings of the 12th symposium on microdosimetry.* Cambridge: Royal Society of Chemistry, 1997; 225-7.
9.   Little MP, Charles MW, Hopewell JW, et al. *Assessment of skin doses.* London: Stationery Office, 1997 (Doc. NRPB 8; no. 3).
10. Draper GJ, Little MP, Soraham T, et al. *Cancer in the offspring of radiation workers: a record linkage study.* Chilton (Oxon): National Radiological Protection Board, 1997 (Doc. NRPB - R298).
11. Phipps AW, Silk TJ, Fell TP, Jarvis NS. *Dose coefficients for workers and members of the public for a range of aerosols using the new ICRP model for the respiratory tract.* Chilton (Oxon): National Radiological Protection Board, 1996 (Doc. NRPB - M279).

12. Stather JW, Phipps A, Khursheed A. *Radiation doses to the embryo and fetus following intakes of radionuclides by the mother.* In: *Proceedings of the 9th International Congress on Radiation Protection: Vienna: April 1996.* Siebersssdorf: International Radiation Protection Association, 1996.

13. Hart D, Jones DG, Wall BF. *Coefficients for estimating effective doses from paediatric X-ray examinations.* Chilton (Oxon): National Radiological Protection Board, 1996 (Doc. NRPB R279).

14. Gies HP, Roy CR, McLennan AM, et al. UV protection by clothing: an intercomparison of measurements and methods. *Health Physics* 1997; **73:** 456-64.

(f) United Kingdom Transplant Support Service Authority

The UK Transplant Support Service Authority (UKTSSA) was established as a Special Health Authority on 1 April 1991 to provide a 24-hour support service to all transplant units in the UK and the Republic of Ireland, taking over the work of the UK Transplant Service. Its main functions include the matching and allocation of organs for transplantation on an equitable basis and in accordance with agreed methodologies; the provision of support and quality assurance to local tissue-typing laboratories; the maintenance and analysis of the national database of transplant information; and the production of audit reports on the status of transplantation and organ donation and use.

The UKTSSA also provides a forum at which transplant and organ donation issues can be discussed and is responsible for the maintenance of the NHS organ donor register, which was established in 1994. By December 1997, over 4.65 million people had registered their willingness to donate their organs in the event of sudden death.

Two more in the series of audit reports prepared on behalf of the transplant community of the UK and the Republic of Ireland, based on data submitted to the National Transplant Database, were published in August[1,2], as was the sixth annual report of the UKTSSA[3].

References

1. UK Transplant Support Service Authority. *Multi-organ retrieval 1994-1996.* Bristol: UK Transplant Support Service Authority, 1997.

2. UK Transplant Support Service Authority. *Liver transplant audit: liver transplants 1985-1995.* Bristol: UK Transplant Support Service Authority, 1997.

3. UK Transplant Support Service Authority. *Transplant activity 1996: incorporating the sixth annual report of the Special Health Authority April 1996 - March 1997.* Bristol: UK Transplant Support Service Authority, 1997.

(g) Public Health Laboratory Service Board

The Public Health Laboratory Service (PHLS) was established under the National Health Service Act 1946[1]. The PHLS Board was formally constituted as a non-Departmental Public Body in 1960 to exercise functions which are embodied in statute in the National Health Service Act 1977[2], as amended by the Public Health Laboratory Service Act 1979[3], and is accountable to the Secretary of State for Health and the Secretary of State for Wales.

The PHLS exists to protect the population of England and Wales from infection by maintaining a national capability for the detection, diagnosis, surveillance, prevention and control of infections and communicable diseases.

During 1997, the PHLS continued to implement major organisational changes, enhanced its support for public health professionals and successfully helped to protect public health through prompt identification of potential hazards and advice on control. The year included:

- the establishment of a new structure to enhance delivery of services in London by placing several strategically located collaborating centres within National Health Service (NHS) microbiology departments by use of funds released by the withdrawal from two laboratories at Tooting and Whipps Cross (the new centres will be at the North Middlesex, University College, the Royal London and St George's Hospitals);

- the setting up of a new single-site food, water and environmental testing laboratory, based at the Central Public Health Laboratory, Colindale, to serve the whole of London; *and*

- publication of an important study of the control of hospital infection in England and Wales[4], followed by guidelines based on the findings of the study[5].

The PHLS continued to be in the forefront of work on antibiotic resistance, and provided evidence on antibiotic-resistant bacteria and on food safety to the House of Lords Select Committee on Science and Technology and the House of Commons Select Committee on Agriculture. It has also been in detailed discussions with DH on the relations of the Service with the planned Food Standards Agency.

References

1. *The National Health Service Act 1946.* London: HMSO, 1946.
2. *The National Health Service Act 1977.* London: HMSO, 1977.
3. *The Public Health Laboratory Service Act 1979.* London: HMSO, 1979.
4. Public Health Laboratory Service. *Hospital-acquired infection: surveillance policies and practice.* London: Public Health Laboratory Service, 1997.
5. Public Health Laboratory Service. *Preventing hospital-acquired infection: clinical guidelines: a supplement to hospital acquired infection: surveillance policies and practice.* London: Public Health Laboratory Service, 1997.

(h)   Microbiological Research Authority

The Microbiological Research Authority is a Special Health Authority which directs the work of the Centre for Applied Microbiology and Research (CAMR) at Porton Down, Salisbury. The CAMR's special resources include containment facilities for the handling of the most dangerous pathogens and biological toxins. The CAMR Research Steering Group provides a systematic assessment of the research work commissioned and funded by DH and its membership comprises representatives from the PHLS, DH and independent external assessors. Projects cover research into infectious diseases, vaccines, animal cell technology and biotherapeutics. These are assessed individually - for example, in terms of the scientific quality, relevance to policy, achievement towards targets and value for money. Included in the current public health research programme are projects related to HIV, *Campylobacter*, *Salmonella* and vaccine development, such as vaccines against meningococci and pneumococci.

(i)   Gulf War syndrome

Despite increased efforts to investigate the range of illnesses and symptoms experienced by former servicemen and servicewomen who served in the Gulf in 1990 and 1991, there is as yet no clear medical or scientific consensus on the existence or aetiology of a disease or diseases linked to service in the Gulf.

The Ministry of Defence (MoD) Gulf Veterans' Medical Assessment Programme (MAP), which has been running since 1993 and is now based at St Thomas' Hospital, London, received 577 referrals from general practitioners (GPs) during 1997. All patients so referred are examined by a consultant physician and given clinical tests; results, and any recommendations regarding treatment, are sent back to their own doctor. GPs were reminded by the Chief Medical Officer about the existence of the MAP, and encouraged to make appropriate referrals, in November[1].

In July, three separate epidemiological studies co-ordinated by the Medical Research Council (MRC) got under way. One, based at the London School of Hygiene and Tropical Medicine, is investigating the reproductive health and the health of children of all 52,000 Gulf veterans and a comparison group of 52,000 service personnel who did not go to the Gulf. The others, at the University of Manchester and King's College School of Medicine, London, will investigate a wide range of symptoms and diseases to try to establish whether they are more common among Gulf veterans than in control groups.

Reference

1.   Department of Health. Gulf Veterans' Medical Assessment Programme. *CMO's Update* 1997; **16**: 2.

(j)   Bioethics

(i)   *Research ethics committees*

Following a largely supportive consultation exercise[1], arrangements to streamline the ethical review of health-related multi-centre research across the UK were introduced during 1997. A Multi-centre Research Ethics Committee (MREC) has been set up in each of the eight English health regions and one in Scotland; Wales and Northern Ireland will also have MRECs in due course. Principal researchers are now required to submit proposals for research that involve five or more Local Research Ethics Committee (LREC) areas to an MREC, which advises on the science and ethics of such proposals. Once MREC approval is given, local researchers at the sites involved will seek LREC advice on purely local factors.

In March, DH published a briefing pack for members of research ethics committees[2]. Arrangements were made to review the system of research ethics committees as a whole during 1998.

(ii)   *Bioethics in Europe*

The Council of Europe's Convention on Human Rights and Biomedicine[3] was opened for signature in April 1997. Its safeguards for the protection of research subjects have aroused some public concern. The Government consulted on the acceptability of these provisions in the Green Paper published in December, *Who decides?*[4], in relation to decision-making for mentally incapacitated people.

A protocol to the Convention prohibiting the cloning of individual human beings was developed[5], and will be opened for signature in 1998.

Cloning of human beings was also prohibited in the United Nations Education, Scientific and Cultural Organization (UNESCO) Declaration on the Human Genome and Human Rights[6], adopted in November. This Declaration contains provisions that prohibit unjustified discrimination, emphasise consent and confidentiality, and encourage the development of educational activities to improve public awareness of the implications of developments in genetics.

The cloning of human individuals cannot take place under UK law (see below).

(iii)   *Human genetics and the Human Genetics Advisory Commission*

The Human Genetics Advisory Commission (HGAC), chaired by Professor Sir Colin Campbell, Vice-Chancellor of the University of Nottingham, held its first meeting in February. The Commission, which reports to Ministers in DH and the Department of Trade and Industry, has a brief to review scientific progress in human genetics; to report on issues that arise from new developments likely to have wider social, ethical and/or economic consequences; and to advise on ways to build public confidence in, and understanding of, the new genetics. The HGAC's initial priorities were cloning and the implications of genetic testing for insurance.

In May, the HGAC established a working group, chaired by Professor Cairns Aitkin, Emeritus Professor of Rehabilitation Studies at the University of Edinburgh, to consider the detailed implications of genetic testing and insurance. The working group's work was informed by responses to a consultation document published in July[7], and by meetings with representatives of insurance organisations, patient groups and geneticists. The HGAC considered and approved the group's report, which was published and submitted to Ministers in December[8]; this report called for a two-year moratorium on the use of genetic tests by the insurance industry.

The first HGAC meeting coincided with the announcement of the first successful cloning of a sheep from an adult cell[9], which led the HGAC to work on the human implications of cloning technologies. The Committee established a joint working group on cloning with the Human Fertilisation and Embryology Authority (HFEA) to prepare a consultation paper on the issues arising from mammalian cloning for human genetics.

The HGAC has also begun to develop its role in communicating with the public about new developments in genetics, and held consultative meetings with scientists, the media, industrialists and others with an interest in the social and ethical issues raised by advances in the understanding of human genetics.

(iv)   Advisory Committee on Genetic Testing

The Advisory Committee on Genetic Testing (ACGT), chaired by the Reverend Dr John Polkinghorne, was established in 1996 to advise Health Ministers on developments in genetic testing and testing services. During 1997, the full Committee met four times, and other meetings were held of its two sub-groups on genetic testing for late-onset disorders and on genetic testing services supplied direct to the public. Priority was given to the issue of a code of practice on genetic testing services supplied direct to the public[10], a subject highlighted in the 1995 report of the House of Commons Select Committee on Science and Technology[11]; the code and guidance was published in September. In November, a consultation document on genetic testing for late-onset disorders was published[12].

During the year, the ACGT began work with the HFEA to consider pre-implantation genetic diagnosis, with a view to public consultation on this topic during 1998.

(v)   Gene Therapy Advisory Committee

Professor Norman Nevin, Professor of Medical Genetics at the University of Belfast, was appointed Chairman of the Gene Therapy Advisory Committee (GTAC) on 1 January.   During 1997, the number of new applications to the Committee doubled with a continued increase in the number of applicants wishing to amend approved protocols.   Research into cancer therapeutics, in keeping with the trend set in 1996, has been the main focus of interest.

The GTAC met five times during 1997 and assessed 13 protocols and amendments.   The Committee approved six new protocols and three amendments; three protocols are still under consideration and one protocol was withdrawn.

In March, the Committee held a public workshop entitled 'Gene therapy: myth and reality; hype and practicality' to assess the achievement of gene therapy, its future developments and potential barriers to advancement.   In view of the rapid pace of change in these areas of research, the GTAC established a standing sub-group to examine the potential clinical and ethical implications of new gene technologies.   This group met for the first time in November to examine in-utero gene therapy.

(vi)   Assisted conception

The HFEA was established by the Human Fertilisation and Embryology Act 1990[13,14].   It is responsible principally for the regulation of certain techniques for the treatment of infertility, including in-vitro fertilisation (IVF), and research on embryos.   The HFEA published its sixth annual report in November[15].

A consultation document[16] was issued in September as part of the review of the written consent requirements in the 1990 Act being conducted for Ministers by Professor Sheila McLean, Professor of Law and Ethics in Medicine at the University of Glasgow; 116 responses were received and a report is expected during 1998.

A review of certain aspects of surrogacy arrangements was established under Professor Margaret Brazier, Professor of Law at the University of Manchester, working with Professor Susan Golombok, Professor of Psychology at City University, London, and Professor Alastair Campbell, Professor of Ethics in

Medicine at the University of Bristol. A consultation paper[17], published in October, elicited 369 responses; a report to Ministers will be made in Summer 1998.

In its response[18] to the House of Commons Science and Technology Committee Report, *The cloning of animals from adult cells*[19], the Government re-affirmed its view that the deliberate cloning of human individuals is ethically unacceptable and that under UK law such cloning cannot take place. However, the Government is not opposed to the use of cloning techniques which do not involve human reproductive cloning in research into serious illnesses in human beings.

(vii)   Protection and use of patient information

Following the publication in March 1996 of guidance for the NHS on the protection and use of patient information[20], a working group chaired by Dame Fiona Caldicott was set up to review the uses of patient information within the NHS for purposes other than direct care, medical research or those required by Statute. Its report[21] was published in December 1997.

The group looked at existing data flows to see whether transfers of patient information were justified by their purposes. It concluded that the flows of information identified could be justified, but that in some areas more data than were strictly required were being transmitted. Two particular areas of concern were identified: a variable awareness of guidance about the confidentiality requirements for personal health information outside a clinical setting, and the need to ensure that information which can readily identify individuals is kept to a minimum. These recommendations are being implemented within the NHS.

(viii)   Consent issues

During the year, the legal position of patients without capacity to give valid consent was considered in case law[22] and in the publication of a Green Paper[4].

The Court of Appeal clarified the relevant common law in relation to several court cases concerning caesarean sections, some involving women who had temporarily lost capacity to give valid consent[22]. The procedures it laid down for seeking a declaration that a caesarean section would be lawful were subsequently notified to the NHS[23].

Following the Law Commission's 1995 report[24], the Government published a Green Paper[4] about decisions concerning the health, welfare and financial affairs of adults without capacity to give valid consent. Views were sought on a number of issues, including the appointment of someone to take health care decisions for an incapable person and the use of an independent second opinion procedure and/or the Court in certain more serious medical interventions such as organ or tissue donation or sterilisation. The Green Paper[4] considered whether people incapable of consent should be included in research projects and whether there should be a committee to oversee such involvement, and sought views on whether advance refusals of treatment, which already have full effect at common law, should be put onto a statutory footing.

The question of taking gametes (eggs or sperm) for storage or posthumous use in assisted reproduction raises particular legal and ethical issues which were highlighted by the case of *R v HFEA, ex parte Blood*[25]. The removal of gametes from an incapable person is subject to the same common law provisions as other medical interventions, but the Human Fertilisation and Embryology Act 1990[13,14] requires the written consent of the donor to storage or use of gametes. A review of the consent provisions in the 1990Act[13,14] was established.

References

1. Department of Health. *On the State of the Public Health: the annual report of the Chief Medical Officer of the Department of Health for the year 1996.* London: Stationery Office, 1997; 242.

2. Department of Health. *Briefing pack for research ethics committee members.* London: Department of Health, 1997.

3. Council of Europe. *Convention for the protection of human rights and dignity of the human being with regard to the application of biology and medicine: convention on human rights and biomedicine.* Strasbourg: Council of Europe, 1996 (ETS 164).

4. Lord Chancellor's Department. *Who decides? Making decisions on behalf of mentally incapacitated adults: a consultation paper.* London: Stationery Office, 1997 (Cm. 3803).

5. Council of Europe. *Additional protocol to the convention for the protection of human rights and dignity of the human being with regard to the application of biology and medicine, on the prohibition of cloning human beings.* Strasbourg: Council of Europe, 1997.

6. United Nations Educational, Scientific and Cultural Organization. *Universal Declaration on the Human Genome and Human Rights.* Paris: United Nations Educational, Scientific and Cultural Organization, 1997.

7. Human Genetics Advisory Commission. *The implications of genetic testing for life insurance.* London: Human Genetics Advisory Commission, 1997.

8. Human Genetics Advisory Commission. *The implications of genetic testing for insurance.* London: Human Genetics Advisory Commission, 1997.

9. Wilmut T, Schnieke AK, McWhir J, Kind AJ, Campbell KHS. Viable offspring derived from fetal and adult mammalian cells. *Nature* 1997; **385**: 810-3.

10. Advisory Committee on Genetic Testing. *Code of practice and guidance on human genetic testing services supplied direct to the public.* London: Department of Health, 1997.

11. House of Commons Select Committee on Science and Technology. *Human genetics: the science and its consequences: Session 1994-95.* London: HMSO, 1995 (HC 41; vol I).

12. Advisory Committee on Genetic Testing. *Consultation report on genetic testing for late-onset disorders.* London: Department of Health, 1997.

13. *The Human Fertilisation and Embryology Act 1990.* London: HMSO, 1990.

14.	*The Human Fertilisation and Embryology Act 1990 (Commencement no. 2 and Transitional Provision) Order 1991.* London: HMSO, 1991 (Statutory Instrument: SI 1991; no. 480c10).

15.	Human Fertilisation and Embryology Authority. *Sixth annual report 1997.* London: Human Fertilisation and Embryology Authority, 1997.

16.	McLean S. *Consent and the law: a review of the current provisions in the Human Fertilisation and Embryology Act 1990 for UK Health Ministers: consultation document and questionnaire.* London: Department of Health, 1997.

17.	Brazier M, Golombok S, Campbell A. *Surrogacy: review for the UK Health Ministers of current arrangements for payments and regulation.* London: Department of Health, 1997.

18.	Department of Trade and Industry, Office of Science and Technology. *The cloning of animals from adult cells: Government responses to the fifth report of the House of Commons Select Committee on Science and Technology: Session 1996-97.* London: Stationery Office, 1997 (Cm. 3815).

19.	House of Commons Science and Technology Committee. *The cloning of animals from adult cells: fifth report: Session 1996-97.* London: Stationery Office, 1997 (HC 373; I-II). Chair: Sir Giles Shaw.

20.	Department of Health. *The protection and use of patient information.* London: Department of Health, 1996 (Health Service Guidelines: HSG(96)18).

21.	Department of Health. *Report on the review of patient-identifiable information.* London: Department of Health, 1997. Chair: Dame Fiona Caldicott.

22.	Re MB (An adult: medical treatment) [1997] 2 FCR 541.

23.	Department of Health NHS Executive. *Consent to treatment: summary of legal rulings.* Leeds: Department of Health, 1997 (Executive Letter: EL(97)32).

24.	Law Commission. *Mentally incapacitated adults and decision-making: an overview.* London: Law Commission, 1995 (LC 231).

25.	R v Human Fertilisation and Embryology Authority, Ex parte Blood. [1997] 2 All ELR 687.

## (k)	Complaints

The new NHS complaints procedure, introduced on 1 April 1996 as described in last year's Report[1], is now established. In his annual report for 1996/97[2], the Health Service Commissioner for England, for Scotland, and for Wales, Mr Michael Buckley welcomed the new procedures, acknowledging the emphasis on early resolution and the added degree of independence. He recognised, as does the NHS, that it has taken some time for the Service to adjust to the new procedure; DH will continue to play a key role in training NHS staff, including the impact of the Health Service Commissioners (Amendment) Act 1996[3], which extended the remit of the Health Service Commissioner to include complaints about matters arising from the exercise of clinical judgment and about family health services.

Work also progressed on the development of a research brief for a formal, UK-wide evaluation project of the new NHS complaints procedure which will go out to tender early in 1998. This extensive evaluation will examine all aspects of the procedure to identify any problems that may adversely affect its effective operation; make suggestions to overcome such challenges; and highlight examples of good practice which can be shared with the NHS as a whole. The project will run for approximately two years, but it hoped that its structure will allow practicable changes to be made as the need for them is identified.

References

1. Department of Health. *On the State of the Public Health: the annual report of the Chief Medical Officer of the Department of Health for the year 1996.* London: Stationery Office, 1997; 246.
2. Health Service Commissioner. *The Health Service Commissioner for England, for Scotland and for Wales: annual report for 1996-97: Session 1997-98.* London: Stationery Office, 1997 (HC 41).
3. *The Health Service Commissioners (Amendment) Act 1996.* London: Stationery Office, 1996.

(l)   Research and development

Collaboration with other research funders

The Department's research and development (R&D) strategy promotes strong links with the science base and with other major research funders. A national forum of research funders has provided an important means to establish closer working links between research interests in the NHS and elsewhere, including the Research Councils, the Association of Medical Research Charities, industry and universities. It meets twice a year to exchange and share information on activities and priorities to improve understanding and co-ordination.

Collaboration between the UK Health Departments and the MRC is formalised in a Concordat. Concordats have also been established with the Engineering and Physical Sciences, the Biotechnology and Biological Sciences and the Natural Environment Research Councils; a new Concordat with the Economic and Social Research Council is being finalised.

European research

During the Fifth Framework Research Programme the EU will focus on certain key actions. Four of these - food, nutrition and health; control of infectious diseases; environment and health; and the ageing population - have implications for public health. The key action on food, nutrition and health will support research towards a safe, healthy, balanced and varied food supply for consumers; that on infectious diseases will seek to develop new and improved strategies for their treatment, prevention, management and surveillance; that on environment and health aims to enhance understanding of the interactions between the genetic, physiological, environmental and social factors involved in sustaining good health, and so reduce the adverse impact on health of changes in the environment and the workplace; and that on ageing will use research to underpin the development of policies and interventions to extend the quality of life and independence of older people.

(m)   Use of information technology in clinical care

During 1997, the Clinical Systems Group (jointly chaired by the Chief Medical and Nursing Officers) reviewed the strategic information issues arising from the 'Service with ambitions' initiative[1], and set up projects to examine how communication of clinical information could be improved. Mr Frank Burns, the Chief Executive of the Wirral NHS Trust and a member of the Clinical Systems Group, was invited to review the existing NHS information management and technology (IM&T) strategy.

Work to implement the IM&T strategy continued during the year, and some important developments were seen. Virtually all hospitals have basic departmental information technology (IT) systems, and linkage of order-communications systems to patient administration systems is proving to be a helpful step towards the development of electronic patient-based records. The electronic patient record programme at Wirral NHS Trust and at Burton NHS Trust has continued to show practical benefits to be derived from such integration of information in the setting of acute clinical care. Work at the Winchester NHS Trust indicates what can be achieved by improving IT communications between hospital-based and community-based staff. *Benefits of using clinical information*[2], comprising 30 case studies of the use of IT in acute, community and primary care, was published in August with a foreword from the Chief Medical and Nursing Officers.

The report of the committee chaired by Dame Fiona Caldicott to review the many non-clinical requirements for patient-identifiable information within the NHS was published in December[3]. In addition to some administrative and technical recommendations, this report stressed the need to promote cultural change in the NHS where confidential patient information is concerned.

The IM&T training programme for clinicians continued to develop IM&T as an integral part of clinical training programmes, in pre-registration and post-registration training alike. In the NHS, over 80% of GP practices now conduct business electronically with their health authority for patient registration purposes, which provides the foundation to meet the challenge of extending the use of electronic links to other functions. Following the introduction of the new NHS number, it is now in use by health authorities and computerised practices have implemented it. Progress was made to connect all NHS Trusts to the

NHSnet, to provide the basis for enhanced communications and more effective health care. Work also progressed on health care resource and health benefit groupings and the health care thesaurus of clinical terms with Read codes (see page 149). Advice was issued in October[4] to help to minimise any potentially disruptive effects to patients of the 'Year 2000' problem, in which some computer programmes that use double-digit year codes may not make the change from '99' to '00' correctly[4].

References

1. Department of Health. *The National Health Service: a service with ambition*s. London: Stationery Office, 1996 (Cm. 3425).
2. Department of Health NHS Executive, Information Management Group. *Benefits of using clinical information: case studies of the successful use of clinical information by practising clinicians.* Bristol: Information Management and Training Development, 1997.
3. Department of Health. *Report on the review of patient-identifiable information.* London: Department of Health, 1997. Chair: Dame Fiona Caldicott.
4. Department of Health NHS Executive. *The year 2000 problem.* Leeds: Department of Health, 1997 (Executive Letter: EL(97)59).

(n)   Dental health

(i)   *Dental health of the nation*

Results from surveys conducted for health authorities in 1996/97 show a mean of 40.8% of 12-year-old children in England had some experience of dental caries, compared with 50% in 1993. The mean number of decayed, missing or filled permanent teeth (DMFT) among 12-year-old children was 1.0 in 1996, compared with 1.2 in 1993. There was no reduction in the mean number of decayed permanent teeth among 12-year-old children in England between 1993 and 1996, but the average number of filled permanent teeth in this age-group fell from 0.7 in 1993 to 0.5 in 1996. Wide regional variations were still evident, with a mean DMFT of 0.66 in South Thames compared with 1.38 in the North West.

(ii)   *General dental services*

On 30 April, 19,341,446 adult patients were registered with an NHS general dental practitioner in England, some 10% below the peak number of 21,617,725 reached in December 1993. However, much of the difference between the two figures stems from operational factors, in particular improved procedures that the Dental Practice Board for England and Wales has implemented to eliminate duplicate registrations. Following the implementation of further improvements to these procedures - in which 373,300 more records were 'cleaned' in the 12 months to April 1997 than in the previous year - adult registrations fell by 441,000 in the 12 months to April 1997.

The Government is committed to reduce inequities in oral health status and access to NHS dental services. Although NHS dentistry is available for much of the population, there are places where acute or long-term problems of access exist, and steps have been taken to improve access to NHS dentistry in such areas. *Investing in dentistry*[1], launched in September, set out a range of possibilities - including the availability of grants to dentists in areas of poor service availability and oral health to expand existing or to set up new practices, in return for long-term commitment to the NHS. Newly qualified dentists, and those who have temporarily left the profession (for example, to bring up families) but now wish to return, are eligible to apply. Up to £9 million (including treatment costs) have been made available under this initiative for 1997/98. Although it is too early to judge the impact of such schemes, which are being continually assessed, imaginative local proposals have come forward for consideration and several have been approved.

The National Health Service (Primary Care) Act 1997[2] received Royal Assent in March. This Act provides the legislative framework for pilot studies of personal dental services (PDS), which will allow dentists, NHS Trusts and health authorities the opportunity to develop new ways to deliver dental services which address local service needs and local oral health priorities. Such an approach should encourage partnerships between health authorities and dentists to explore more flexible ways to provide primary oral health care in response to local needs and oral health targets. Further information about the PDS scheme was given in *A guide to personal dental services pilots under the NHS (Primary Care) Act 1997*[3]. The NHS Executive invited expressions of interest to pilot these schemes; 101 responses had been received by the deadline of 31 October, 25 of which were given funding to develop full proposals. The first PDS pilot schemes will come into operation from October 1998.

(iii)   Community dental services

Health authorities in England were reminded of their responsibility for all primary care dentistry in guidance issued in March[4], which emphasised that the community dental services (CDS) should continue to provide a full range of services for patients who experience difficulty in obtaining treatment from the general dental services (GDS) - the 'safety net' function - in addition to the provision of services for patients with special needs, whose oral health requirements would not otherwise be met within the GDS, and redefined the role of the CDS accordingly.

At 30 September 1996, there were 580 senior professional staff working in dental public health and community dental health in England, including district dental officers, assistant district dental officers, senior dental officers and consultants in dental public health, and 800 other dentists in the CDS - of whom about 15% were employed directly by health authorities, and about 85% by NHS Trusts with which health authorities had contracts for the provision of such services.

(iv)   Hospital dental services

The number of hospital dentists in England rose by 2% from 1,364 to 1,390 between September 1995 and September 1996. In September 1996, there were 450 consultants in post, an increase of 1% over the previous year. Over the same period the number of senior registrars rose by 11% from 99 to 110, and the number of registrars fell by 2% from 153 to 150; the number of senior house officers rose by 8% from 370 to 400. (Figures refer to whole-time equivalent posts.)

In 1996/97, there were 636,039 new outpatient referrals to consultant clinics - 442,764 in oral surgery, 114,180 in orthodontics, 57,125 in restorative dentistry and 21,970 in paediatric dentistry. There were 1,929,951 repeat attendances at outpatient clinics - 721,315 in oral surgery, 741,333 in orthodontics, 385,970 in restorative dentistry and 81,333 in paediatric dentistry. The basis for reporting outpatient activity in dental hospitals has been revised in line with a national agreement to assure more comparable inter-hospital data, so there can be no direct comparison with figures reported in previous years.

(v)   Continuing education and training for dentists

There were 555 trainees in 47 regionally based vocational training schemes (45 in the GDS, one in the CDS and one in the Dental Defence Agency) in England on 1 September 1997; there were also 30 trainees in two general professional training pilot schemes.

The National Centre for the Continuing Professional Education of Dentists (NCCPED) was established as a three-year pilot project to manage and monitor the national budgets for the provision of continuing professional education (CPE), vocational training, general professional training pilot schemes, peer review and clinical audit in the GDS on behalf of the NHS Executive. The NCCPED will evaluate the effectiveness of use of these budgets and co-ordinate the development and assessment of new systems to provide CPE. It will work closely with the postgraduate dental deans and directors of dental education, the Committee for Vocational Training for England and the Central Audit and Peer Review Assessment Panel.

The following priority areas were identified for the training of general dental practitioners in 1996/97: informatics skills; reinforcement of the concepts of preventive dentistry and nutrition as set out in the oral health strategy; 'hands-on' experience (in respect of phantom heads, typodonts, and pigs' jaws, as well as patients); the management of elderly or disabled patients and those with special needs; instruction in sedation techniques, pain control and the management of anxious patients; promotion of distance learning initiatives; courses for those who are, or intend to be, trainers, advisers or examiners; training for those who wish to carry out clinical research relevant to general dental practice and evidence-based dentistry; the training and development of practice support staff; the promotion of peer review and clinical audit in general dental practice; and training in purchasing and contracting skills for use in the NHS.

During the year, DH continued to fund the development, production and distribution of distance learning material for general dental practitioners which can be obtained free of charge from dental postgraduate deans or via the Internet (at: www.dentanet.org.uk); some 22 different computer-assisted learning programmes have been developed and distributed, or are in development. A videotape entitled 'Oral health strategy until 2003: your patients' oral health and you' was distributed to NHS general dental practices in England in January.

(vi)   Dental research

During 1997, the fourth national decennial survey of dental health was commissioned by the Department to be carried out in 1998 by a consortium from the Office for National Statistics and the Universities of Birmingham, Dundee, Newcastle upon Tyne and Wales. This survey will mainly focus on trend data on the hard tissues of the mouth, with reference to UK surveys in 1978[5] and 1988[6]; a report is due in Autumn 1999.

Field work for the oral health component of the National Diet and Nutrition Survey of those aged 4 to 18 years was completed.

The project board for the NHS research and development programme in primary dental care was convened, and invited applications for research in various areas including: dental auxiliaries; the view of recipients of dental care; general anaesthesia; dental materials; oral health promotion; orthodontic needs; the interface between primary and secondary care; and quality issues. It is expected to start to commission successful applications during 1998.

References

1.   Department of Health NHS Executive. *Investing in dentistry.* London: Department of Health, 1997 (Health Service Guidelines: HSG(97)38).
2.   *The National Health Service (Primary Care) Act 1997.* London: Stationery Office, 1997.

3.   Department of Health NHS Executive. *A guide to personal dental services pilots under the NHS (Primary Care) Act 1997.* London. Department of Health, 1997.

4.   Department of Health NHS Executive. *Primary care dental services.* London: Department of Health, 1997 (Health Service Guidelines: HSG(97)4).

5.   Todd JE, Walker AM, Dodd P. *Adult dental health: United Kingdom: 1978 (vol 2).* London: HMSO, 1982.

6.   Todd JE, Lader D. *Adult dental health: 1988: United Kingdom.* London: HMSO, 1991.

CHAPTER 10

INTERNATIONAL HEALTH

(a)   England, Europe and health

Many of the health challenges encountered in England and the United Kingdom (UK) as a whole are also found in the rest of Europe; diseases have no respect for national boundaries. The pace of technological advance, ageing populations and rising expectations are leading to growing demands on health care services throughout Europe and beyond. The challenges of drug dependence and other lifestyle-related health problems are common to many countries.

The opportunity to work together on common problems within the European Community (EC), and in international bodies such as the World Health Organization (WHO) and the Council of Europe, brings great benefits. The UK has much expertise to offer, but can also benefit greatly from the knowledge of others, the insight provided by international comparisons, and the greater resources that international co-operation can bring into play.

(i)   The European Union

The Health Council

The Council of Ministers is a key decision-making body of the European Union (EU), in which all Member States are represented. Councils of Ministers with particular responsibilities, such as health, meet regularly to deal with relevant EC business.

1997, the Health Council held general meetings on 5 June and 4 December. It reached a common position on a proposed Directive on tobacco advertising and on the creation of a network for the epidemiological surveillance and control of communicable diseases.

Negotiations on the proposal to establish a programme of action on health monitoring were concluded and the programme is now under way. Discussions on proposals for three new programmes of Community action on rare diseases, injury prevention and pollution-related diseases were continuing at the year's end; decisions on these programmes are expected in 1998.

The Council adopted conclusions on the EU-United States Task Force on communicable diseases. Resolutions were agreed on the European

Commission's report on the state of women's health; migrant doctors; health-related aspects of drug use; and on cross-border co-operation on the supply of organs and tissues of human origin.

The Council took note of developments on transmissible spongiform encephalopathies (TSEs) and agreed to keep the subject under review. It discussed the public health aspects of food safety and took note of a proposal for a recommendation on the suitability of blood and plasma donors and the screening of donated blood.

High Level Committee on Health

The European Commission's High Level Committee on Health met twice during the year. It gave advice on the possible shape and scope of a future framework for Community action on health, and considered the public health implications of enlargement of the EU.

Meetings of European Chief Medical Officers

The Chief Medical Officers of the Member States meet informally twice a year to exchange professional views on Community health policy, and on relevant WHO and Council of Europe programmes. Their meetings, which are attended by representatives of the WHO and the Council of Europe, provide an ideal opportunity to promote closer collaboration between the EC, the WHO and the Council of Europe.

Other European Community programmes

The European Commission held meetings of experts in the field of blood safety and the health risks of exposure to electromagnetic fields to assist in the preparation of Community measures. The Commission brought forward measures to implement the five public health programmes adopted by the Council and the European Parliament in the context of the current framework for Community action in public health, including the new programme on health monitoring.

Free movement of people

Health professionals

The number of health professionals from other Member States of the European Economic Area (EEA) working in the UK is small and most come for short periods of time to gain experience. In 1997, 1,860 doctors with recognised qualifications from other Member States obtained full registration with the General Medical Council, 360 dentists with the General Dental Council, and 46 pharmacists were registered with the Royal Pharmaceutical Society of Great Britain. In addition, 1,392 nurses and 46 midwives were accepted by the UK Central Council of Nursing, Midwifery and Health Visiting, and 59 individuals with the Council for the Professions Supplementary to Medicine (comprising one chiropodist, 11 dietitians, 11 occupational therapists, 34 physiotherapists, and two radiographers).

Patients

EC Social Security Regulation 1408/71 continued to operate satisfactorily, co-ordinating health care cover for people moving between EEA Member States. The main categories covered were temporary visitors, detached workers and pensioners transferring their residence to another Member State. In addition, during 1997, 837 applications by UK patients for referral to other Member States specifically for treatment of pre-existing conditions were approved by the Department of Health (DH); 847 citizens of other Member States were treated in the UK on the same basis.

(ii)   Council of Europe

During 1997, the Council's European Health Committee took forward work on xenotransplantation, liver transplantation from living related donors, quality improvement systems in health care (especially waiting times for treatment), blood and blood transfusion, and a number of issues related to patients' rights and patients' choice. It also discussed equity in health care for vulnerable groups, such as those in prison, older people and the chronically ill.

The Committee collaborated with the WHO on a range of issues, including the European Network of Health Promoting Schools.

(iii)   Relations with Central and Eastern Europe

The plan of co-operation with Hungary, by which support is given to short-term exchanges and visits by health professionals, was renewed.

Work continued in relation to the applications from ten countries in Central and Eastern Europe to join an enlarged EU.

(b)   The Commonwealth

A Commonwealth Health Ministers' Meeting was held on 4 May, immediately before the World Health Assembly. Dr Jeremy Metters, the Deputy Chief

Medical Officer, led the British delegation to the meeting, and presented a paper on the impact of the environment on health and the UK National Environmental Health Action Plan (NEHAP); this presentation was well received, with many delegates asking for further information about the UK NEHAP. The Chief Nursing Officer chairs the Commonwealth Nurses Federation Agenda for Action Steering Group.

Other issues discussed at the meeting included AIDS, child survival and women and health. It was agreed that the 12th triennial meeting of Commonwealth Health Ministers should be held in Barbados in 1998, with the theme of "Health sector reform in the interests of 'Health for All'".

(c)   World Health Organization

(i)   European Regional Committee

The 47th session of the European Regional Committee was held in Istanbul in September. The Chief Medical Officer led the UK delegation and, as chair of the Environment and Health Committee, reported on progress on Member States' implementation of NEHAPs and on plans for the third European Conference on Environment and Health, due to be held in London in 1999.

The UK delegation supported a European Regional Action Plan for a Tobacco-Free Europe, which was endorsed by the meeting. During the debate, the Committee were informed of the Government's new public health policy and, in particular, the high priority that would be given to achieving a reduction in smoking prevalence in the UK.

The meeting also discussed a new draft of the 'Health for All in the 21st Century' strategy. Further discussions would take place during 1998, before a further draft would be issued to the 48th session of the Regional Committee in September 1998.

Dr Jeremy Metters, the Deputy Chief Medical Officer, was elected to the Standing Committee of the Regional Committee for a three-year term of office.

(ii)   Executive Board

The 99th meeting of WHO Executive Board took place in January. The Chief Medical Officer attended the meeting as a Board member. Resolutions were adopted on budgetary reform, efficiency savings, a mechanism for priority setting, and a review of WHO regional arrangements.

Discussions were held on a successor to the WHO 'Health for All' strategy. The Chief Medical Officer made a presentation to the Board on this future strategy which was very well received. The WHO Secretariat was asked to produce a draft strategy which, after further discussions, would be submitted to a future World Health Assembly for endorsement.

In May, following the World Health Assembly, the 100th meeting of the Executive Board agreed priorities for the WHO for the following year, taking into account resolutions passed at the Assembly.

(iii)   World Health Assembly

The 50th World Health Assembly, the annual meeting of the Member States of the WHO, took place in Geneva in May. The UK delegation was led by Dr Jeremy Metters, the Deputy Chief Medical Officer, and included the Chief Nursing Officer and other officials from DH, the Department for International Development and the UK Mission to the United Nations in Geneva.

The World Health Report 1997[1], which focused on chronic non-communicable diseases, was commended. The WHO Director General, Dr Hiroshi Nakajima, described how chronic diseases killed more than 24 million people annually, and the role WHO would play in trying to fight these diseases. Delegates also heard a speech read out on behalf of the newly appointed Minister of State for Public Health, Ms Tessa Jowell MP, which set out the new Government's priority to tackle the root causes of ill-health in the UK.

Resolutions were passed on a range of issues including WHO Collaborating Centres; the promotion and sale of medical products through the Internet; the prevention of violence; malaria prevention and control; and the eradication of dracunculiasis.

Reference

1. World Health Organization. *The world health report 1997.* Geneva: World Health Organization, 1997.

APPENDIX

Appendix Table 1: *Population age and sex structure, England, mid-1997, and changes by age, 1981-91, 1991-92, 1992-93, 1993-94, 1994-95, 1995-96 and 1996-97.*

Recent changes in the population age structure are described in Chapter 1 (see page 65).

Appendix Table 2: *Five main causes of death for males and females at different ages, England, 1997.*

This Table contrasts the main causes of death in different age-groups for males and females alike.

It should be noted that the rankings are dependent upon how diseases are grouped. The International Classification of Diseases (ICD) is divided into 17 broad chapters, covering different types of diseases - for example respiratory diseases. Within these chapters, individual diseases or groups of diseases are given a 3-digit code, which in most cases can be further broken down into 4-digit codes. For the purposes of producing these Tables, distinct diseases have been used in most cases - vague remainder categories have been avoided, even if there were a higher number of deaths, in order to make the data more meaningful and useful. However, for the 1-14 years age-group, where the numbers of deaths are very small, the rankings are based on whole chapters of the ICD.

At the age of 35 years and over, the major burden of mortality derives from circulatory disease and malignant neoplasms. At the age of 75 years and over, respiratory diseases also contribute strongly. At ages 15-34 years, suicide and undetermined injury and motor vehicle traffic accidents are the leading causes of death for males and females alike. The leading causes of death among children are external causes of injury and poisoning (mostly accidents) and neoplasms.

Appendix Table 3: *Relative mortality from various conditions when presented as numbers of deaths and future years of 'working life' lost, England and Wales, 1997.*

The total number of deaths at all ages attributed to selected causes are given. The percentage distribution of deaths demonstrates the major impact of circulatory disease and cancer in both sexes. In 1997, over 80% of deaths occurred at the age of 65 years and over.

Years of 'working life' lost between the ages of 15 and 64 years indicate the impact of various causes of death occurring at younger ages. For this Table, a death occurring under the age of 15 years accounts for the loss of the full 50-year period between the ages of 15 and 64 years, whereas a death at age 60 years contributes a loss of only 5 years of 'working life'. Thus weight is given to the age at death as well as the number of deaths, and emphasis is given to the burden of deaths occurring at younger ages.

For males, although circulatory disease and cancer still contribute substantially to loss of 'working life', other causes become more prominent. These include accidents and suicide and undetermined injury, and also those deaths occurring early in life - particularly infant deaths, which account for about 15% of years of 'working life' lost.

For females, the total years of future 'working life' lost from all causes combined is much less than for males, reflecting considerably lower death rates in females. Cancer - particularly of the breast, cervix, uterus and ovary - is a major contributor to loss of life in females aged under 65 years. In 1997, cancer accounted for 22% of all female deaths, but 39% of years of 'working life' lost. By contrast, although causing 41% of the total number of deaths, circulatory disease accounted for only 16% of the years of 'working life' lost. In other respects, the pattern is broadly similar to that for males, although accidents and suicide account for a smaller proportion of deaths among females.

Appendix Table 4: *Trends in 'avoidable' deaths, England, 1979-97.*

The concept of 'avoidable' deaths was discussed in detail in the Report of 1987[1]. These indicators - developed in this country by Professor Walter Holland and his colleagues[2] - have been chosen to identify selected causes of mortality amenable to health service intervention, either preventive or curative. They might best be called 'potentially avoidable' deaths as, while it might not be possible to prevent every death deemed avoidable, it is expected that a substantial proportion could be prevented. The indicators are now published as part of the Public Health Common Data Set.

The Table presents recent secular trends of nine categories of 'avoidable' deaths. The data are presented as age-standardised mortality ratios, which adjust for differences in the age structure in the years compared. During the period 1979-97, substantial declines are evident in all of the categories presented. The age-standardised mortality ratio for all 'avoidable' deaths combined has fallen by 50% since 1979.

Appendix Table 5: *Live births, stillbirths, infant mortality and abortions, England, 1960, 1970, and 1975-97.*

Trends are discussed in Chapter 1 (see page 66).

Appendix Table 6: *Congenital anomalies, England, 1987, 1992, 1996 and 1997.*

This Table shows the numbers of babies notified with selected congenital anomalies. In the past, the Table referred to the number of mentions of selected anomalies, but this was difficult to interpret as a baby can have more than one congenital anomaly. The data for 1987 and 1992 have been re-calculated to enable comparisons over time, but it should be noted (see Chapter 1, page 70) that changes to the notification list in January 1990 affected the following groups: ear and eye malformations, cardiovascular malformations and talipes.

Appendix Table 7: *Cancer registrations by age and site, males, England and Wales, 1992.*

The Table indicates the distribution of cancer registrations in men at different ages. At all ages combined, cancers of the lung, large intestine (including rectum) and prostate account for about half of the registrations. In childhood, a high proportion of cancers are attributable to leukaemias, lymphomas, tumours of the central nervous system, and embryonic tumours such as neuroblastomas and retinoblastomas. At older ages, cancer of the lung is the major cause registered. However in the oldest age-group presented (85 years and over), prostate cancer accounts for substantially more registrations than lung cancer.

Appendix Table 8: *Cancer registrations by age and site, females, England and Wales, 1992.*

In childhood, the pattern of female cancers is broadly similar to that in males. However, in the 25-44 years age-group cancers of the breast (42%) and cervix (16%) predominate. At older ages, breast cancer continues to account for many registrations, although cancers of the lung, large intestine and skin (non-melanoma skin cancers are not included in the Table) also occur in substantial numbers.

Appendix Table 9: *Immunisation uptake, England, 1980-1996/97.*

The information presented in this Table is discussed in Chapter 6 (see page 203).

Appendix Table 10: *Cumulative total of AIDS cases by exposure category, England, to 31 December 1997.*

Recent trends in AIDS cases are discussed in Chapter 6 (see page 189).

Appendix Table 11: *Expectation of life at birth, all-cause death rates and infant mortality, England and other European Union countries, circa 1995-96.*

This Table includes two key overall measures of general health: expectation of life and infant mortality. Recent data are presented for various European countries. Although problems often exist with regard to comparability of data, international comparisons provide an important perspective to the assessment of overall progress. In particular, such comparisons can highlight the scope for improvement and help to stimulate action to achieve progress.

In 1996, average life expectancy at birth in England was 74.6 years in males. Recent figures from our European neighbours ranged from 71.2 years in Portugal to 76.3 years in Sweden. The equivalent figure for females in England was 79.7 years, which compares with a European Union (EU) range from 78.2 years in Ireland to 82.8 years in France.

The infant mortality rate is also often used as a key descriptor of the overall health of a country. In 1996, the rate in England was 6.1 per 1,000 live births. This figure was approximately average for EU countries at that time, contrasting with higher rates of 8.2 in Belgium in 1992 - other sources however suggesting that this rate has fallen substantially in subsequent years - and 7.3 in Greece in 1996. Some countries have achieved considerably lower rates, notably Finland and Sweden, where rates have fallen to 4.0 per 1,000 live births.

Additional information is presented on the age-standardised all-cause mortality rates for EU countries, with particular reference to deaths occurring under the age of 65 years. For males, the English death rate is well below the EU average and is only bettered by Sweden and the Netherlands. However, for women the English mortality rate is above the EU average.

Appendix Table 12: *Age standardised death rates per 100,000 men aged 35-64 years by social class and employment status, England and Wales, 1976-81, 1981-85, and 1986-92.*

This Table is described in Chapter 1. More detailed information is presented elsewhere[3].

268

Appendix Table 13: *Standardised mortality ratios by country of birth and social class for men aged 20-64 years, England and Wales, 1991-93.*

This Table is described in Chapter 1. More detailed information is presented elsewhere[3].

Appendix Figure 1: *Weekly deaths, England and Wales, 1996 and 1997, and expected deaths, 1997.*

This Figure illustrates the week-by-week registrations of deaths from all causes at ages one year and over for 1997. These are compared with the observed values in 1996 and expected values in 1997. The expected numbers of deaths for 1997 are calculated as an average of the deaths registered in the same week over the previous five-year period, 1992-96.

References

1. Department of Health and Social Security. *On the State of the Public Health: the annual report of the Chief Medical Officer of the Department of Health and Social Security for the year 1987.* London: HMSO, 1988: 4, 72-82.
2. Charlton JR, Hartley RM, Silver R, Holland WW. Geographical variation in mortality from conditions amenable to medical intervention in England and Wales. *Lancet* 1983: **i:** 691-6
3. Drever F, Whitehead M, eds. *Health inequalities: decennial supplement: Office for National Statistics.* London: Stationery Office, 1997 (Series DS; no. 15).

Table A.1: *Population age and sex structure, England, mid-1997, and changes by age, 1981-91, 1991-92, 1992-93, 1993-94, 1994-95, 1995-96 and 1996-97*

Age (in years)	Resident population at mid-1997 (thousands)			Percentage changes (persons)						
	Persons	Males	Females	1981-91	1991-92	1992-93	1993-94	1994-95	1995-96	1996-97
Under 1	616	316	300	10.9	-1.0	-3.6	0.2	-3.1	-1.9	2.2
1-4	2490	1278	1213	15.2	1.2	0.2	-0.4	-0.4	-1.8	-2.1
5-15	6964	3574	3390	-13.1	1.2	1.8	1.6	1.0	0.9	0.8
16-29	9149	4690	4459	4.7	-2.0	-2.5	-2.5	-1.9	-1.6	-1.5
30-44	11036	5601	5435	11.5	-0.1	0.8	1.5	1.7	1.9	1.8
45-64/59*	10090	5602	4488	-0.2	3.0	2.3	1.8	1.4	1.2	1.0
65/60-74†	5338	1921	3417	-3.2	0.3	0.7	0.5	-1.8	-1.2	-0.8
75-84	2670	1027	1643	17.6	-1.3	-2.7	-2.4	3.5	2.4	1.6
85+	931	243	688	49.2	4.7	5.1	3.0	3.4	2.2	2.0
All ages	49285	24251	25034	3.0	0.4	0.3	0.4	0.4	0.4	0.4

* 45-64 years for males and 45-59 years for females.
† 65-74 years for males and 60-74 years for females.

Note: Figures may not add precisely to totals due to rounding.

Source: ONS

Rank	All ages - 1 & over		1-14 years		15-34 years		35-54 years		55-74 years		75 years & over	
	Males	Females	Males	Females	Males	Females	Males	Females	Males	Females	Males	Females
1	410-414 Ischaemic heart disease — 25%	410-414 Ischaemic heart disease — 19%	E800-E999 External causes of injury & poisoning — 29%	140-239 Neoplasms — 21%	E950-E959 Suicide and undetermined injury† — 22%	E950-E959 Suicide and undetermined injury† — 12%	410-414 Ischaemic heart disease — 23%	174 MN of female breast — 18%	410-414 Ischaemic heart disease — 29%	410-414 Ischaemic heart disease — 19%	410-414 Ischaemic heart disease — 24%	410-414 Ischaemic heart disease — 20%
2	480-486 Pneumonia — 9%	430-438 Cerebrovascular disease — 12%	140-239 Neoplasms — 17%	E800-E999 External causes of injury and poisoning — 21%	E810-E819 Motor vehicle traffic accidents — 18%	E810-E819 Motor vehicle traffic accidents — 10%	150-159 MN of digestive organs and peritoneum — 9%	179-189 MN of genito-urinary organs — 9%	162 MN of trachea, bronchus & lung — 11%	150-159 MN of digestive organs and peritoneum — 9%	480-486 Pneumonia — 13%	480-486 Pneumonia — 15%
3	430-438 Cerebrovascular disease — 8%	480-486 Pneumonia — 12%	320-389 Diseases of the nervous system and sense organs — 14%	320-389 Diseases of the nervous system — 14%	E850-E869 Accidental poisoning by drugs, medicaments & biologicals — 7%	200-208 MN of lymphatic and haematopoietic tissue — 5%	E950-E959 Suicide and undetermined injury† — 7%	150-159 MN of digestive organs and peritoneum — 7%	150-159 MN of digestive organs and peritoneum — 10%	162 MN of trachea, bronchus and lung — 8%	430-438 Cerebrovascular disease — 10%	430-438 Cerebrovascular disease — 14%
4	150-159 MN of digestive organs and peritoneum — 8%	150-159 MN of digestive organs and peritoneum — 6%	740-759 Congenital anomalies — 10%	740-759 Congenital anomalies — 12%	200-208 MN of lymphatic and haematopoietic tissue — 3%	174 MN of female breast — 5%	162 MN of trachea, bronchus & lung — 6%	410-414 Ischaemic heart disease — 7%	430-438 Cerebrovascular disease — 6%	430-438 Cerebrovascular disease — 8%	490-496 Chronic obstructive pulmonary disease and allied conditions — 7%	415-429 Diseases of pulmonary circulation & other forms of heart disease — 6%
5	162 MN of trachea, bronchus & lung — 7%	415-429 Diseases of pulmonary circulation & other forms of heart disease — 6%	460-519 Diseases of the respiratory system — 9%	460-519 Diseases of the respiratory system — 9%	001-139 Infectious and parasitic diseases — 3%	001-139 Infectious and parasitic diseases — 5%	571 Chronic liver disease — 6%	162 MN of trachea, bronchus & lung — 6%	490-496 Chronic obstructive pulmonary disease and allied conditions — 6%	174 MN of female breast — 7%	150-159 MN of digestive organs and peritoneum — 6%	150-159 MN of digestive organs and peritoneum — 5%
Remainder	43%	45%	21%	24%	47%	63%	50%	53%	38%	48%	40%	39%
All causes	246412	271595	931	633	5878	2455	17992	11880	90439	62020	131172	194607

MN = Malignant neoplasm.

†Suicide and undetermined injury=(E950-E959)+(E980-E989) excluding E988.8.

Note: percentages may not add up to 100 due to rounding.

Table A.3: *Relative mortality from various conditions when presented as numbers of deaths and future years of 'working life' lost, England and Wales, 1997*

Cause (ICD9 code)	Males				Females			
	Number of deaths (thousands)		Years of 'working life' lost (thousands)		Number of deaths (thousands)		Years of 'working life' lost (thousands)	
	All ages	(%)	Age 15-64	(%)	All ages	(%)	Age 15-64	(%)
All causes, all ages	266		864		292		512	
All causes, 28 days and over	265	(100)	794	(100)	291	(100)	456	(100)
All malignant neoplasms* (140-208)	70	(27)	171	(22)	65	(22)	178	(39)
Trachea, bronchus and lung cancer (162)	19	(7)	36	(5)	11	(4)	20	(4)
Breast cancer† (174)	0	(0)	0	(0)	12	(4)	48	(11)
Genito-urinary cancer (179-189)	13	(5)	15	(2)	10	(3)	31	(7)
Leukaemia (204-208)	2	(1)	12	(2)	2	(1)	9	(2)
Circulatory disease* (390-459)	110	(42)	181	(23)	120	(41)	72	(16)
Ischaemic heart disease (410-414)	67	(25)	117	(15)	56	(19)	29	(6)
Cerebrovascular disease (430-438)	22	(8)	25	(3)	36	(12)	21	(5)
Respiratory disease* (460-519)	42	(16)	47	(6)	51	(18)	32	(7)
Pneumonia (480-486)	22	(8)	23	(3)	35	(12)	14	(3)
Bronchitis, emphysema and asthma (490-493)	3	(1)	7	(1)	2	(1)	6	(1)
Sudden infant death syndrome (798.0)	0	(0)	11	(1)	0	(0)	6	(1)
All accidental deaths* (E800-E949)	6	(2)	123	(15)	5	(2)	33	(7)
Motor vehicle traffic accidents (E810-E819)	2	(1)	63	(8)	1	(0)	17	(4)
Suicide and undetermined injury(E950-E959 plus E980-E989 excluding E988.8)	4	(1)	86	(11)	1	(0)	24	(5)

* These conditions are ranked as well as selected causes within the broader headings.　　† Not calculated for male breast cancer.

Deaths under 28 days excluded, except from 'All causes, all ages'.

Source: ONS

Table A.4: Trends in 'avoidable' deaths, England, 1979-97. Age-standardised mortality ratios (1979 = 100)

Condition	SMR[1] 1979	1986	1987	1988	1989	1990	1991	1992	1993	1994	1995	1996	1997[3]	Actual number of deaths[2] 1979	1997[4]
Hypertension/cerebrovascular (ages 35-64)	100	73	69	63	60	57	58	55	52	49	49	49	47	8811	4202
Perinatal mortality[5]	100	65	61	60	57	56	55	52	52[6]	52[6]	51[6]	49[6]	48[6]	8839	4264[6]
Cervical cancer (ages 15-64)	100	96	90	86	81	78	72	68	64	54	56	57	51	1060	562
Hodgkin's disease (ages 5-64)	100	75	84	74	65	60	58	57	60	39	49	41	38	340	141
Respiratory diseases (ages 1-14)	100	41	44	42	41	39	42	28	44	47	36	36	42	308	135
Surgical diseases[7] (ages 5-64)	100	71	58	75	51	58	58	61	55	45	52	50	58	247	143
Asthma (ages 5-44)	100	114	114	110	94	86	91	70	68	66	47	61	64	231	160
Tuberculosis (ages 5-64)	100	60	67	56	57	48	46	47	52	51	56	43	51	208	110
Chronic rheumatic heart disease (ages 5-44)	100	35	34	20	28	23	19	14	17	19	17	13	14	118	20
Total 'avoidable' deaths	100	70	66	63	60	57	57	54	53	50	50	49	48	20138[8]	9722[8]
All causes: ages 0-14 years	100	74	73	72	67	64	59	52	52	49	49	49	48	10502	5155
All causes: ages 15-64 years	100	86	84	82	80	79	76	74	73	70	70	69	68	119158	82080
All causes: all ages	100	89	86	85	85	82	82	79	81	77	78	77	76	554840	521598

1 The standardised mortality ratio (SMR) for a condition is calculated by dividing the observed number of deaths by the expected number of deaths based on 1979 death rates.
2 Excluding deaths of visitors to England.
3 The 1997 SMR has been calculated using the mid-1996 population as the 1997 estimates are not yet available.
4 From 1993 the mortality data for some causes of death are not directly comparable with those for 1992 and earlier years as a result of coding changes.
5 Stillbirths are included in the figures for perinatal mortality and total 'avoidable' deaths, but not in deaths from all causes.
6 The definition of stillbirth changed on 1 October 1992 to include 24 to 27 weeks gestation; to provide a comparable trend, these stillbirths are excluded from the figures for 1993 (848), 1994 (832), 1995 (842), 1996 (892) and 1997 (842).
7 Appendicitis, abdominal hernia, cholelithiasis and cholecystitis.
8 Figures for total 'avoidable' deaths take account of deaths from asthma in the 5-14 years age-band which are also included in the figures for respiratory diseases.

Source: Department of Health (SD2F), from data supplied by ONS

273

Table A.5: *Live births, stillbirths, infant mortality and abortions, England[1], 1960, 1970 and 1975-97*

Year	Live births Number	Stillbirths Number	Stillbirths Rate[2]	Early neonatal mortality (deaths under 1 week) Number	Early neonatal mortality Rate[3]	Perinatal mortality (stillbirths plus deaths under 1 week) Rate[2]	Post-neonatal mortality (deaths 4 weeks to under 1 year) Rate[3]	Infant mortality (deaths under 1 year) Rate[3]	Abortions[1] Rate[4]
1960	740859	14753	19.5	9772	13.2	32.5	6.3	21.6	-
1970	741999	9708	12.9	7864	10.6	23.4	5.9	18.2	87.6
1975	568900*	5918	10.3*	5154	9.1	19.3*	5.0	15.7	149.9
1976	550383*	5339	9.6	4468	8.1	17.6	4.6	14.2	148.7
1977	536953	5087	9.4	4070	7.6	16.9	4.5	13.7	152.7
1978	562589	4791	8.4	3975	7.1	15.4	4.4	13.1	157.7
1979	601316	4811	7.9	4028	6.7	14.6	4.6*	12.8	158.8
1980	618371*	4523	7.3	3793	6.1	13.4	4.4	12.0	164.5
1981	598163	3939	6.5	3105	5.2	11.7	4.3	10.9	168.8
1982	589711	3731	6.3	2939	5.0	11.2	4.5	10.8	171.1
1983	593255	3412	5.7	2746	4.6	10.3	4.2	10.0	169.2
1984	600573	3425	5.7	2640	4.4	10.0	3.9	9.4	177.3
1985	619301	3426	5.5	2674	4.3	9.8	3.9	9.2	177.6
1986	623609	3337	5.3	2640	4.2	9.5	4.2	9.5	183.5
1987	643330	3224	5.0	2518	3.9	8.9	4.0	9.1	187.7
1988	654363*	3188	4.8	2543	3.9	8.7	4.1	9.1	196.6
1989	649357	3056	4.7	2368	3.6	8.3	3.7	8.4	200.0
1990	666920	3068	4.6	2382	3.6	8.1	3.3	7.9	199.0
1991	660806	3072	4.6	2260	3.4	8.0	3.0	7.3	194.4
1992	651784	2777†	4.2†	2174	3.3	7.6†	2.3	6.5	190.1
1993	636473*	3621*	5.7	2074*	3.3	8.9	2.1	6.3	190.8
1994	628956*	3583*	5.7	2011*	3.2	8.8*	2.0	6.1	191.4
1995	613257	3406	5.5	1991	3.2	8.8	1.9	6.1	193.4
1996	614184	3345	5.4	1980	3.2	8.6	2.0	6.1	206.4
1997	607216	3250	5.3	1856	3.1	8.4	2.0	5.9	-

1 Relates to England residents. 2 Per 1,000 live births and stillbirths. 3 Per 1,000 live births. 4 Per 1,000 conceptions (live births, stillbirths and abortions).

* These figures have been incorrectly cited in previous Reports.

† 1992 figures exclude 198 stillbirths of between 24 and 27 completed weeks gestation registered between 1 October 1992 and 31 December 1992, following the introduction of new legislation (see Chapter 1), and are consistent with those for earlier years. The figures for later years are on the new (wider) definition of stillbirths.

Source: ONS

Table A.6: Congenital anomalies, England, 1987, 1992, 1996 and 1997 *

ICD codes	Anomaly	Live births† 1987	1992	1996	1997¶	Stillbirths§ 1987	1992	1996	1997¶
	Babies born with anomalies								
	Number	12650	5637	5129	4837	262	138	157	165
	Rate	196.6	86.5	83.5	79.2	4.1	2.1	2.5	2.7
320.0-359.9, 740.0-742.9 (Q00.0-Q07.9)	**Central nervous system**								
	Number	401	235	186	148	80	45	50	38
	Rate	6.2	3.6	3.0	2.4	1.2	0.7	0.8	0.6
360.0-379.9, 743.0-743.9, 744.0-744.3 (Q10.0-Q17.9)	**Ear and eye**								
	Number	755	206	207	203	16	7	6	4
	Rate	11.7	3.2	3.4	3.3	0.2	0.1	0.1	0.1
749.0-749.2 (Q35.0-Q37.9)	**Cleft lip/cleft palate**								
	Number	780	678	520	527	17	12	13	7
	Rate	12.1	10.4	8.5	8.6	0.3	0.2	0.2	0.1
390.0-459.9, 745.0-747.9 (Q20.0-Q28.9)	**Cardiovascular**								
	Number	829	393	435	412	24	7	23	16
	Rate	12.9	6.0	7.1	6.7	0.4	0.1	0.4	0.3
752.6 (Q54.0-Q54.9, Q64.0)	**Hypospadias/epispadias**								
	Number	1073	521	497	437	-	1	-	1
	Rate	16.7	8.0	8.1	7.2	-	0.0	-	0.0
755.2-755.4 (Q71.0-Q73.8)	**Reduction deformities of limbs**								
	Number	282	168	182	123	13	4	9	2
	Rate	4.4	2.6	3.0	2.0	0.2	0.1	0.1	0.0
754.5-754.7 (Q66.0, Q66.1, Q66.4, Q66.8)	**Talipes**								
	Number	2070	736	565	571	21	4	10	7
	Rate	32.2	11.3	9.2	9.3	0.3	0.1	0.2	0.1
758.0-758.9 (Q90.0-Q99.9)	**Chromosomal**								
	Number	544	467	398	321	21	16	24	19
	Rate	8.5	7.2	6.5	5.3	0.3	0.2	0.4	0.3

Note: From January 1990 certain minor malformations are no longer notified, and have been excluded from the figures shown. For example, club foot of positional origin is now excluded from the category 'Talipes', ICD9 codes 754.5-754.7. This change in notification practice largely accounts for the decrease in numbers of malformations reported in some categories. From 1995, ICD10 codes (in brackets) are in use.

* Provisional. †Rates per 10,000 live births. § Rates per 10,000 total births. ¶Data as at 22 May 1998.

Source: ONS

275

Table A.7: *Cancer* registrations by age and site, males, England and Wales, 1992*

| | Numbers and percentages | | | | | | | | | | | | | | | |
| | Age-group (years) | | | | | | | | | | | | | | | |
	All ages	%	0-14 years	%	15-24 years	%	25-44 years	%	45-64 years	%	65-74 years	%	75-84 years	%	85 years and over	%
Eye, brain, and other nervous system	2288	2	155	24	82	11	319	7	879	3	584	2	242	1	27	0
Mouth and pharynx	2237	2	4	1	8	1	175	4	921	4	662	2	383	1	84	1
Oesophagus	3350	3	1	0	0	0	79	2	989	4	1201	3	862	3	218	3
Lung	24770	23	0	0	5	1	276	6	5750	22	9916	27	7245	23	1568	19
Stomach	6255	6	1	0	2	0	112	2	1425	5	2207	6	1985	6	523	6
Pancreas	3022	3	0	0	0	0	73	2	779	3	1013	3	886	3	271	3
Large intestine and rectum	14669	14	0	0	11	1	352	8	3896	15	5059	14	4249	14	1102	13
Prostate	15792	15	1	0	2	0	12	0	1702	7	5468	15	6541	21	2066	25
Bladder	8528	8	0	0	7	1	164	4	1987	8	2991	8	2670	9	709	9
Skin (melanoma only)	1625	2	3	0	27	4	334	7	658	3	327	1	226	1	50	1
Leukaemias and lymphomas	8780	8	325	50	296	39	991	22	2399	9	2301	6	1942	6	526	6
All other cancer†	16910	16	166	25	312	41	1658	36	4745	18	5069	14	3896	13	1064	13
Total cancer†	108226	100	656	100	752	100	4545	100	26140	100	36798	100	31127	100	8208	100

* Cancer = malignant neoplasm.

† Excludes figures for non-melanoma skin cancer (ICD 9 code 173), which are greatly under-registered.

Note: Percentages may not add up to 100 due to rounding.

Source: ONS

Table A.8: Cancer* registrations by age and site, females, England and Wales, 1992

Numbers and percentages

	All ages	%	0-14 years	%	15-24 years	%	25-44 years	%	45-64 years	%	65-74 years	%	75-84 years	%	85 years and over	%
Eye, brain, and other nervous system	1857	2	146	30	58	8	261	3	594	2	449	2	288	1	61	0
Mouth and pharynx	1296	1	6	1	14	2	106	1	376	1	373	1	273	1	148	1
Oesophagus	2359	2	0	0	0	0	23	0	387	1	624	2	904	3	421	3
Breast	31526	28	1	0	20	3	3515	42	13890	42	6507	23	5187	19	2406	20
Lung	12255	11	2	0	5	1	217	3	2889	9	4569	16	3634	13	939	8
Stomach	3852	3	1	0	2	0	76	1	490	1	974	3	1486	5	823	7
Pancreas	3176	3	1	0	3	0	50	1	547	2	906	3	1155	4	514	4
Large intestine and rectum	14535	13	1	0	8	1	312	4	2851	9	4061	14	4848	17	2454	20
Ovary	5272	5	5	1	38	6	386	5	2044	6	1433	5	1056	4	310	3
Cervix	3597	3	1	0	54	8	1328	16	1058	3	607	2	428	2	121	1
Other uterus	4237	4	0	0	5	1	151	2	1617	5	1245	4	874	3	345	3
Bladder	3497	3	3	1	3	0	56	1	653	2	1042	4	1205	4	535	4
Skin (melanoma only)	2439	2	6	1	89	13	581	7	785	2	453	2	365	1	160	1
Leukaemias and lymphomas	7429	7	192	39	242	35	659	8	1644	5	1811	6	1991	7	890	7
All other cancer†	13769	12	123	25	145	21	692	8	2864	9	3654	13	4179	15	2112	17
Total cancer †	111096	100	488	100	686	100	8413	100	32689	100	28708	100	27873	100	12239	100

* Cancer = malignant neoplasm.

† Excludes figures for non-melanoma skin cancer (ICD9 code 173), which are greatly under-registered.

Note: Percentages may not add up to 100 due to rounding.

Source: ONS

277

Table A.9: *Immunisation uptake (percentage of children immunised by their 2nd birthday and of children given BCG vaccine by their 14th birthday), England, 1980-96/97*

Year	Diphtheria	Tetanus	Polio	Whooping cough	Measles	Mumps/ rubella	BCG[1]	Haemophilus influenzae b (Hib)
1980[2]	81	81	81	41	53	-	82	-
1981[2]	83	83	82	46	55	-	78	-
1982[2]	84	84	84	53	58	-	75	-
1983[2]	84	84	84	59	60	-	76	-
1984[2]	84	84	84	65	63	-	71	-
1985[2]	85	85	85	65	68	-	77	-
1986[2]	85	85	85	67	71	-	76	-
1987/88[2]	87	87	87	73	76	-	76	-
1988/89	87	87	87	75	80	7	71	-
1989/90	89	89	89	78	84	68	36[3]	-
1990/91	92	92	92	84	87	86	90[3]	-
1991/92	93	93	93	88	90	90	86[3]	-
1992/93	95	95	95	92	92	92	74	-
1993/94	95	95	95	93	91	91	79	75
1994/95	95	95	95	93	91	91	52[4]	91
1995/96	96	96	96	94	92	92	95[4]	94
1996/97	96	96	96	94	92	92	81	95

1 Estimated percentage of children given BCG vaccine by their 14th birthday.

2 Estimated percentage immunised by the end of the second year after birth (excludes BCG).

3 The school BCG programme was suspended in 1989 because there were insufficient supplies of BCG vaccine; figures for the subsequent two years were relatively higher as a result.

4 The school BCG programme for 1994-95 was delayed because of the measles/rubella immunisation campaign.

Sources: 1980-87/88: Form SBL 607; 1988/89 onwards: Form KC51 (except BCG), Form KC50 (BCG)

Table A.10: *Cumulative totals of AIDS cases by exposure category, England, to 31 December 1997*

(Numbers subject to revision as further data are received or duplicates identified)

How persons probably acquired the virus	Number of cases			
	Male	Female	Total	%[§]
Sexual intercourse:				
Between men	9757	-	9757	70
Between men and women				
Exposure to				
'high risk' partner[*]	45	158	203	2
Exposure abroad[†]	1014	797	1811	13
Exposure in the UK	81	87	168	1
Investigation continuing/closed	32	16	48	<1
Injecting drug use (IDU)	430	183	613	4
IDU and sexual intercourse				
between men	250	-	250	2
Blood factor treatment				
(eg, for haemophilia)	554	5	559	4
Blood or tissue transfer				
(eg, transfusion)	47	72	119	<1
Mother to infant	117	126	243	2
Other or investigation continuing/				
closed	124	20	144	1
Total	12451	1464	13915	100

[*]   Partner(s) exposed to HIV infection through sexual intercourse between men, IDU, blood factor treatment or blood/tissue transfer.

[†]   Individuals from abroad and individuals from the UK who have lived or visited abroad, for whom there is no evidence of 'high risk' partners.

[§]   Total does not add up to 100 because of rounding.

Source: CDSC/PHLS

Table A.11: Expectation of life at birth, all-cause mortality rates and infant mortality, England and other European Union countries, circa 1995-96

Country	Year	Expectation of life at birth		All cause mortality rate*		Infant mortality rate†
		Males	Females	Males	Females	
England	1996	74.6‡	79.7‡	276.4§	168.7§	6.1§
United Kingdom	1995	74.1	79.5	294.5	178.5	6.2
Austria	1996	74.1	80.4	330.8	157.2	5.1
Belgium	1992	73.1	79.9	338.9	175.3	8.2
Denmark	1996	73.1	78.4	343.9	217.3	5.6
Finland	1995	72.9	80.4	364.8	148.3	4.0
France	1994	74.4	82.8	356.8	146.1	5.9
Germany	1995	73.4	80.0	347.2	166.2	5.3
Greece	1996	74.9	81.2	298.9	118.8	7.3
Ireland	1993	72.6	78.2	330.2	184.7	6.1
Italy	1993	74.6	81.1	302.3	145.2	7.1
Luxembourg	1996	73.3	80.9	360.1	159.2	4.4
Netherlands	1995	74.7	80.6	269.4	160.8	5.5
Portugal	1996	71.2	78.6	416.5	175.6	6.9
Spain	1995	74.4	81.8	327.7	131.4	5.5
Sweden	1995	76.3	81.8	238.1	139.2	4.0
EU average	*1995-96*	*74.1*	*80.7*	*325.6*	*157.4*	*6.0*

* Per 100,000 population aged 0-64 years, age-standardised.

† Per 1,000 live births.

‡ Figures for England calculated by Government Actuary's Department by slightly different methodology to WHO figures.

§ England data provided by Office for National Statistics (ONS).

Source: WHO European Office 'Health for All' statistical database

Table A.12: *Age standardised death rates per 100,000 men aged 35-64 years by social class and employment status, England and Wales, 1976-81, 1981-85 and 1986-92*

Social class	Employed			Unemployed		
	1976-81*	1981*-85	1986-92	1976-81*	1981*-85	1986-92
I/II	611	530	448	850	836	782
IIIN	845	647	472	1362	876	711
IIIM	777	676	611	1234	941	1041
IV/V	921	809	725	1264	984	1333
Non-manual	728	589	460	1106	856	746
Manual	849	742	668	1249	962	1187
Rate ratio manual vs non-manual	1.17	1.26	1.45	1.13	1.12	1.59

*1981 refers to Census day in the first time period and post Census day in the second time period.

Source: ONS

Table A.13: *Standardised mortality ratios by country of birth and social class for men aged 20-64 years, England and Wales, 1991-93*

Social class	Country of birth				
	England and Wales	Caribbean	Indian sub-Continent	Scotland	Ireland (all parts)
All causes					
I/II	71	83	96	82	95
IIIN	100	84	112	121	127
IIIM	117	105	120	169	166
IV/V	135	99	158	186	173
All*	100	89	107	129	135
Deaths	175847	1680	4114	4596	5994
Ischaemic heart disease					
I/II	71	51	132	84	92
IIIN	107	84	179	114	124
IIIM	125	69	183	157	155
IV/V	137	69	223	163	148
All*	100	60	150	117	121
Deaths	52219	369	1736	1253	1706
Cerebrovascular disease					
I/II	68	103	138	54	93
IIIN	96	133	93	79	111
IIIM	118	205	135	190	172
IV/V	149	193	326	141	174
All*	100	169	163	111	130
Deaths	8350	160	299	189	288
Lung cancer					
I/II	58	37	30	82	88
IIIN	87	68	51	114	156
IIIM	138	66	55	221	216
IV/V	151	72	90	225	214
All*	100	59	48	146	157
Deaths	16082	114	171	479	693
Accidents and injuries†					
I/II	56	91	62	69	79
IIIN	74	48	75	83	121
IIIM	106	136	99	233	185
IV/V	138	123	91	315	280
All*	100	121	80	177	189
Deaths	10769	83	172	363	371

* Includes unclassified deaths.

† Excludes suicides and undetermined deaths.

Source: ONS

Figure A.1: *Weekly deaths, England and Wales, 1996 and 1997, and expected deaths, 1997*

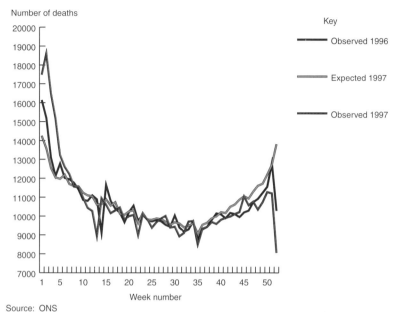

Source: ONS